"Altruistic love should ideally be a permanent state of mind, an unconditional wish that all beings may find happiness and the causes of happiness. It embraces all beings without exception. When altruistic love encounters suffering, it becomes compassion, which springs from the same benevolence, but more specifically wishes that beings may be free from suffering and from the many possible causes of suffering. Paul Gilbert and Choden's *Mindful Compassion* is a precious and most welcome contribution toward bringing about a more compassionate society."

—**Matthieu Ricard**, Buddhist monk and author of
Happiness: A Guide to Developing Life's Most Important Skill

"An inspiring book that will be deeply appreciated by many therapists, teachers, and those who come to them for help with their suffering. Gilbert is internationally recognized for his contribution to the understanding and treatment of emotional disorders. His genius is being able to bring compelling theory together with practical application. Choden is widely known as a wonderful teacher, deeply based on his own long practice of mindfulness. In this book they come together to offer us keys that can both unlock our understanding and motivate our practice—showing how mindfulness and compassion realize their deepest potential when cultivated together. A book full of wisdom that will be a wonderful resource for a whole generation."

—**Mark Williams**, professor of clinical psychology at the
University of Oxford and author of *The Mindful Way through
Depression and Mindfulness: A Practical Guide to Finding Peace
in a Frantic World*

"This book is a brilliant synthesis of two grand psychological traditions—mindfulness and compassion. In clear, compelling prose, Gilbert and Choden illustrate how the human brain gets us into trouble time and time again. Then, they explain why we need both compassion and mindfulness to liberate ourselves from unnecessary suffering, and they offer elegant exercises to train the mind in those vital human capacities. Wise and hopeful, this landmark contribution to mindfulness literature is a modern reevaluation of human nature and the path to emotional freedom and cultural sanity."

> —**Christopher Germer, PhD**, clinical instructor at Harvard Medical School, author of *The Mindful Path to Self-Compassion*, and coeditor of *Wisdom and Compassion in Psychotherapy*

"*Mindful Compassion* is a perfect mix of heart and smart. Gilbert and Choden blend sensibilities from evolutionary science with practices derived from ancient spiritual traditions. Their book offers an alternative to the driven, competitive, and often destructive forces that shape the modern world. *Mindful Compassion* is soul-soothing science."

> —**Kelly G. Wilson, PhD**, associate professor of psychology at the University of Mississippi and coauthor of *Acceptance and Commitment Therapy*

"Packed full of useful resources for therapists and coaches, this book is for anyone interested in the links between evolutionary science, compassion, and mindfulness. It is especially of interest to those who wish to know more about Buddhist perspectives on mindfulness."

> —**Russ Harris**, author of *The Happiness Trap*

"The growing interaction between Western psychology and Buddhism has great significance to our contemporary understanding of what leads us to suffer in our lives and what can lead to happiness. In this book, Paul Gilbert and Choden create a rich blend of Buddhist and Western thinking around the importance of compassion at the heart of our lives and our emotional health. They offer invaluable insights into the way our minds creates our reality and how we can wake up to what leads to suffering and what can bring us happiness and peace of mind. *Mindful Compassion* is an illuminating, readable, and necessary background of Western and Buddhist understanding that will support and deepen the current application of mindfulness. It can also be a valuable resource for anyone wishing to deepen their own personal journey of awakening."

—**Rob Preece**, author of *The Wisdom of Imperfection* and *The Courage to Feel*

"The wise and powerful lessons contained in this book hold many keys to our liberation from suffering. Reading the kind words of these authors, it feels as though the reader is receiving a direct, personal transmission from learned experts. Grounded in the state of the art of our science and steeped in the wisdom of Buddhist psychology, *Mindful Compassion* is often the first book I will recommend to people who seek to deepen their personal practice."

—**Dennis Tirch, PhD**, adjunct assistant clinical professor at Weill Cornell Medical College and author of *The Compassionate-Mind Guide to Overcoming Anxiety*

MINDFUL COMPASSION

how the science of compassion can help you
understand your emotions, live in the present,
and connect deeply with others

PAUL GILBERT, PHD
and CHODEN

New Harbinger Publications, Inc.

Distributed in Canada by Raincoast Books

Copyright © 2014 by Paul Gilbert and Pema Choden
New Harbinger Publications, Inc.
5674 Shattuck Avenue
Oakland, CA 94609
www.newharbinger.com

First published in the UK by Constable, an imprint of Constable & Robinson Ltd, 2013

Cover design by Amy Shoup
Text design by Tracy Marie Carlson
Acquired by Tesilya Hanauer
Edited by Elisabeth Beller

Library of Congress Cataloging-in-Publication Data

Gilbert, Paul.
  Mindful compassion : how the science of compassion can help you understand your emotions, live in the present, and connect deeply with others / Paul Gilbert, PhD, and Choden.
    pages cm
  ISBN 978-1-62625-061-1 (pbk. : alk. paper) -- ISBN 978-1-62625-062-8 (pdf e-book) -- ISBN 978-1-62625-063-5 (epub) 1. Compassion. 2. Mind and body. I. Title.
  BJ1475.G46 2014
  155.2'32--dc23

                              2014000027

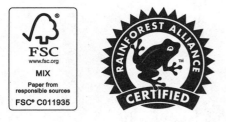

Printed in the United States of America

20   19   18

10   9   8   7   6   5   4

CONTENTS

Part I
THE ISSUES

Part II
THE PRACTICES

PREFACE

Writing this book together has been a fascinating journey. We would like to share a little of how it began and unfolded.

Our mutual colleague Dr. Alistair Wilson is a consultant psychiatrist with a long-term interest in how Buddhist practices of mindfulness and compassion can be integrated with Western scientific understanding of mental processes. In 2008, Alistair organized a conference on neuroscience and compassion that took place at the Buddhist retreat on Holy Isle, off the island of Arran on the west coast of Scotland. It was at this meeting that we first met. We have very different backgrounds and life experiences, so we'll describe them briefly here.

Paul

I grew up in Nigeria in the 1950s and lived there until I was twelve years old. Living far away from any major towns, I had a fantastic sense of freedom, but I also saw a lot of suffering: poverty, and people with leprosy and other illnesses, all struggling to survive. I recall being quite distressed by a man asking me for money; his face and fingers were eaten away by leprosy. I spent my adolescence in a rather harsh boarding school in Britain, disconnected from my family and previous lifestyle. My first degree was in economics, but as I had always wanted to work closely with people, I did a second degree, eventually qualifying as a clinical psychologist in 1980.

I was very interested in how and why our minds evolved and came to function in the way they do. My focus was on depression, which can be so destructive that it can even lead people to kill themselves. Many early psychotherapists, such as Freud and Jung, realized that we need to understand the mind against an evolutionary background. When looked at through the lens of evolution, we can see something that most people often don't recognize, which is that this brain of ours is wonderful and complex but not that well put together. In fact, our brains are very "tricky" to handle and come with a lot of glitches and difficulties. It turns out that the way our minds and brains evolved can set us up for a lot of suffering. As I began to realize this, it was like a light coming on. It made sense of so much. In 1989, I published a book called *Human Nature and Suffering*, exploring these ideas.

I had always been very interested in nature programs, and I remember seeing one on how turtles scrambled from their sand nests trying desperately to reach the sea, only to be picked off by seabirds, foxes, and many other predators in the first hours of life—most of them wouldn't make it to adulthood. I think that David Attenborough and his team's wonderful work has perhaps done something that he may not have anticipated, which is to bring home the harshness and cruelty of nature: most life-forms must eat other life-forms to survive, the young are common targets for predators, and viruses and bacteria are life-forms that kill and maim and cause suffering to many other life-forms in a narrow pursuit of their own welfare. Then there is the small matter of recognizing that our own lives are very limited, and we will, like all other living things, flourish, decay, and die.

On becoming aware of these issues, I, like many of my generation, developed an interest in Buddhism in the late 1960s and the 1970s and dabbled in some meditation. But it was becoming aware of the deeper teachings that inspired me.

About 2,500 years ago, the Buddha worked out that life is about suffering, partly because everything is impermanent: all living things come into existence, flourish, decay, and die. The Buddha, of course, knew nothing about the scientific processes that lie behind the way things are, such as the Big Bang theory of the universe, the workings of our genes, and the processes underlying the flow of life, but he was able to focus on a very simple but profound observation—everything changes and nothing lasts. Despite this impermanence (which is obvious to anyone who thinks about it for a moment), we have minds that seek permanence and stability; and yet these very same minds are chaotic and consumed by easily activated passions, desires, fears, and terrors. The solution, the Buddha suggested, is to develop a clear insight into the nature of our predicament and tame the grasping mind so that we are less pulled this way and that.

This is fascinating stuff, and evolutionary psychology has added this insight: our brains and bodies evolved as survival and reproducing vehicles for genes. No wonder we have such a problem. *It really is not our fault.* As I spoke to my Buddhist colleagues about these insights, something seemed to strike a chord in them. Many acknowledged that they had never really thought about it like that. They said that sometimes it's very easy to convey the idea that we have a chaotic mind and that we are suffering because we've done something wrong or haven't done something right. Evolutionary understanding completely removes that kind of blaming and shaming. I've spent many years trying to understand shame and to help people who suffer from it, so marrying evolutionary understanding with Buddhist insight and training became something of a mission for me.

So at that lovely conference on the beautiful Holy Isle, Choden and I had the opportunity to walk, taking in the beauty of the island, and to talk in depth about our different approaches. (We also took swims in the cold Scottish sea that were quite invigorating, to say the least!) We shared many similar ideas about the problems of the human mind and the difficulties of training it. He noted that when people begin to practice mindfulness and compassion in depth, it can actually bring up very painful and difficult feelings. (He describes his own experience of this in chapter 6.) So it wasn't long before we both recognized that it would be a tough but exciting project to try to write something together, integrating our different understandings and experiences: mine from the perspective of clinical and evolutionary psychology and Choden's from a Buddhist tradition.

Although I had explored the concept of training minds in compassion in an earlier book (*The Compassionate Mind,* 2009), we wanted to include mindfulness as a basis for training in compassion; explore some of the obstacles that people encounter when they begin to train the mind; and, in particular, develop a step-by-step set of practices rooted in Choden's training and my experience of developing practices for people struggling with mental health problems.

You will see some differences in writing style that we have tried to smooth out, but we are not trying to disguise the source of the writing. I saw my task as building the insights from the science of mind and mind training and Choden's as bringing ancient practices to life for the Western mind. The last few years have certainly been an opportunity of great learning for me; and I express considerable gratitude for Choden's patience and perseverance in explaining things. I have been inspired by his knowledge and openness to think deeply about certain practices and to not be afraid to think of things in new ways. I've also been impressed by his openness and preparedness to engage in personal exploration of some very difficult issues (which he tells us about in chapter 6). And of course I have valued his friendship.

We've also had the opportunity of running some compassion-focused retreats together where we could develop and refine the practices in part II. The retreats involve periods of silence, reflection, and inner practice for building skills to cultivate our compassionate minds and engage more effectively with the world. These have generally proved very beneficial for people and certainly have been for me as a participant. We hope to continue these in the future.

Choden

My journey into Buddhism and intensive meditation practice took a somewhat unusual route. I grew up in Cape Town in the dying days of the apartheid era. I was privileged to lead a middle-class life and got pretty much everything I wanted at a material level. But I was not happy. Some big part of me felt unborn and unlived. Part of this was to do with living in a divided society. It affected us all. As a white person, I felt separated from the instinctual power of black Africa and felt condemned to live in the sanitized world of white privilege and prosperity. So despite enjoying good material circumstances, there was always a deep, nagging sense of dissatisfaction in me. Is life just about getting a house, a job, a partner, going on lavish holidays—is there not something else too? These questions lay unformed in my young mind.

Later, when I became a Buddhist monk, this resonated with the story of the Buddha who, despite being a prince with great affluence and prestige, felt somehow deeply out of accord with his life. Upon seeing how material prosperity did not deal with the deep questions of life and the suffering he saw around him, the Buddha renounced his affluence and privilege. As described later in this book, he deserted his palace and went alone into the wilds to seek out the roots of suffering and the causes of genuine happiness and peace.

Something that shocked me when I was still young was the murder of my primary-school headmaster by thieves who broke into his house one night and raped his wife. At a stroke, some part of my childhood safety was shattered. What struck me much later when looking back is how precious and fleeting this life is and how so many people live in a private, inner world filled with shame and secret pain, yet so little is spoken about it in this world and so few skills are provided for navigating this inner terrain.

After leaving school, I spent five years studying law, then graduated, and worked at a small law firm in Cape Town doing my legal internship. I spent most of my time at the debtors' court applying for orders to seize the property of people who could not pay their debts. I felt like a cog in the capitalist machine bringing more misery to people who were already oppressed and exploited. At this time I met Rob Nairn, a well-known meditation teacher and former professor of Criminology at the University of Cape Town. He had just given up his professorship and had founded a Buddhist retreat center in Nieu Bethesda in the semidesert region of the Karoo. He taught me meditation and became a close mentor and friend.

After I completed my articles, I was admitted to the sidebar of the Supreme Court as an attorney in 1985. I always knew deep within myself that this was not my destiny; it was instead a powerful part of my conditioning and a way of living out my father's dream of becoming a lawyer. I was then conscripted into the army for two years in the last days of apartheid and felt even more intensely the polarization within South African society. During basic training, I used to sit in a disused toilet and do my meditation practice. One night the duty corporal ran into me on the parade ground and seeing that I had a small Tibetan rosary in my hand, accused me of smoking a joint. I said, "No, I am saying my mantra." He was so dismayed and it was so far outside his field of perception that he completely avoided me after that. I think he thought I might cast a spell on him!

Soon after my national service was complete, I decided to leave South Africa and follow Rob Nairn to Scotland. My father had always said that I should complete my studies and then "go and meditate in the Himalayas." He always thought that my spiritual calling would be a temporary phase and that I would soon return and take up my career as a lawyer, marry, and have a family. But this was not to be. I had never left the country before, but after I did leave in 1990, I did not return for seven years.

First, I worked at Samye Ling monastery in southern Scotland, studying and practicing meditation. Then in 1993, I undertook a three-year, three-month meditation retreat. This was a huge experience in my life and a big turning point. The retreat was completely secluded and set in the rolling green hills of Scotland. Most of the time the weather was wild and stormy, and in the winter time, it snowed so often that the roads were frequently impassable. There was a strict regime of meditation from 4:30 in the morning till 10:00 at night. We were learning and practicing the deep tantric methods of Tibetan Buddhism that were about transforming our mind at its deepest level. The group was international and comprised Italians, Spaniards, Americans, and English, but very few Scots. During the retreat, we lived in very small and austere rooms with little more than a shrine, a small cupboard, and a box for meditating and sleeping in.

My father came to visit me just before I went to the retreat and asked me where the bed was. I said, "Dad, there is no bed. We sleep in a meditation box!" At that moment, one of the monks started blowing a long Tibetan horn designed for the Himalayas, and it let out a shrill, deafening sound, whereupon my father, not known for his spiritual austerities, said, "Get me out of here—I need to go to the pub and have a strong whisky!" But he was amazingly tolerant of my unusual journey, especially given that he had paid for my expensive school and legal training.

There was a six-month period during the retreat when we were not able to go outdoors and were completely silent—it was just ourselves, our minds, and the wild Scottish winter. But it was an extraordinary and transformative experience, especially looking back now. Unsurprisingly, when I came out of the retreat, it took some time to readjust to the outside world. When we had started the retreat, there was no such thing as the Internet or e-mail, so when we emerged in March 1997, we were all intrigued to know what this new cyber world was all about. Soon after coming out, I took robes and, all in all, I was a monk for seven years including the retreat.

Despite the fact that I deeply resonated with the tantric practices of Tibetan Buddhism and felt its transformative potential, I realized that not many people would embark on such an austere journey and subscribe to an ancient spiritual tradition from the East. So I began to work with Rob Nairn on developing a more straightforward approach that involved teaching people simple skills to work with stress and depression. For most people, the idea of becoming enlightened is a mere daydream, and a more pressing reality is to stabilize and gain insight into our wild minds and learn to cultivate skillful ways of thinking and behaving. This became known as *mindfulness meditation*, a secular approach to working with the mind that does not involve joining any religious tradition.

In 2008, I met Paul Gilbert on Holy Isle. We had invited him to present at a conference on neuroscience and compassion. He and I made an immediate connection. What struck me from the start about Paul was his focus on self-compassion and how important this is in accompanying mindfulness and working with the mind. Also what struck me was his notion of *affiliate connection*—how we are biologically set up to connect and relate with others, and if we are starved of these connections, our lives are greatly impoverished. This resonated with my background of Mahayana Buddhism in which compassion is at the forefront of training the mind. So we began to have many fascinating discussions, and out of these dialogues, the idea of writing a book together was born.

In 2009, Rob Nairn and I played a key role in launching an MSc program in Mindfulness with Aberdeen University in Scotland, though the ideas of Paul Gilbert strongly shaped our approach to working with mindfulness and compassion together. In fact, this is the first Master's program in the UK that actively involves the teaching of compassion within a mindfulness training context. So the focus is not only on learning to be present and centered, but also on being kind and caring to ourselves as well as working directly with the self-critical mind.

We hope this book will provide readers with new insights into the relationship between mental health problems, our evolutionary history, and how easily our minds can be shaped by the environment in which we grow up. One of this book's themes is that many of the problems we have with our minds are not our fault but that, nevertheless, we need to take responsibility for training our minds. After all, it might not be your fault if a lightning bolt destroys your roof, but it is your responsibility to repair it—and learning how to do that skillfully is not a bad idea. Mindfulness and compassion are both means for doing just this and healing some of the other problems that nature has unwittingly bestowed upon us. While the struggle of evolution has built complex minds with complex motives and emotions, only humans have the potential to understand their own minds, train them, and make wise choices as to what kind of person they want to become.

ACKNOWLEDGMENTS

Paul

I'm delighted to be able to say that I owe a debt to so many. First, of course, to my family, especially Hannah (who promotes compassion with her own website, http://www.compassionatewellbeing.com) and James for their support and encouragement, with special loving appreciation to Jean (who usually wakes alone to my early morning writing). I now use speech software (I can't type to save my life), so she hears me chattering away. Heartfelt appreciation to the support and work of Chris Irons, Kirsten McEwan, and Corinne Gale for being wonderful research colleagues over many years—people I've been lucky enough to publish with, who did the clever bits. Special thanks to Andrew Gumley and Christine Braehler in developing and testing the compassion approach to psychosis.

Many thanks to all the colleagues and friends at our charity the Compassionate Mind Foundation (http://www.compassionatemind .co.uk), in particular: Diane Woollands, Chris Gillespie, Jean Gilbert, Mary Welford, Deborah Lee, Chris Irons, Michelle Cree, Ken Goss, and Ian Lowens. In America, Lynne Henderson, Dennis Tirch, and Russell Kolts have trained with me, bringing their many years of experience in meditation and clinical psychology to developing and advancing compassion-focused therapy and writing their own books on shyness, anxiety, and anger. Mauro Galluccio has been exploring the compassion approach for the conduct of international negotiations, and we now have many colleagues throughout Europe and indeed in other parts of the world who are using the model in their own inspiring ways. From the work of many, evidence is gradually emerging for the value of compassion-focused approaches to many aspects of life. Following the scientific, evidence-based approach is something that both Choden and I are deeply committed to.

Much appreciation goes to Chris Germer for his inspirational work on mindfulness and self-compassion and his preparedness to share so much and advise so kindly and wisely. Matthieu Ricard has been inspirational for us too. We are immensely grateful for some of the practices, the many discussions, his taking time to read some of this book and offer us his wisdom and kindness. You can see many of his ideas on compassion by following him on YouTube. Kristin Neff has also been a pioneer with her focus on self-compassion.

For many years, we have been keen to advance training in compassion-focused therapy, and so many thanks to Paul Lumsdon and Guy Daly, who together enthusiastically made possible the finances and organization to start the first postgraduate training in Compassion Focused Therapy in January of 2012 as a collaboration between the Derbyshire Healthcare Foundation Trust and the University of Derby. At the university, Linda Wheildon, Michael Townend, and especially Wendy Wood, the program leader, have been extraordinarily hard working in getting the process of the postgraduate training organized. Wendy's experience and enthusiasm have provided delight and great relief.

When I started clinical work in 1976, I had little idea at all of the importance of teaching people with mental health difficulties the value of developing compassion. Special thanks must go to the many people I have worked with over the last thirty years. They have not only taught me the importance of compassion but also about the real struggles and difficulties, fears, sadness, and yearning that can come with engaging compassionate feeling. Without them, their courage, insights, and support, we would understand far less.

Last but not least, I offer much gratitude and friendship to Choden for his enthusiasm in engaging in this project, keeping going when it became very tiring, and working to try to balance the importance of scientific insight with personal practice. I have certainly learned a lot and have been changed in the process. I hope to continue doing so.

Choden

I would like to acknowledge and thank Lama Yeshe Rinpoche, my spiritual teacher, for his wise and compassionate support over many years of guiding me on the Buddhist path.

I also want to thank Rob Nairn for his friendship and wisdom in shaping our particular approach to mindfulness training. Our partnership resulted in the formation of the Mindfulness Association, which is committed to teaching a compassion-based mindfulness training.

I would like to acknowledge the Mindfulness Association as being the source of the mindfulness teachings and practices that inform chapters 7 and 8 of the book. For anyone wanting to practice a compassion-based mindfulness training drawn from these chapters, see http://www.mindfulnessassociation.net.

Thanks also to the core team of the Mindfulness Association, who have shaped our compassion-based mindfulness training: Heather Regan-Addis, Norton Bertram-Smith, Vin Harris, Annick Nevejan, Fay Adams, Kristine Jansen, Clive Holmes, and Angie Ball.

I would like to thank Dr. Charlotte Procter for her work on the Mindfulness Scotland Manual, which influenced our mindfulness training, some of which is reflected in chapter 7 of the book.

Last, but certainly not least, I would like to thank Paul for his support and kindness over the last few years. He has been a great friend.

Both of us wish to thank all the folks at Constable & Robinson for their hard work, in particular, Fritha Saunders for her continuing encouragement and enthusiasm. She is a delight to work with, and we have been most fortunate in having her as our editor.

INTRODUCTION

Have you ever thought about how wonderful it would be if we could cure cancer, prevent children from dying of starvation, build a more just world, and help people find peaceful ways to resolve conflicts? If so, you are already on the path of compassion. Focusing on the wish for others to be free of suffering and its causes, and *being happy* when this comes about, might not normally be considered as the very basis of compassion, but in fact, it is, and shortly we will explain why.

Within Christian traditions, having a compassionate and kind orientation to those less fortunate than ourselves, the sick and poor, is the central focus for life.[1] Commonly compassion is defined as "being sensitive to the suffering of self and others with a deep commitment to try to prevent and relieve it."[2] This definition is interesting because, if we think about it for a moment, we can see that this simple statement points to two very different mental abilities or psychologies. The first is being open and receptive to suffering, not shutting it out. Indeed, the word "compassion" comes from the Latin word *compati*, which means "to suffer with." So we can ask ourselves what special attributes and skills we need in order to move *toward* suffering. The second mental ability, or "psychology," is about how we then respond to suffering in ourselves and others. In this book, we will explore these two abilities in depth and suggest methods for training in them.

If compassion is only "to suffer with," then it comes down to things like sympathy and empathy, which are important but only part of the story. What is also needed is to do something to alleviate suffering (and indeed prevent it if we can); this is linked to the second part of the definition. This calls on a very different part of our minds that is linked to the abilities to be kind, supportive, understanding, and motivated for action. Now these might require actually learning how to be mindful and accepting rather than hating or fighting with suffering. We might also need to go more deeply into it—just like somebody who has an anxiety condition such as agoraphobia might have to learn to go out, face, and tolerate anxiety rather than trying to get rid of it. But the important point we wish to make is that our abilities to engage with, tune in to, and try to understand the sources of suffering are *different* from those associated with the alleviation and prevention of suffering.

Imagine the scenario of a doctor seeing a new patient. First, doctors must pay attention to the pain and suffering of their patients in order to identify where the pain is and what its causes are. There is no point in trying to treat the wrong condition. However, once they've pinpointed the malady, they don't stay focused on the pain but turn their attention to what will relieve it. They draw on their knowledge and experience in order to prescribe a treatment that will bring about healing. In addition, they might take their patient's hand with a reassuring smile and understanding that kindness helps settle fear.

Developing our inner compassion is like becoming our own doctors and healers. We develop the ability to engage with what is painful and seek to understand its roots, but we also need very different qualities linked to the desire to engage wisely, supportively, and kindly. Compassion involves understanding and acceptance of suffering but not just sitting in it—like sitting in one's own dirty bathwater and believing that acceptance means you shouldn't do anything. Indeed acceptance is an act of courage that calls for wise action (see chapter 8). So if we *only* focus on the ability to engage and understand pain we actually miss half of the story.

Training the Mind

Both of these processes require training. We need to work on the process of tuning in to and being moved by and empathic toward pain and difficulties we or others may be experiencing. And similarly, we need to work on cultivating the qualities of wise engagement and kindness. The only way a doctor can become a healer is to study and understand the nature of disease. Then he is in a position to facilitate healing. When it comes to our own minds, it's the same. We need to understand the nature and causes of suffering so we can engage with it in effective and caring ways. And given that one source of much of our suffering is to do with how our minds and emotions work, we need to study our minds to become aware of the forces at play. Learning how to observe carefully what goes on in our minds is a very important skill; it is known as *mindfulness*, and it is something we will be focusing on in depth in this book (see chapter 7).[3, 4]

So compassion is not about being overwhelmed or sinking into our own or other people's pain; it is not about being superficially nice so people will like us; it is not weakness, softness, or letting people off the hook if they cause harm. The key to compassion is tuning in to the nature of suffering, to understand it in the depths of our being, and to see clearly into its source; but equally important is to be committed to relieve it and to rejoice in the possibility of the alleviation of suffering for all.

Matthieu Ricard, a long-term Buddhist monk and French translator for the Dalai Lama, worked together with Tania Singer, a neuroscientist, to try to understand what goes on in the brain when we feel compassion. Their research led them to the conclusion that if you just have empathic concern for suffering (e.g., for the children who are dying in agony for lack of medicine or food, or the plight of the abused, tortured, and diseased) without engaging in some positive feelings associated with trying to do something about it, it can become a dark journey indeed. We could be left with feelings of rage or even hopelessness.[5] An example of this second aspect of compassion is evidenced by the tearful celebration that erupted among medical scientists in October 2011 when they looked at their data on a malaria vaccine and realized that it had worked and that they could now save thousands of children's lives.

Anger can be an important emotion to wake us up to the fact that compassionate action is needed. Paul often acknowledges that his interest in compassion arose from a mixture of anger and sadness that so many people's short lives are miserable; that vast amounts of the world's research resources are spent on weaponry and defense; that the bulk of the wealth of the world is held in the hands of a few; and that we seem locked into a competitive psychology in our economies that is driving us all crazy.[6] In 1984, Bob Geldof and Midge Ure became so moved by the famine in Ethiopia and frustrated and angry by government prevarications that they raised huge sums of money through Band Aid and Live Aid. So anger at injustice and suffering can move us to action. However, of course, anger can also be quite destructive and so, while understandable and a spark to action, mindful compassion offers a more skillful and assured way of engaging suffering and taking action.

Sadness too is an emotion that connects us to suffering. In Buddhist traditions, sadness is often an emotion that moves us to compassionate action (see chapter 6). Again, however, mindful compassion helps us not wallow in sadness but rather use it as a call to action.

Another crucial element to compassion is the concept of *flow*—again, a key theme we will be returning to in more detail later. We can be compassionate *to other people*, and it's this outward flow of feeling that is generally the main focus in the literature on compassion. But, again, this is only part of the story—that one-way flow. We also need to be open and receptive to the compassion *from other people toward us*. We can notice how other people's kindness supports us and affects us emotionally, and we can learn to be mindful of that too. Another aspect of the flow of compassion is learning to be compassionate toward ourselves, something that at times could be emphasized more in the Buddhist and Christian literature. It's simply not possible to develop deeper levels of compassion if you're not open to compassion coming toward you and if you are resistant to developing self-compassion.[7] For example, if there are things in you that you block or detest, then you're going to struggle to empathize about similar things in other people.

Our Multiple Selves

Gardeners and farmers love to see things grow. Most parents know the pleasures of seeing their children flourish. However, even though we can be sensitive to other's people's feelings and struggles and reach out to help them, there is a big "yes, but" to our deeply felt compassionate motive "to relieve suffering in ourselves and others." It is a fact that compassionate desires and motives compete with many other motives in our minds: to get on in the world, to compete and outperform others, to get rich, to get "laid," or to defend our religious or ethnic group. We are a species with many contradictory and conflicting parts. We can even experience joy when we see enemies being destroyed and rejoice in tyrants getting a bullet in the head. Our entertainment industry revolves around "good" guys killing "bad" guys with justification and pleasure; and, sadly, games for children exploit these aspects of our minds.

So the human mind is full of competing motives. If we live in a threatening world where people don't value compassion, and where instead we have to compete with others and worry all the time about keeping our jobs or preventing our houses from being repossessed, then these are not the conditions for nurturing a compassionate mind. In this case, our inner capacity for compassion can become like a forgotten garden that is overgrown with brambles. Worse still, people can start to think that compassion is a weakness—some kind of soft fuzzy thing that is all about self-indulgence or submissive kindness.[8, 9] It is absolutely not those things. As we will see, compassion requires strength, determination, and courage within an emotional context of kindness and connection with others. These are like seedlings in the ground waiting to be nurtured and allowed to grow.

Understanding the Mind

Most of us learn a lot about mathematics or history but very little about how our minds work. Societies that are only interested in whether people can toil from dawn until dusk don't tend to help people understand themselves better. They seek to foster aspirations of becoming an engineer, tennis player, pilot, or shop worker. At no time are Western children taught that our minds can be *very difficult and tricky to cope with*—riddled with passions and feelings emanating from a brain that has been evolving over millions of years. Little or nothing is taught about becoming mindful and compassionate toward what's going on in our minds, and how this can really help when we are struggling with anxiety, anger, depression, and self-doubt. Given the huge advances in psychology and our understanding about our minds, this is nothing short of a tragedy. However, it highlights just how much we orient education toward each of us becoming a productive unit.

While we recognize the central importance of compassion to spiritual systems such as Christianity, and indeed refer to them from time to time, in this book we are going to be focusing more on certain Buddhist ideas that derive from an Eastern philosophical system. We do this because Buddhism has been one of the few spiritual traditions that have argued that *far* more time needs to be given to becoming familiar with and training our minds because without insight and training, our minds can easily become chaotic, dangerous, and prone to fear, rage, and despair. In fact, Buddhist texts suggest that the untrained mind can verge on insanity because it cannot regulate its own passions and wild emotions, and for this reason there are so many terrible cruelties and injustices throughout the world.

However, we wish to make it clear that we are not adopting these ideas as a religion, but as a psychological system. Indeed, Paul does not buy into some of the metaphysical beliefs underpinning Buddhism, such as the need to earn a good rebirth and the idea that pain and suffering can be related to unskillful behaviors in a previous life—common though these are to most Buddhist schools.[10] According to some commentators, the Buddha himself never strayed into those metaphysical speculations. The Dalai Lama has frequently spoken about the importance of distinguishing Buddhist psychology from its more metaphysical dimensions.

The reason that Buddhist psychology is so important is simply because Buddhism has spent thousands of years focusing on the mind: observing how the mind gets itself in various tangles and learning to understand and train it so that we can live more peaceful and balanced lives. Our Western traditions of psychology and psychotherapy are also beginning to reveal important insights about how our minds work, and increasingly these two traditions are coming closer together as scientific studies substantiate much of what the Buddha taught thousands of years ago in terms of the importance and effectiveness of observing and training one's mind. The excitement for us in writing this book is to bring these two traditions together.

The Self We Might Choose

Compassion requires us to cultivate an inner capacity and become a certain type of person, referred to as a *bodhisattva* in the Buddhist tradition—someone who is committed to understanding suffering and relieving it wherever possible. For this we must train. Just like a marathon runner puts in hard work to train every morning even when it's cold because they are committed to taking part in a marathon, so too we need to actively cultivate the qualities of the compassionate mind, especially when the journey gets tough and we are up against all manner of challenges.

Coming face to face with the pain and suffering of life is difficult. We know that the reality of our lives is that we are born, flourish for a while, spread a few genes around, and then decay and die. This is the lot of all living beings. Life doesn't last that long. Today, middle-class people can expect somewhere between 25,000 and 30,000 days with a bit of help from modern medicine and healthy living. If you are born into poverty, it could be much less. And, of course, during these 25,000 days, all kinds of illnesses and tragedies can strike us and those close to us.

Being prepared to face the reality that we are part of a life that has multiple diseases and ways of dying in pain—and that we can be our own worst (intensely cruel) enemy—can be distressing and even traumatic. It might make us angry or anxious—but being confronted by suffering calls upon something very deep within us. It is actually a wake-up call and requires courage. This is a key element of the compassionate mind and one of the hallmarks of a *bodhisattva*: being prepared to face the reality of life and find ways to engage with it based on courage, kindness, and commitment.

Now, to be honest, it's probably not a good start to talk about waking up to suffering when you want to sell a self-help book on compassion! We usually look to self-help books to promise that we'll feel better if we just follow the various recipes. So how can "waking up to suffering" do that? Well, the point is, it's not just waking up to suffering but what we do *next* that is crucial. Not surprisingly, we are going to argue that this will involve harnessing and developing the qualities of the compassionate mind, which begins the process of gradually transforming our inner world and awakening our capacity to care for ourselves, other people and life-forms, and the environment we live in. So even though things are difficult, awakening compassion changes our *relationship* to ourselves and our world, and this makes all the difference.

The Importance of Wisdom

Running throughout the path of development of compassion is wisdom. Now wisdom is not a mysterious or mystical thing It is simply knowledge plus experience that gives rise to insight.[11]

Knowledge + Experience = Insight

We have to build our wisdom; it does not just arise by itself. We have to work at gaining knowledge and developing insight into the causes of suffering. In our view, the *type of wisdom* you develop really depends on your *motive*—and this is where compassionate motives become crucial because there are so many different motives and hence different types of wisdom. For example, if we are oriented toward a compassionate approach *to suffering*, wisdom is about understanding suffering so that we can alleviate it. So our motive is crucial in determining the kind of knowledge we seek and how our knowledge and experience is applied.

The Lotus in the Mud

The metaphor for this book is "the lotus in the mud." We have chosen this because it resonates with a core wisdom of the link between pain and suffering and compassion. It is drawn from an ancient myth within the Mahayana Buddhist tradition. Basically, the mud represents our darker side: our self-centeredness, aggression, fears, and cruelty, the things we might prefer to avoid and push under the carpet. It also represents the stark reality of evolved life: the struggle and pain of life that all things are impermanent, and we just find ourselves in the flow of life for a short while with many of the motives for self-survival and prosperity that other animals share (we explore this in chapter 2). And at times any of us can be hit by tragedies and feel we are "sinking." Mud of course prevents clarity of vision. Yet the mud is the sustenance for the lotus; without it, the lotus could not emerge. Therefore, it is the relationship between the mud and the lotus that is absolutely crucial. Similarly, compassion evolves from the evolution of caring behavior. It is an evolutionary development and could not have arisen without the struggle of life.

The lotus cannot separate itself from or get rid of the mud because it depends on it—it is the same for us. Compassion awakens as we are touched by our suffering and that of those around us. The lotus symbolizes the awakening mind of compassion, the shift from self-focused pleasure-seeking to addressing the core issue of suffering. With it comes motivation and commitment to enter the mud (suffering) and cultivate the positive qualities of love, care, understanding, and joy through which we open out and respond to the pain of life in ourselves and others. This is a key theme of the book, and it is something we explore in more depth in chapter 6.

Key Points

- There are two distinct "psychologies," or mental abilities, that make up compassion: one that helps us to *engage* with suffering, to understand it; and another that arises from our skillful actions and our efforts to *alleviate* it.

- The human mind is full of competing motivations and potentials. For the compassionate mind to arise and make a difference in our lives, we need to actively train in both these psychologies.

- While many spiritual traditions provide great teachings on love and compassion, Buddhism is a unique resource because it offers practical methods for training the mind in compassion.

- Western science too is now revealing ways in which we can begin to train our minds with the aim of creating improved well-being and compassionate living for all.

Part I

THE ISSUES

1

WAKING UP

Understanding our minds is perhaps one of the greatest challenges for modern science and each of us personally. You don't have to think about this very much to recognize that the human mind generates outstanding achievements in science, medicine, and institutions for justice, but it is the same mind that can produce the most awful atrocities and acts of greed. For all the challenges that we face in the world, from the injustices of rich versus poor; the need to address global warming and nurture our planet; the need to reduce exploitation of young, weak, and poor; to the need to develop universal health care systems—the common denominator in all of these is our minds. It's our minds that will create grasping selfishness, pitting group against group, or an open, reflective, cooperative, and sharing approach to these difficulties. And, of course, it is our minds that are the source of our own personal experiences of happiness and joy, or anxiety, misery, and despair.

So this book is a story about how our minds came to be the way they are, what we now know about how they work, and, most importantly, how we can train them to rise to the challenges we face in the external world and also within ourselves, in the ebb and flow of our emotions and feelings. Indeed, we suggest that the more we understand our minds, the more we will be able to understand how and why we need to train them (which is what we set out to do in part II).

Many Eastern and Western philosophers, not to mention religions, have struggled with the issues of the nature of our minds and the nature of suffering in the world. In this book, we will explore insights generated from modern psychological research but also much older traditions, including Buddhism. The reason that there is now so much Western interest in Buddhism is because, for thousands of years, Buddhist scholars and devotees studied and developed practices of *introspective and reflective psychology* and an ethic based on compassionate insights—ways by which individuals can become very familiar with their minds, learn to stabilize and organize them for their well-being, and cultivate key qualities that are associated with personal and social health. We can explore Buddhism as a psychology of introspection and ethics that has given rise to insights about how tricky and difficult our minds can be and what we can do about it. So let's start at the beginning and think about what led the Buddha to become so interested in trying to understand the roots of suffering as arising from our own minds.

We start with an important story that comes from the early life of the Buddha. It is said that he was born into a family that ruled parts of a district that is now in Nepal. His name was Siddhārtha Gautama, but he was to become known as the *Buddha* later in his life; this means the "awakened one." The exact date of his birth is unknown, but it is believed to be around 563 BC or 623 BC. He died at about eighty years old, a very good age for that time.

His father, the king, was by various counts an ambitious fellow and very keen for Siddhārtha to become a great king in his own right. At his birth, many wise men foretold to the king that his son would indeed be a great leader and would be known throughout the world for many centuries. However, they prophesied that he would either be a great king or a great spiritual adept (or expert), depending upon the circumstances he encountered in his life. The latter possibility caused the king great anxiety, and, desperate to prevent it, he shielded his son from all forms of suffering and provided him with every pleasure conceivable. He built Siddhārtha a golden palace (maybe more than one) with beautiful gardens, and provided him with plenty of distractions in the form of the finest foods, wines, and young ladies.

The king gave strict instructions that everything had to be kept beautiful so that Siddhārtha would never discover the reality of poverty and suffering that lay beyond his palace gates, and would therefore never want to go on any spiritual quest. But curiosity got the better of Siddhārtha, and one night he sneaked out of his gilded palace. There he discovered a totally different world—one of immense poverty and suffering, of disease, decay, death, and cruelty. It is said he saw a man beating a horse and was overcome by his first encounter with cruelty. He saw beggars thin and dying in the street and was shocked to see death and poverty. Perplexed and distressed, he fled the palace under the cover of night, leaving behind his wife and child, and set out on the dusty roads of India, determined to understand the causes of suffering and attain enlightenment. Unlike some spiritual teachers who came from positions of hardship and struggle, Siddhārtha came from a life of luxury.

The way he dealt with this traumatic shock is a very important part of the story, with something to teach us too, because it's quite possible he could have thought to himself: "Oh, my goodness, it is terrible out there. I am really much better off staying where I am. I think I'll just go back and enjoy my life, count the money, and keep the wine and the women flowing." How many of us in his position would have done just that and stayed in our bubble of pleasure? In fact when you think about it, this is a parable for *our lives*—most of us prefer to live in our own comfortable bubble and hope life is not too harsh with us. Part of the problem is that the longer we live in the bubble and become accustomed to turning a blind eye to the harshness of life, the more we can become desensitized to it until something knocks on our door and brings us face to face with reality.

In Siddhārtha's time, India was awash with gurus and sages of all types practicing various chanting meditations, yoga, cleansing rituals, and much else besides—basically offering solutions to the endemic problem of suffering. He was to sample many of them. He tried the ascetic life of giving up all desires because desires were seen as the source of suffering. The problem was that he nearly died of malnutrition in the process, and realized that this wasn't a solution at all but simply a strategy of avoidance.

One story tells of how, when he was close to death from extreme fasting, he saw a musician floating past on a boat. The musician was tuning his instrument a little tighter and then a little looser, until exactly the right pitch was obtained, so that he could play the right note. Siddhārtha immediately recognized that *balance* was the crucial ingredient for so much of life as this provides the condition for something new to emerge and flourish. In this way he came to recognize the importance of the *Middle Way*—a path of balance between the extremes of indulgence and denial.

Once he had given up the ascetic life and had begun to eat again, he knew that he needed to find another way—this was the path of *closely observing his own mind*. In the depths of his renunciation and despair, he had realized that his own mind held the answer to the timeless riddle of happiness and suffering. He saw that how he related to his mind, and what arose within it, determined whether he would be happy or not. So in this way he came to see his own mind as the greatest teacher of all. It was a source of his happiness or misery.

The Four Noble Truths and Modern Psychology

The Buddha's story is interesting for a number of reasons. First is the way he approached the problem of suffering in the world, trying to understand its root causes; and second is what he decided to do about it, namely find a path that uprooted these causes of suffering. You can immediately see that if the Buddha started with a theistic view that suffering was in the world because some gods had ordained it that way, then this avenue of personal research would never have got off the ground. His completely open approach to suffering was a revolutionary way to break free from the idea that things are *ordained* to be the way they are. Siddhārtha was to put our own minds at the center of the story in a way that makes him like a modern psychologist.

Siddhārtha's deep insights were expressed in his first teaching on the *Four Noble Truths*. He taught that these truths are self-evident if you spend time considering them for yourself. In fact, the Four Noble Truths are very compatible with the basic scientific approach to things in the world. Geshe Tashi Tsering, who wrote a very insightful and authoritative book on the Four Noble Truths, points out that they are completely compatible with secular scientific approaches.[1] Simply put, the Four Noble Truths come down to this: we can recognize that suffering exists; it has various causes; once we understand what those causes are, we can do something about them; the possibility of freedom from suffering exists by finding ways to prevent these causes from re-occurring.

In principle this is no different from any scientific endeavor, such as researching and treating cancer. Two thousand years ago, people simply died of mysterious conditions and nobody knew why. But now we know that there is such a thing as cancer; this leads us to study its causes; this offers the possibility of being free of the disease; and this leads us to apply the appropriate treatments and do the things that prevent cancer from arising (e.g., antismoking campaigns).

The Buddha applied the Four Noble Truths to the understanding of suffering, and this is what we will now explore.

The First Noble Truth

The First Noble Truth is that suffering exists. As Geshe Tashi Tsering points out, there are many different types of suffering, such as the suffering associated with old age, illness, injury, and death; the suffering associated with encountering aversive things; the suffering associated with not being able to have pleasant things; and the suffering linked to the way our minds operate.[2]

Now, in the original Pali language, the term used is "dukkha." This has a far wider and more subtle meaning than "suffering." It refers to a pervasive sense of unease in which we sense in our very gut that our lives are precariously rooted in the shifting sands of impermanence and we cannot keep hold of what we like or keep away what we do not like. In their very accessible introduction to Buddhism for Western readers, *Buddhism for Dummies*, Bodian and Landaw put it simply when they say that *dukkha* arises from meeting things that you don't want or like (e.g., running into a hated enemy in the street); being parted from things that you do want and like (e.g., the death of a loved one or losing your job); and failing to get what you want (e.g., being rejected by someone you have fallen in love with). And then, as they point out, the Buddha asks us to reflect on how much our lives are ruled by these three things; how much they cause our minds to react with emotions of fear, anger, and sadness; and how we come to discover that we are not in control of what happens in our lives.[3]

In Buddhist texts, *dukkha* is described as operating on three levels. First, there is the "suffering of suffering"—the actual experience of pain and dissatisfaction. One example, often cited, is eating poisoned food and then experiencing the pain of being sick. Second, there is the "suffering of impermanence." The Buddha taught that the very act of being born creates *dukkha* because all living things are destined to flourish for a short while and then decay and die. Incidentally, this is true for all things in the universe. Even our sun will one day use up its nuclear fuel, become a red giant, and then collapse and explode, showering new elements into the universe that may one day become the building blocks for life on some other planet. A more personal example of the suffering of impermanence is that while we are eating poisoned food, we may be enjoying it very much but are unaware of the poison that has not yet taken hold—the suffering was avoidable (had we known the food was poisoned) but unintentional (because we didn't know). Third, there is the "suffering of the composite"—that all things are composed of other things; and this includes our bodies, which are made up of many parts that change and decay. This is the most subtle level of *dukkha*—that pain is built into the very fabric of being alive. It is part of the deal, and it is something that we cannot escape, yet it is something we can learn to come to terms with. An example of this form of suffering is that we have a body that feels pain and gets sick so eating poisoned food can affect us adversely.

Modern science is adding to our understanding of the causes of pain in ways that would have amazed the young Siddhārtha. It has revealed that some of the sources of illness are partly our genes and partly viruses and bacteria that depend on living things like us for their own survival. They inhabit this earth with us and, like us, they evolve, change, and multiply. In 1348–1350, Europe was hit with the bubonic plague, caused by the bacterium *Yersinia pestis*. It is estimated that this wiped out 40–60 percent of the European population in two years. When Europeans turned up in the Americas, many of the indigenous peoples were not immune to European diseases such as measles or chickenpox, and more serious illnesses such as syphilis and smallpox were alien to them. These diseases accounted for the huge decline in their populations at this time. Furthermore, it's extraordinary but true that the influenza outbreak that lasted from June 1917 until December 1920 killed more people than died in the First World War—50–100 million by some estimates—making it one of the deadliest pandemics ever. And, of course, viruses are just one of a multitude of ways in which our lives are brought to a premature end; there are also earthquakes, tornadoes, floods, tsunamis, and countless other events.

While the focus of science has been on understanding and alleviating the physical nature and causes of pain, spiritual traditions like Buddhism have tended to focus more on alleviating suffering—that is, working with how the mind reacts to pain. Nonetheless, the Dalai Lama has always been a keen advocate of scientific research because the rationale behind the Four Noble Truths is to understand and alleviate suffering *in any ethical way possible*, not just through working with our minds. He has often noted that meditating is not enough—we need action! For science to address suffering is clearly a compassionate endeavor. It is linked to the Second Noble Truth.

The Second Noble Truth

The Second Noble Truth is that *dukkha* has a cause, or more accurately a series of causes, and when we properly understand and address these causes, *dukkha* can end. At this point it is important to make a clear distinction between pain and suffering—*dukkha* relates more to the experience of suffering than the reality of pain. In Buddhist texts, suffering primarily concerns the way our mind reacts to pain and the meanings we put onto things. The Buddha never said we can put an end to *pain*; rather, if we understand the causes of pain, then we can take actions to avoid it. For example, if you know that smoking causes lung cancer, then stopping smoking may prevent the onset of this disease.

But let's consider the case where you *are* actually dying from cancer. In this event, not only is there the pain of dying, but there are also the meanings you give to the pain and the experience of dying, which then become the focus of your suffering. Now, supposing you could control your pain through modern medicine and you knew you would not die in agony, and you saw your life as meaningful and perhaps believed that you would go to heaven to meet all your dead relatives for a happy reunion. In this case, your level of suffering would be much less than another scenario in which you felt that you could not bear the pain, you were frightened of it, you saw your whole life as pointless, and death was the end of the road with no life hereafter. Even though the basic event is the same—dying of cancer—how we experience it and attribute meaning to it varies greatly according to how our mind relates to it. Western philosophers and psychologists have also spent time thinking about how we give meaning to events and how that process then shapes our emotions and actions.

One of the central tenets of Buddhism is that it's our wish for things to be different from the way they are that can set us up for *dukkha*. We all tend to have strong ideas about what we want and what we do not want, but reality seldom accords with our preferences. It is not just a life free of pain that we want; we want so many other things too. We want to find people who will love us and whom we desire; we want to be free from hunger or cold; we want secure, well-paid jobs, nice houses, and top-of-the-range cars; we want holidays, TVs, iPads; and the list goes on endlessly. Although wanting is part of how our minds are and the way we live our lives, the problem is that wanting can become insatiable because we are a species that always tries to improve and get more. The Buddha was not being unkind when he said that it is our attachments to all of these desires that cause us trouble. He was simply pointing to the fact that if we feel we've "got to" or "must have" these things, and we "can't bear it" if we don't, this sets us up for suffering.

In fact there are many modern psychologists who argue exactly the same thing. They say that it's our inner imperatives of "got to, must, mustn't, should, and ought" that bind us to the path of *dukkha*.[4] Cognitive therapies, for example, point out that we often tell ourselves: "I *can't bear* it that I feel this way" or "I *must* have somebody to love me" or "'She *should not* do that to me" or "I *must* have A or B." So what really drives *dukkha* is this intense emotional craving—the sense that we *have* to have things the way we want them. This holds us chained to the wheel of suffering. This is similar to what many psychologists mean when they say that it's not so much attachment that causes us problems, but more the motivational state of craving and "musting"; or, as the late American therapist Albert Ellis would say, "musterbation."[5] Again, it's not so much wanting things that is the issue; it's how we go about trying to secure what we want and how we react if we can't get what we want that are crucial.

The Buddha argued that because we are so driven to pursue pleasure and avoid pain, we are vulnerable to the destructive emotions of greed and hatred, and under the power of these emotions, we can inflict terrible suffering on other living creatures. For example, the way we produce food to feed ourselves now causes terrible suffering to billions of animals we share this planet with. This points to a deeper meaning within the Second Noble Truth, which is that the more self-focused we become in trying to avoid pain and service our pleasures, the more we fall victim to greed and not sharing, and one of the consequences of this is living in a world where some people have billions of dollars while many others are starving and don't even have 50 cents. In fact, a root cause of suffering, according to the Buddha, is our fierce sense of self-centeredness.

Interestingly, modern science and evolutionary psychology reveal that being self-focused and driven by our likes and dislikes is partly to do with genes—we are set up by evolution to experience strong likes and dislikes as this is what enables us to survive and reproduce. Imagine if overnight something happened to our genes and we gave birth to children who didn't want anything: they were not bothered about eating, learning to walk, socializing, developing friendships, or having sex. No species survives without genes building highly motivated organisms to pursue these things. When you think about it, this is just common sense, but it has serious implications for how these gene-built systems play out in our minds. As we will see later, though, the cultures we live in and also the choices we make are highly influential on the kind of motives we pursue.

This leads to an extraordinarily important insight and an important corollary to the teaching of the Buddha: it is *not our fault* that we are the way we are with all our drives, passions, and aversions. All of the drives of wanting pleasure and avoiding painful things, desiring nice food, comfortable houses to live in, and loving sexual partners, are built into the very fabric of our genes. The key point, however, is that these basic motivations can take control of our minds in very self-focused ways, and if we do not become aware of them, they will run the show of our lives (we will explore this in the next chapter). This is analogous to having a garden and not paying it any attention—it will grow in all directions, but we might not like the result. So just as we can learn how to cultivate our garden and make choices as to what we want to grow, so too we can learn to cultivate our minds and make wise choices about the qualities and habits we want to cultivate and make manifest.

The Third Noble Truth

The Third Noble Truth is cessation—*dukkha* can end, or at least it can be significantly reduced. Bear in mind, though, this does not mean we will never again experience pain. What it means is that we can move toward developing an inner peacefulness and stability even in the presence of great pain and difficulty. The Buddha said that we can find ways to gradually let go of our attachment to things, even though we are still actively involved with our lives. *Dukkha* (but not pain necessarily) can gradually be reduced as we learn to live with things *as they really are*, moment by moment.

The method by which we begin to recognize the way our desires and emotions grab hold of our mind is by learning to observe our mind in action, and becoming very familiar with it. We have a capacity for self-awareness and reflective thought that other animals do not. Right now you can stop reading this book and become aware of yourself: you are aware that you exist, aware that you're sitting somewhere reading, aware that you are having thoughts and feelings about what you are reading, and you can decide whether to continue reading to follow the story, even though you're tired and don't feel like continuing. It's amazing what our minds can do! And, most significantly, you have an *awareness of being aware*. You can be aware that you are thinking all these things. It's like mirrors within mirrors within mirrors. This capacity for awareness of what's going on inside ourselves is the basis of *mindfulness*. It is a mental capacity that enables us to stand back and look at the moment-by-moment processes and dramas of the mind and experience what it is like to become an impartial observer.

For many people, this initiates the beginning of an important shift within themselves—instead of being caught in the storylines that are easily triggered by our desires or emotions, such as reliving an argument from the night before, we touch the momentary liberation of looking at this story from the outside, realizing that we don't have to fuel it. We take a view "from the balcony" with respect to what's going on in our minds. This can gradually diminish the power of the "have to" and the "must" mentality.

This is the potential path to liberation that the Buddha was pointing to with the Third Noble Truth. It takes birth in the *small* moments of our lives. When we pay attention to these moments through practicing mindfulness, it has the potential to awaken an entirely different dimension of awareness within us. The Buddha also taught that through observing the mind, it becomes quieter, and when it does, insight naturally arises into how it works. So when the mind is no longer caught up, moment by moment, in the tumble dryer of emotions, desires, views, and worries, it settles. It's like a person sitting in a muddy pool; if she can just sit still, the mud will gradually settle and the water will become clear. This will enable her to *see into the depths of the water*.

Modern psychology is also trying to find better ways of helping people settle their minds and develop clearer insights into the nature of their problems. But Buddhism goes one step further. It focuses on insight into the nature of mind itself. When our mind settles and becomes calm, we can begin to see how we are living in a world full of mind-created illusions. With a clear mind we can recognize how our sense of an individual mind is itself a temporary creation. It has been formed from the genes of our parents, shaped by the world we inhabit, and lasts for a relatively short time until the body it inhabits decays and dies. But this is not the end of the story. As our insight deepens, we can gain insight into a different level of mind, referred to as "big mind" in Zen Buddhism—a quality of unbounded awareness that is free from the limited creations of our biological mind and is characterized by the full development of our innate qualities of wisdom and compassion. So the Third Noble Truth points to the cessation of one type of mind and an initiation into a much deeper experience of who we can be.

The Fourth Noble Truth

The Fourth Noble Truth points to a path to freedom from *dukkha*—how we can come to grips with *dukkha* and gradually soften and loosen it.[6] Siddhārtha understood that if we want to bring about change at the deepest level, we need to develop skills for working with all the different parts of ourselves in a sustained and coordinated way. This is something we will be coming back to when we describe the compassionate attributes and skills in chapter 4.

The path of awakening set in motion by the Buddha went through various phases after his death, generally referred to as the *Three Turnings of the Wheel of Dharma*, but two skills for training the mind run throughout these phases of teaching: mindfulness and compassion. These skills are the main focus of our book, but they are approached from a secular perspective, both acknowledging their Buddhist source while also applying the latest insights from neuroscience and psychology.[7]

When we really come down to it, what the Buddha was saying in his teaching on the Four Noble Truths is that it is the mind that gives rise to the experience of *dukkha*—suffering only arises because we have minds that enable it to arise. We could imagine computers or robots doing similar things to humans, but they don't suffer because they don't have feelings or conscious awareness, and they don't have a mind that wishes to be happy and free of suffering. And since the mind is the root of *dukkha*, learning to train the mind to behave differently is crucial for alleviating it.

It naturally follows then that the first skill is to become more familiar with the workings of our mind by observing it in action. In fact the word "meditation" simply means familiarization. Today, all over the world, people are practicing "mindfulness meditation," which is the practice of paying attention to the moment-by-moment flow of our thoughts and emotions in a nonjudgmental way.

However, it has been understood within the Mahayana Buddhist tradition for a long time that what really changes the mind is the practice of compassion, which is the second main skill. Furthermore, in order for deep change to take root, we need to apply both mindfulness and compassion together, as these skills work together like the two wings of a bird. This is also the understanding that is emerging from both neuroscience and psychology—that compassion transforms the mind, but mindfulness provides the basis and stability for such change. This is a theme we will be exploring throughout this book.

Emergence and Interconnectedness

Although we are going to focus on training our own individual minds, we also want to make a strong point here about *interconnectedness* and our relationship to other minds and the societies we cocreate. Western philosophies, stretching as far back as the Stoics and early Christianity, as well as more recent sciences such as sociology and anthropology, all stress the importance of seeing ourselves as highly interconnected beings—our very sense of self depends on each other. An important principle that is at the heart of Western science and Buddhism is that everything co-arises—everything is based on relationships. All the molecules in our body are determined by the relationships of the atoms that make them up. There is no grand designer putting the atoms together to make molecules, or building molecules into proteins or proteins into bodies, and so on. Instead, due to the operation of the laws of nature, molecules emerge out of atoms, proteins emerge out of the combination of molecules, and bodies emerge out of the relationship of proteins (and other substances of course). Taking another example, anthills are not built by any designer directing other ants and making architectural drawings but simply through the interactions of individual ants going about their instinctual business. In a similar way, genes build our bodies simply through a process of interaction.[8]

In this way, we can see that everything emerges through patterns of relationships. Moreover, anything new is dependent upon preexisting processes and the laws of their interaction. This applies to our personal relationships too. It is now well understood by modern psychology that we are mutually interdependent and influence each other.[9] This is not a metaphysical sense of connectedness but the way we have been built, the way we have evolved as a species. We know that the love children receive when they are young influences the genes that become expressed[10] through them and how their brains develop.[11] But whether or not parents are able to love their children may be linked to what happened *to them* in their own childhood and the *intergenerational flow* of love or abuse and neglect. Furthermore, having friendships and supportive relationships, in contrast to being bullied or isolated, can have a huge impact on people's physiological states, vulnerability to illnesses, and susceptibility to mental health problems. In fact, the way we relate to each other influences our physiological states moment by moment.[12]

Our identity is also linked to our connections with others and the social conditions we grew up in. This is illustrated by an example that we will use a number of times throughout this book: if we had been kidnapped as babies and brought up in violent drug gangs, the chances are we would now be violent ourselves; we might have killed or tortured people, or perhaps we might be dead or languishing in prison. This is a tragedy because we know that this is the destiny of many young males who grow up in these environments. In this instance, there would be no possibility for the version of ourselves as a long-term Buddhist and long-term clinical psychologist to come into existence. Even more tragic is that if we had been adopted into rival gangs, we might have tortured or killed each other, and the friendship and mutual learning that we now have would be a completely unlived potential. To think about it from the mindset of the kinds of people we are now is of course extremely distressing—but it's important because it shows how fragile the sense of self is.

Consider also that if we were living in Rome 2,500 years ago, we might be looking forward to the Roman games this weekend. In the first three months of the opening of the Colosseum, over ten thousand people lost their lives just for entertainment. The Roman Empire lasted for around 700 years, so the number of deaths for violent entertainment is probably incalculable. Also, crucifixions—a dreadful way to die—were standard practice at that time and so too was horrific torture. But the Romans were not aliens with different genes or different brains; in essence they were exactly the same as you and me. What was different was that the culture they were part of and the values that underpinned it condoned acts of great cruelty and this then shaped the relationships that arose in this culture. So, for example, it might have been a respectful job at that time to be an organizer of gladiatorial shows.

Although some people remain fascinated by sadism and modern television wants to sell us more and more violent TV shows, as a culture we have nonetheless moved away from the horrific values of times gone by. The reason many of us have the values we do and enjoy lives that are relatively free of fear is because of the cultural values and institutions we have built up to contain the destructive potentials within us. It is because of the courageous efforts of those long dead that we now can live lives of relative freedom.

Therefore, every facet of our lives, from the way our brains are organized to our cultural values, is part of a complex, interconnected web that not only operates in the here and now, but is linked to generations long gone and will ripple on into generations to come. The American psychologist Philip Zimbardo has spent a lifetime understanding how good people can end up doing bad things. He called it the Lucifer effect.[13] We are very vulnerable to behaving well or poorly because we are deeply social beings. Perhaps one of the greatest enemies of compassion is conformity; a preparedness to go along with the way things are, sometimes out of fear, sometimes complacency, and sometimes because we do what our leaders tell us to do.

We can also recognize just how much everything around us depends on the actions of others. Consider your car. Its creation depended on generations of inventors, people who are prepared to mine the iron that made the steel, people who work in the factories to assemble the parts, and people who risk their lives in deep sea oil wells. There is nothing around us—from the food we eat to the clothes we wear to the houses we live in and to the hospitals we go to when we are sick—that does not depend on the actions of others. Sometimes we kid ourselves that we are single, encapsulated selves that are completely self-reliant, but this is mere illusion and fantasy.

Within this context, it's extraordinary how often we don't notice the everyday kindness of people who go out of their way to be helpful and considerate, and who go the extra mile to make sure they do a good job. It's so important that we pay attention to the kindness and compassion coming *toward* us because the news media constantly pulls our attention to the tragic and destructive stories such as rape, murder, and bombings. But the fact of the matter is that we have evolved as a species to be emotionally oriented toward cooperating and helping each other, and a large part of our happiness comes from these relationships of love and care.[14, 15] Indeed, this brings us back to a key theme of this book, which is that compassion is not just about tuning in to the details of suffering, but is also very much about appreciating and being grateful for those living beings that surround us and whose actions make our very survival and well-being possible. There are some psychologists who suggest that every day we should bring to mind what we are grateful for—not in a guilty way, but simply paying attention to the helpfulness of others—as there is now good evidence that focusing on gratitude can be very helpful for our well-being.

All this is also very relevant to our modern era because, although we seem to be becoming less cruel and violent[16] due to social change, we are allowing tendencies to emerge, driven by political and economic pressures, that are overly focused on competitiveness, selfishness, and greed, and this is causing serious trouble for so many people.[17] Frankly, we are driving ourselves crazy![18] The drive for increased efficiencies is now recognized to be turning the British National Health Service (which should be at the heart of compassion) into an uncompassionate service.[19] We may get efficiencies but we will create a world that is just cold and heartless to live in. Efficiency often means streamlining so that two jobs are collapsed into one, or people are given more and more responsibilities and duties until the job is too big and they struggle to maintain quality. If we are to create compassionate societies we need to understand these processes and to work out how to neutralize social forces that are pushing us toward greater competition, greed, and exploitation. We need to wake up and, as the Buddha did, come out of our golden palaces. In this way, mindful compassion needs to address the fact that our lives are interconnected with the lives of others and that we cocreate the world we live in.

The Buddha's Story and Us

Stories that last for centuries usually do so because they point to a fundamental insight about our lives. The Buddha's story is an archetypal one of waking up to a certain reality and then, just like the heroes of old, rising to the challenge of going out and gaining knowledge and wisdom for the quest so as to reach the goal—for the Buddha it was liberation from suffering. In many ways the Buddha's story is the story of all of us who, to some degree, live in our gilded palaces. If we are lucky enough to grow up in loving families, then our parents will try to protect and care for us so that we can enjoy our childhoods, and we will grow up with more or less the same aspirations that they have, and live similar lives. Also, in our production-focused society in the West, we feel so proud of having developed our science and technology to such an extent that we are relatively free from famine, and, for the most part, enjoy the comforts of warm houses, running water, and sanitation. Our science has served us greatly and has cushioned us somewhat from the harsh realities of life that existed just a few hundred years ago. Anesthetics and pain control, coupled with palliative care, ease the passage of those who are dying. Modern medicine can even cure many diseases and injuries that would have killed us less than a hundred years ago. There is much to celebrate and be deeply grateful for in modern science and in those who have dedicated their lives to these causes.

But, in our quieter moments, most of us glimpse a darker truth. We sense that despite our best efforts the reality of pain and suffering is a constant glimmer on the horizon, sometimes far away yet at other times, very close. There are many things that medicine and our world of gadgets cannot protect us from. So we try to keep ourselves constantly distracted with our iPods, BlackBerries, multichannel TVs, and so on. In fact, the whole capitalist system seeks to hold us addicted and needy of things and possessions—enticing us to buy more, have more, and enjoy the pleasures of life. It needs this to keep functioning like a serpent eating its own tail, more and more, faster and faster, cheaper and cheaper. In this way it subtly encourages us to close our eyes to the suffering beyond our gates and the reality of our own lives, and indeed of life itself. Mindful compassion, however, is not about turning a blind eye; it is not about dishonesty and greed; it is not about hiding through fear. It is about seeking the truth of how we create suffering within our own minds and how we create suffering in the social systems we are part of.

Just like the Buddha, our first step is to understand the causes of suffering and to seek the knowledge that will equip us to understand our minds better. Therefore, the next two chapters will focus on how our minds are constructed, enabling us to gain this knowledge and, in so doing, show how the Buddha's Second Noble Truth is still very relevant today.

It might be useful to engage in the following reflections in order to convert some of the knowledge in this chapter into personal wisdom.

Reflection One

Sit quietly where you will not be disturbed and consider how different you might have been if you had grown up in a different environment. Choose any environment provided it's very different from the one you grew up in. Perhaps think of one of great wealth or one of great poverty or one that is violent. What would it be like to give up the identity you have right now? If this feels difficult, remind yourself that this is a reflection exercise designed to provoke insight. Notice how this resistance affects you. Try to be curious, open, even playful if that helps. The point of the exercise is just to notice your resistance without feeling guilty or ashamed. Paul has often reflected on the fact that giving up the identity of "being a psychologist" would be extremely tough indeed! There is no blame here, just mindful fascination of why it's so important.

Reflection Two

The next reflection is to think about how you would feel if you lost the material things around you. Again this may be difficult. For example, Paul is very attached to his house and to his guitars, even though he doesn't play them very well! Again, this exercise is not to encourage you to give things up, but simply to help you notice your resistance to losing them and how this feeds into holding onto and needing to maintain a certain lifestyle. When we begin to think about the suffering this would cause us, we might give a thought to what happens to somebody in a war situation who sees their house blown up or perhaps swept away by a tsunami—by being in touch with our own distress we can feel that of others.

Both these reflections can help us understand how attached we are to so much that has been created around us but also how tragic it is that some people who lose these things can lose their very sense of identity too; or worse still, they remain in destructive relationships and life situations because their sense of identity depends on them.

Reflection Three

Now, without needing to change your identity too much, imagine what it would be like to start every day thinking of yourself as a deeply compassionate person; that you are going to train and practice every day, even for just a few minutes; that you are on this mysterious journey of life, in a world full of pain and suffering, and your principal job is to do what you can while you're here. We are going to look at this in detail in the practice section of the book, but for the moment, think about whether this shift in orientation might open you up to wanting to know more about the nature of life and how you can respond more skillfully to the struggles and difficulties that occur. Focus on the joyfulness of this reflection.

Key Points

- The Buddha realized that our minds are a major source of our own fulfillment and happiness but so too of our unhappiness and despair. Therefore, learning to understand and train our minds is crucial. This was expressed in his teaching of the Four Noble Truths.

- In the Fourth Noble Truth, the Buddha set out a path to ending suffering and the causes of suffering. Two key skills that are part of this path are mindfulness and compassion. Learning to understand these skills, what blocks them and how to train in them, is the focus of this book.

- Not only do we inhabit individual minds that are very tricky, but we are part of relationships and social systems that can be a source of happiness or suffering depending upon many conditions that lie beyond our control.

- Mindful compassion helps us wake up to what we are caught up in. It is about seeking the truth of how we create suffering within our own minds and how we create suffering in the social systems we are part of. With this wisdom about suffering we can set out to alleviate and prevent it.

2

EVOLVED MIND AND MOTIVATIONS

Suffering arises precisely because we have biological bodies and minds, with nerve cells and brain systems that can feel pain and emotion. These have evolved and emerged over many millions of years in what we call the *flow of life*. This is the story of how our world gave birth to the simplest of single-cell organisms in the sea (called *prokaryotes*) some three to four billion years ago and how those life-forms gradually evolved and transformed into all of the species we see on Earth today.

It is important for us to understand how our bodies and minds were designed in the flow of life, and how they function, so that we can begin to cultivate them in ways that are conducive to mindful compassion. Understanding how our minds have evolved offers deep insight into the major problems we are going to face when trying to cultivate a wise, mindful, and compassionate mind.

Understanding Our Origins— The Flow of Life

Over the last two to three thousand years, many thinkers and philosophers have realized that our minds are tricky and troublesome, and riddled with problems. For example, our capacity for reason struggles to restrain many of our motives and emotions, and we can find ourselves doing things because powerful irrational forces control the inner show, such as seeking out sexual partners, falling in love, wanting children, and, more destructively, defending our status or identity, joining tribes and groups, and then rushing off to war to protect our particular group. These motives are not based on reason or logic. Many early Greek philosophers argued that reason is the faculty that we should cultivate so we can avoid getting lost in the chaos of our passions and instinctual drives. But, while reason is helpful to us, we can also reflect more on what our motivations really are and which of them will help us grow, develop, and prosper. So given the various motivations that can take hold of us, our task is to be reflective enough to choose wisely which motivations to cultivate and which to be wary of. This book will argue that the cultivation of motives based on mindfulness and compassion can have far-reaching consequences for our own well-being, mental health, and relationships, our sense of the person we are and the meaning in our lives, and for the world that we are part of and want to create.

While some spiritual traditions have tried to focus us on universal love, forgiveness, and the brotherhood of humanity, these motives, noble as they are, run up against opposing motives that are about getting ahead, securing power, destroying our enemies, or behaving with excessive cruelty to those around us. Even today, thousands of people are suffering from the terrors of war and torture, starvation stalks the lives of millions, and human wealth is held by a small minority who are reluctant to share. Consequently, compassionate motives are up against an evolved mind that is riddled with conflicting motives and desires that are propelled by powerful emotions. These are not new insights, of course, but what many early thinkers on the human condition could not know was exactly *why* we are "up against it," *why* our minds are so chaotic and driven by passions, and *why* it is so hard to apply our reason or take a compassionate position. This knowledge has only become available relatively recently with our understanding of evolution.

The Evolutionary Journey

The person most associated with uncovering how we are all part of the flow of life is Charles Darwin (1809–1882). He was the son of an affluent landowner and tried his hand at medicine before deciding to go into the church. However, he had a fascination for the natural world and jumped at an opportunity in 1831 to set sail on the HMS *Beagle* as the ship's naturalist. He was to spend eighteen months at sea exploring diverse lands in South America and the Galapagos as the *Beagle* engaged in its activities of surveying the southern hemisphere. Darwin encountered many species that were alien to Europe, and this prompted him to inquire how such variety could come into being. His insights into how the great variety of life came about transformed our understanding of life on Earth. Species change, he said, because they are constantly confronted with challenges for food, survival, and reproduction, and those best fitted to survive do so and pass their characteristics on to their offspring. This groundbreaking insight gave birth to the concept that species change by natural selection and evolution, although Darwin himself never used the term "evolution."

So relentless is the struggle for survival that 99 percent of all species that ever existed are now extinct—a sobering thought. The Neanderthals became extinct about 250,000 years ago during the last ice age, and now only their bones and artifacts are proof that they ever existed at all. We will never know exactly how they thought or what they loved, or the feelings they had for their children and their families, and their hopes for the future. But, as Buddhist philosophy points out, all things change and nothing is permanent—especially life-forms and their genetic combinations and mutations, which we now know are constantly changing in ways that are quite surprising.[1]

Precisely *how* characteristics (e.g., running speed, color of fur, body mass, or human brains) were passed from one generation to another was unknown because Darwin knew nothing about genes. The first clue of *genetic transmission* came from Gregor Johann Mendel (1822–1884), an Austrian scientist and friar. He experimented on thousands of pea plants and explored how characteristics could be passed from one generation to the next. His important observation, that you could deliberately cultivate and transfer specific characteristics of a pea, was overlooked until 1890. Nonetheless, *Mendelian inheritance*, as it became known, formed the basis for looking for the means whereby information was transferred from one generation to the next.

In 1953 at Cambridge, Francis Crick and James Watson published their discovery of this mechanism of gene transfer and called it *DNA* (short for *deoxyribonucleic acid*). Over the next sixty years, scientists who were part of the genome project, tried to code all of the genes that we inherit. Originally, it was thought that we would have hundreds of thousands of genes, but in fact we have only 25,000 to 30,000. Even more fascinating is that we share many genes with other species. We have 70 percent of our genes in common with mice, 80 percent with cows, and 98–99 percent with chimpanzees. Of course this does not mean that a mouse is 70 percent human or a chimpanzee is 98 percent human. This is because genes work very differently in combination, and many genes appear to be "silent."

In fact, it is the way genes interact and the way they build our bodies and brains that is the key to understanding our minds. What is interesting is that much of our DNA shows evidence of the remnants of viruses that have deposited their DNA in us. This may be one way in which our genes get mutated and changed. What is also important is that some genes can get turned on and off according to the environments (from the womb to early life experiences) in which we live. We now know that even if you carry genetic sensitivity to certain conditions like depression, those conditions don't necessarily manifest but depend on certain types of environment (e.g., loving and affectionate ones will literally protect you from the activation circumstance of repressive genes).

The Consequences of Evolution for Mindful Compassion

Genetic evolution actually fits quite well with Buddhist thinking "that everything emerges from preexisting conditions," which is precisely how the evolutionary process works. We would not be here as we are now (you as you and me as me) without all that has gone before, stretching right back to the birth of the universe. Central to this insight is the recognition that there is no pre-design in the evolutionary process, only adaptation and change with "the new" constantly emerging from "the previous."

Precisely because it's a constant process of emergence of what is new from what went before, evolution can't go back to the drawing board and start again but instead adapts previous designs. In this way, what has gone before always exerts a strong influence on what can evolve later. For example, our basic skeleton, with our spine running down the back and our four limbs, was designed in the sea for fish. This works well as a coat hanger suspended in water but becomes more troublesome when creatures move onto land and then much later evolve into mammals and stand upright.

Similarly, evolution cannot design things in advance; rather, designs emerge because they have certain advantages. For example, if you look at the giraffe, it has difficulties getting down to drink, and sex is none too easy either. You'd think: *How on earth did that creature evolve in that way?* But then you discover that actually it can eat from branches that no other animal can reach, so this advantage led to a gradual elongation of its neck *at the cost* of creating other difficulties. These are called trade-offs. Another example commonly cited is the peacock's tail: it's a fantastic display that is designed to entice females, but can be a problem when it comes to running away from predators.

Human bodies and brains are full of all kinds of trade-offs and compromises too. Standing upright rather than being on all fours gave humans the advantage of being able to see into the distance and have both hands free. The downside of this adaptation is that considerable force now goes down through our spinal column, hips, and knees, which were not originally designed to carry a weight like ours today. There have been adaptations to the spine and joints, of course, but because of this original design, many people today get slipped discs and require replacements of key joints because they wear out. Standing upright also affected the female pelvis in such a way that childbirth became more difficult because the fetus can get stuck; and tragically, millions of women and their babies have died because of this evolutionary adaptation—bigger heads to accommodate increasing intelligence running up against constrictions in the birth canal.[2]

We should also consider that many of our basic systems are designed to work within limits. This is especially true for systems in our body that try to protect us. For example, diarrhea and vomiting are the body's normal way of dealing with toxins. For the most part, they work quite well. But there are some illnesses that cause these natural defenses to stay active longer than is needed, and when that happens, people can die from dehydration and loss of nutrients—a very common cause of death for children in the developing world. It's not so much the illness that kills them but the body's own defenses to the illness. There are also a range of autoimmune diseases where basically our immune system fails to recognize our own body as its own and attacks it. Cancer cells are appearing in the body all the time, but it's when the body fails to regulate them that problems arise.[3]

The point of this story is to show how the evolution of our bodily systems is not moving us toward perfection but responding to challenges in ways that, on the whole, are helpful but not always so. In fact, the process of evolution is one reason that we are susceptible to many diseases and injuries and can die in so many different ways. Moreover, we come to see that it is precisely because there is no designer in the way our brains and bodies have evolved that causes us all kinds of difficulties. So when we look at the human brain, we can see that evolution has given rise to an extraordinarily complex but not that well put together organ. Indeed, the first flickers of compassion for ourselves begin when we have compassion for the fact that our brains are very tricky and full of conflicting motives, desires, and emotions that often don't work well together. This is one reason we are so susceptible to anxiety, depression, rages, and paranoia!

As we saw, the Buddhist approach to the dilemma of being alive is based on acknowledging the reality of suffering and trying to understand its causes—and seeking a way out. Science is contributing to this process by showing how the causes of suffering are linked to basic evolutionary process and design. An authentic path of mindful compassion requires us to be aware of the life situation we are in and why our minds are the way they are. Such insight and knowledge become a part of our emerging wisdom, and this wisdom then informs our compassionate response.

Old and New Brains

Using these insights, we can now focus on how our minds came to be the way they are, why it can be so hard for us to find inner peace, and why we can so often become our own worst enemies. The evolutionary model begins with the basic premise that humans are an evolved species and that over many millions of years, the brain has evolved as an organ to coordinate the body's actions in the world. Every function of the body from breathing to heart rate, every movement we make, every emotion we feel, and every thought we have is regulated by the brain. What the sensors pick up, the brain interprets: "Is this food?" "Could that be a predator?" "Could this be a sexual opportunity?" "Is this a storm coming, and do I need to take shelter?" Once the brain has decided that certain signals offer certain possibilities, it needs to direct the body to act accordingly: to approach and eat food, run from a predator, fight with a competitor, mate with a sexual partner, or take shelter. So our brains have mechanisms for dealing with threats and taking advantage of certain opportunities that promote survival and reproduction.

If we look at the natural world around us, for instance by watching wonderful naturalist films by people such as David Attenborough and the BBC cameramen, we see that most animals pursue similar goals to humans. These include finding food, avoiding becoming food, seeking out sexual partners, fighting over status and desirable things, and looking after offspring. We can also see that they display types of emotions similar to ours, such as anxiety, anger and aggression, being satisfied and relaxed, or being high on sexual desire and pursuit. Their brains are built to be motivated in ways that are similar to ours.

The human brain is part of this flow of life and comes with very similar design features. We too have mechanisms in our brains that are oriented to these kinds of goals, and we too can react with anger and anxiety if our goals are threatened or blocked. And, likewise, we can feel joy when things go well. We can call these motives and emotions *old-brain* functions because they have evolved over many millions of years and are common to many other forms of life (see figure 2.1).

Emotions are guides for our motives. We will spend the next chapter looking at emotions in some detail because they play a fundamental role in giving our lives meaning and they underpin compassion; but they also have the potential to cause havoc and block compassion. For the moment, we will note how they are linked to our motives. For example, if you want to pass an exam, make money, ask somebody out on a date, or grow vegetables (all of which are motives), you then make the effort to accomplish these things; if successful, chances are you will experience agreeable emotions such as pleasure, excitement, or satisfaction. In contrast, if you fail the exam, lose money, your date turns you down, and your vegetables get eaten by slugs, your emotions are likely to be unpleasant, and you may well end up feeling frustrated, disappointed, or sad.

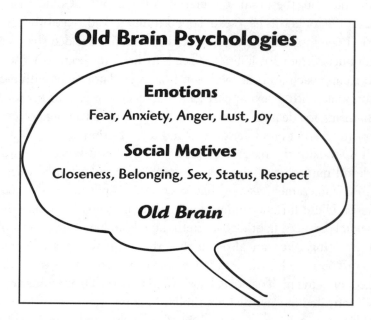

Figure 2.1 The functions of our old brain

In this way, our emotions are inner signals that indicate whether we are accomplishing our motivating goals. This is going to be an important point when we start thinking about what *compassionate motives* are, how they work in us, and what emotions go with them.

The Problems with Humans Getting Smart

What's crucial to our approach is that we need to explore the implications of having newly evolved, specialized brain systems that offer us a whole range of competencies that no other animals possess. Around two million years ago, the human brain started to get smart! Fossil studies tracing human origins have revealed a number of different species going back to ones called *Homo erectus* and *Homo habilis*, allowing us to see a gradual change in brain size and capacity over millions of years. The typical functions that we now have as part of our new "smart" brain are depicted in figure 2.2.

We became able to imagine and fantasize and to think, reason, and plan in ways that animals cannot do. We developed language as a wonderful medium to help us think and communicate with each other. We became able to use symbols that again provide a huge capacity for thinking. But our thinking brain can be a double-edged sword. Consider, for example, that a zebra runs for its life when chased by the lion, but once the chase is over, it quickly returns to grazing on the savannah. But this is seldom the case for humans because we constantly think, analyze, fantasize, predict, and anticipate. These new-brain capacities can cause us to spend half the day dwelling on how terrible it would have been if the lion had caught us. We might run all kinds of images and fantasies through our minds which terrify us. And then we worry about whether something similar might happen tomorrow—what if we don't spot it next time and what if the children go out. And what if and what if…! This is the downside of our new-brain capacities. Other animals do not spend time worrying about putting on weight or what will happen to the children if they aren't able to find a job or whether others like them or not or how to go about developing a good reputation. Getting smart has introduced a completely new dynamic to the flow of life: a thinking, self-aware, and reflective mind; but also one that can get *caught in loops of thinking* about, for example, frightening things that stimulate anxiety, getting more anxious, and then thinking about frightening things again. In his famous book *Why Zebras Don't Get Ulcers*, Robert Sapolsky makes plain that our thinking smart brains can give us all kinds of hassles.[4]

Not only were we able to stand back and think about ourselves in relation to the world we lived in, but at some point we also became able to think about the minds of other people. So we can think about what someone else is feeling, what their motives might be, and why they might be feeling what they are feeling right now. This is quite extraordinary when you consider it. So you can think in this way: *If I tell Sally this, she will probably tell Fred, who would then tell John, but John is unreliable and could well use this information to get back at me.* Thinking in this way gives us insight into ourselves as humans and, together with our ability to communicate, allows us to become fantastic storytellers, novelists, and producers of Hollywood movies.

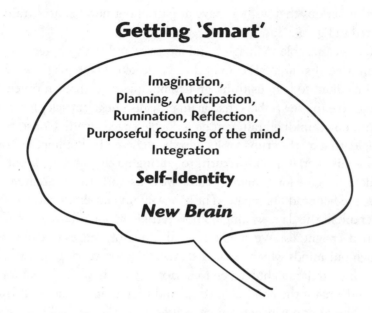

Getting 'Smart'

Imagination,
Planning, Anticipation,
Rumination, Reflection,
Purposeful focusing of the mind,
Integration

Self-Identity

New Brain

Figure 2.2 New-brain competencies and abilities

Our new brain also endows us with the capacity to be *aware of being aware*. We are aware that we exist, that we have a mind, and that our existence will end. We can be aware that we are having the thought that "we are aware," or be aware of the experience of being aware. Thus the *quality* of our awareness is different than that of other animals as well, and this recently evolved capacity "to be aware of being aware" enables us to practice mindfulness. It allows us to observe our minds and then make choices about them. Clearly, no other animal can *choose* to become mindful by training and purposely directing their attention (see chapter 7).

Another quality that makes us different from other animals is that we have a sense of self as being unique and individual. Now the whole emergence of life depends upon individual organisms. When the first life-forms came into being, they had membranes around them that separated the inside (the cell) from the outside. So life itself is a process whereby organisms become individual entities, separated from the environment in which they exist, but at the same time being dependent on that environment too. So the beginning of "individuality" and being a "separate self" is billions of years old.

However, humans have a completely new awareness of what it means to be contained within our own skins with our unique bodies and brains. This awareness and sense of being an individual self enable us to think about the future and the kind of people we want to be (or don't want to be), how we want to feel, and the life we want to live. In contrast, other animals live day to day. They cannot reflect on what it means to be a separate self existing in the world; they simply live out their innate motives and emotions. This process, of course, can be helpful or very unhelpful because clinging to and trying to create certain types of self-identity can cause all kinds of problems. Nonetheless, the desire to become a certain kind of person is also important for developing mindfulness and compassion; and this again highlights the importance of motivation, namely what kind of self we are motivated to try to become.

When we refer to all these abilities as being part of our *new brain* this does not refer to *where* they exist in the brain (although the frontal cortex is important) but simply that they are very *new competencies* on this planet as far as we know. As we have seen, these abilities use our attention, imagination, and ability to fantasize, anticipate, plan, think, and reason. Our new-brain abilities have made the world what it is today with diverse cultures, science, cars, TVs, mobile phones, and medicine, but— and this is a big but—these new-brain abilities can also cause us serious problems and distress. For example, we can reason about conflicts and plan revenge; we can also use our intelligence to work out how to build nuclear weapons. We can ruminate on how unhappy we are and plan to kill ourselves. We can create in our heads a sense of our self as inferior and unloved, or we can feel entitled to have far more resources than other people.

Basically, our new-brain capacities can be hijacked and directed by our old-brain passions, motives, and fears. Our planning, reasoning, and imagining can be directed by the emotions and motives of the old brain. Rather than using our thinking and attention to help us regulate or cope with unpleasant emotions or help us stimulate positive emotions, the old brain can pull us in the direction of threat-based anxiety and anger, and this can become the focus for thinking, dwelling, and ruminating. We get stuck in loops of "thinking stimulating feeling" and "feeling stimulating thinking" and so on. This is an unfortunate consequence of getting smart; and if we do not take responsibility for it, this *evolutionary glitch* can land us in deep trouble. This is depicted in figure 2.3.

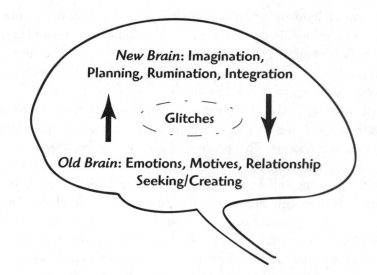

Figure 2.3 Interactions of new- and old-brain psychologies

These are not new insights; over the last two thousand years, Eastern and Western philosophers have understood that we can get caught up in vicious circles in which our emotions stir up our thoughts and our thoughts then further inflame our emotions. For example, if we become anxious, we can start to dwell on anxious thoughts and possibilities, and this can then make us more anxious. Many developments in psychotherapy, especially in the cognitive schools of psychology, have focused on the way our thoughts, motives, and emotions can cause us all kinds of difficulties because of the feedback loops that they create in our minds.

Getting smart also means that, unlike other animals, we are able to think about our own inner emotions and motives, and we can judge them along with our behaviors and efforts too. The problem is, we might not like what we experience inside of us. We might not like the surges of fear or anger or our tendencies to get irritated with people or be submissive to them. We might be alarmed by some of the sexual or aggressive fantasies that flow through us, and instead of having compassion for ourselves for having such a tricky brain, we might become critical and at war with ourselves.

In this respect, many mental health problems are caused by people trying to avoid "feeling their feelings" or experiencing a fantasy life. Clearly, if you're avoiding, suppressing, and dissociating from what's going on inside you, then there is very little chance for understanding your mind and there's little basis for being compassionate toward yourself.[5]

But, of course, our brains have also evolved capacities for enjoyment and happiness, for caring, affection, affiliation, and peacefulness. So we can learn how to use our new-brain abilities to focus on peaceful feelings and to organize our minds in constructive ways. We can learn to pay attention in particular ways and become more mindful of what goes on in our heads. How we go about doing this is a central focus of this book.

How the Brain Coordinates Itself

By now we are beginning to see the problems of why the brain is *so* tricky. It is because it's complex and multilayered and has been put together in bits and pieces over many millions of years.[6] A lot of processing that goes on in the brain doesn't even come into consciousness because consciousness is actually quite a late stage in the processing sequence. Nonetheless, given all our different motives, desires, and possibilities, the brain has to find ways of enabling these different systems and structures to interact in a coordinated way, and this is typically where both helpful adaptations and problems arise.

Key to our human abilities is our capacity for a fantastic *coordination of abilities and competencies*, such as attention, reasoning, facilitating and inhibiting behaviors, and regulating emotions. We are a species that can integrate information at a fantastic level. Take driving a car, for example: you are changing gears with your hands and feet; using your eyes to steer and watch out for cars behind you, in front of you, and to the side of you; talking to your friend next to you; answering your mobile (hands-free of course); keeping an eye on your GPS; and stopping at red lights. And you can do this for hours on end! A chimpanzee, our nearest relative, would never survive more than a few seconds because it could not coordinate anything like that level of activity and attention focusing.

Our body enables a fantastic coordination of processes that allow us to take in and digest food, breaking it down into nutrients that the body can use to build proteins and various chemicals that then give energy to our muscles and so on. So physiological systems need to be very carefully coordinated to function appropriately; and if one aspect gets out of balance, then the body as a whole can suffer. But it's the same with the mind. Our brain needs to coordinate an amazing number of different systems, types, and amounts of information.

Motives Coordinate the Mind

What we focus our attention on and how and what we think, feel, and behave, can all be coordinated by the motives that are operating in us, some of which we might not even be aware of. This is going to be an important insight when it comes to choosing compassionate motives because compassion will also coordinate our mind in a particular way. We can see how powerful motives are for influencing how our minds operate by imagining somebody who is highly motivated to get on in the world, make as much money as possible, grab every sexual opportunity, and live a hedonistic life. Then compare that to somebody who is motivated to understand their own minds and be as thoughtful and compassionate to others as possible. Can you see how focus of their attention, feelings, and behaviors will be organized in different ways according to what they are motivated to become or do? Back in 1989, Paul coined the term "social mentality" to describe the way in which our motives are like the conductors of an orchestra of attention, thinking, and behaving.[7] Becoming more mindfully aware of how our motives are triggered, which then coordinates our thinking, attention, feeling, and behaviors, allows us to stand back and decide if we want to go down that road or not. There is increasing evidence that different motives and social mentalities actually stimulate our brains in different ways. For example, the psychologist Emiliana Simon-Thomas and her colleagues[8] looked at what happens in our brains when we focus on either compassion- or pride-based goals. They found that inducing compassion stimulated areas of the brain that are also activated when people respond to pain in others and are associated with parental caring behaviors. In contrast, inducing pride activates areas in the brain related to thinking about oneself. As with all these things, it is not that one is good and the other bad; it is about finding balance and appreciating the effect of a compassionate focus in our brains.

So we can contrast a caregiving and compassion-oriented motive with a self-focused and competitive one. When we are in a caregiving mode, we focus our attention on the distress or needs of others, feel concern for them, work toward providing them with what they need, and feel rewarded by their recovery or prosperity. In humans this may even become linked to self-identity; for example, "I would like to be a caring person." In contrast, our self-focused, competitive motives would have us focusing on how we can do better than other people, constantly comparing ourselves with others, taking pleasure in being better than them, and not wanting to share our successes. This is outlined in figure 2.4. It is essential then to recognize that our motives can organize so much of what goes on in our minds.

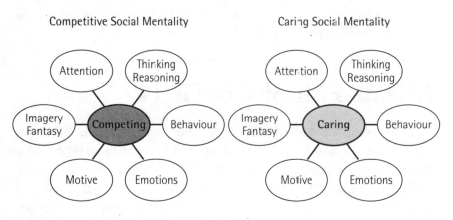

Figure 2.4 Different social mentalities

In general, a social mentality can only develop in relationships. Once a social mentality is activated, it is "looking for" a response from others. If you "seek care," then you need others to provide it; if you make a sexual pass, then you need another person to reciprocate in order to develop a sexual relationship. Receiving certain signals from others enables the social mentality to function in the unfolding development of that type of relationship. This is important because what do you think happens if a social mentality can't elicit certain signals—for example, if every time you seek care, people humiliate or reject you; or if you make a sexual pass at someone and they respond by telling you that you are too old, fat, and ugly? The social mentality is then blocked. Not only can this cause emotional disturbance, but it can also thwart the development of skills associated with the social mentality. So, if your care-seeking is constantly rejected, you might simply close it down or become very unskilled in recognizing and dealing with your need to be cared for. So you can see that our social mentalities are constantly being shaped by our interactions. This is why we call compassion a *social mentality*, because it is focused not just on the self, but also on one's interaction with *others* and how we respond to the ways that they interact with and react to *us*.

At times, then, it's useful to give ourselves the opportunity to pause and reflect on what is actually motivating us: What are our core goals in life? What do we see as being a meaningful life? If we imagined that we were approaching the last days of our life, what would we like to look back on? How would we like to be remembered? What are we doing right now to try to become that person?

Minds Full of Conflicts

By now it is clear that we have many different types of motives that organize our thinking, feelings, and behavior, which are set up to do different things in different contexts. Despite this, it's still something of a shock to recognize just how "multiple" we are. Paul had not been qualified as a clinical psychologist for very many years when these issues really began to hit psychology; in particular, a book that made a big impression on him was Robert Ornstein's *Multimind*. Over twenty-five years ago, Ornstein wrote this:

> The long progression in our self-understanding has been from a
> simple and usually "intellectual" view to the view that the mind
> is a mixed structure, for it contains a complex set of "talents,"
> "modules" and "policies" within.... All these general
> components of the mind can act independently of each other;
> they may well have different priorities.[9]

In fact this is now a pretty standard view in psychology. Twenty years ago, Dennis Coon opened an introductory undergraduate text on psychology with this graphic depiction:

You are a universe, a collection of worlds within worlds. Your brain is possibly the most complicated and amazing device in existence. Through its action you are capable of music, art, science, and war. Your potential for love and compassion coexists with your potential for aggression, hatred...murder.[10]

What Coon and other researchers suggest is that we are not unified selves, despite our experience of being so. Rather, we are made up of many different possibilities for creating meaning and generating brain patterns and states of mind. What is surprising is that this knowledge is still not filtering down into society in a more general way. Perhaps this is because the illusion of being a single self that has control over all aspects of the mind is so powerful and compelling that we don't want to let go of it. As we become more mindful, however, we become more aware of this *family of competing emotions and motives*, or different types of self, that are bubbling away inside us. It is important to remember that these are created because of basic brain design and social context—they are not personal and not our fault—so it's useful to shift more and more to an observing stance and not to overidentify with them. This is why mindfulness is so important in providing the basis from which to cultivate a compassionate motive.

Clearly, motives and social mentalities overlap, and one can suppress another; for example, it can be difficult to be competitively aggressive and caring at the same time. But, of course, people switch between different mentalities and can blend them together. Indeed, the ability to switch between them when we need to is an indication of good mental health.[11] For example, a man may compete in the job market by trying to prove to people how skilled and valuable he is, but when he goes home, a different self may emerge within him; he may be a loving father who does not feel the need to compete with his children for his wife's affection and time. Individuals who become trapped in a particular mentality or motivational system (like being competitive or submissive all the time) can struggle with being cooperative, caregiving, or care-receiving. This can then impoverish their lives in many ways. So these are important questions for all of us: What motives can take control of our minds, under what circumstances is this most likely to happen, and what are the consequences of this happening? How mindful are we of our minds being controlled by these various motives that evolved over many millions of years?

The Affliction of Self-Identity

Not only do motives organize our minds, but also maintaining a sense of self is very important for most of us because it helps us to maintain our self-integrity and our sense of being connected to others. We can find ourselves becoming very distressed if we feel things or behave in ways that do not fit with our sense of who we are.

In her book *Multiplicity*, Rita Carter offers a fascinating overview of how we are a whole host of different selves in one head.[12] There's the self that appears when we are angry, the self that turns up when we get anxious, the sad self, the perfectionist self, the self as romantic lover, the self as a fantastic friend, and the self as loving or irritable parent, and the list goes on—each of these selves having its own individual way of thinking, feeling, and wanting to act. For the most part we are aware that these different feelings, thoughts, and experiences of ourselves are constantly flushing through us on a daily basis. We do our best to feel centered in ourselves and be in control of all our emotions, but deep down we know we are not. The recognition that we have the potential for many different selves within us, and that these selves can be in conflict with each other, is something that has been understood for a long time. One of the founding fathers of modern psychology, William James, wrote about this problem over a hundred years ago:

> I am often confronted by the necessity of standing by one of my
> empirical selves and relinquishing the rest. Not that I would not,
> if I could, be both handsome and fat and well dressed, and a
> great athlete, and make a million a year, be a wit, a bon-vivant,
> and a lady-killer, as well as a philosopher, a philanthropist,
> statesman, warrior, and African explorer, as well as a "tone-poet"
> and saint. But the thing is simply impossible. The millionaire's
> work would run counter to the saint's; the bon-vivant and the
> philanthropist would trip each other up; the philosopher and the
> lady-killer could not well keep house in the same tenement of
> clay. Such different characters may conceivably at the outset of
> life be alike possible to a man. But to make any one of them
> actual, the rest must more or less be suppressed. So the seeker of
> his truest, strongest, deepest self must review the list carefully
> and pick out the one on which to stake his salvation. All other

selves thereupon become unreal, but the fortunes of this self are real. Its failures are real failures, its triumphs real triumphs, carrying shame and gladness with them.[13]

As James explains, one motive for being a certain kind of person can turn off the attributes or qualities needed for another motive. For example, if you are fighting your enemies, then your motivation to care for them, and your feelings of distress at the suffering you are causing them, are all firmly turned off. You might even take pleasure in seeing them suffer. Indeed, this seems the focus of much of our entertainment these days. So the important point here is that there may be some elements of our mind that are not accessible to us because other aspects have turned them off. We may not even stop to think about the distress we cause other people because we are so focused on our annoyance with them or the threat they pose us and our wish to dominate or be heard.

What so often determines the course of action we take is our sense of self-identity, who we take ourselves to be: "the bon-vivant or the philanthropist." Our self-identity is the way we coordinate the multiple influences that have shaped us, the values we have acquired along the way, the things we aspire to and the things we defend.[14] Our identity is simply a way in which we can organize our minds; otherwise it would be almost impossible to know what to think, value, or do in any given situation.

But identity is so often an arbitrary thing. For example, as we mentioned in the previous chapter, if we had been kidnapped as babies and brought up in violent drug gangs, that would become our identity. This background would be our main reference point within that culture, and we might defend our gangster identity with a passion and genuine belief.[15] Unless we had some way of stepping outside of that culture and coming to appreciate just how much the violent gangster identity had been *shaped for us*, we would have no way of choosing to be different.

Consequently, there are many downsides to having a sense of self and self-identity. The American social psychologist Mark Leary has actually referred to the evolution of self-awareness as something of a curse in his book *The Curse of the Self*.[16] It's a compelling read and illuminates just how tricky having a sense of self can be because we can overidentify with its values. We then feel compelled to defend our sense of identity and values, which can make us very aggressive if we feel threatened, or we can become vulnerable to depression if we feel we have lost a sense of self-identity. If identifying with being slim and attractive is a core value that defines who we are, then putting on weight threatens our very self-identity and can plunge us into feelings of shame, self-loathing, and depression.

Another example might be identifying with our self as being a "tough guy." If someone jostles us in the pub one night, this may threaten our self-identity, and we may feel compelled to lash out because we don't want to lose face or appear to be weak—especially in the case of a young male. Our self-identity can also be linked to how we feel we belong to a particular group, for example, a religion, country, or even a football team. This link and "fusion" of us to a group can be so strong that if someone threatens or insults our group, we feel personally threatened or affronted and even can take it as a reason to kill that person. This is particularly true with certain religious groups. What is interesting is that there may be *no material* losses or gains; it all comes down to attachment and clinging to who we think we are. In Buddhism, self-identity is seen as an illusion, and becoming attached and clinging to it as being real is considered a cause of great suffering.

The Shamed Self

One sense of self that we certainly don't choose but many people can get locked into is the shamed self (see chapters 5 and 6). When the Dalai Lama first came to the West, he was reportedly stunned by the level of self-criticism, shame, and self-hatred that afflict so many Western people. Many people with mental health problems are riddled with shame and even kill themselves because of it.[17] We may feel this way because people have been critical in the past or have condemned us. People who have been physically or sexually abused, come from emotionally neglectful backgrounds, or have experienced bullying or acute loneliness can experience strong feelings of shame and unlovability. They believe that they are seen negatively in the minds of others or that if others really knew them well, they would reject them as bad, inadequate, or flawed. They live their lives in hiding, never being able to open up and connect with others because of the fear of being judged and rejected.

When we feel ashamed, we not only fear that people will lack understanding of and kindness toward us, but we also start criticizing and attacking ourselves. What happens then is that our sense of self becomes focused around a shamed identity and feelings of shame with oneself.[18] And just when we need compassion and the support of others to help us with our inner struggles and difficulties, we find the opposite: the negative feelings that we direct toward ourselves are full of disappointment, hostility, and condemnation. As we will see in chapter 5, shame is one of the biggest blocks to developing mindfulness and compassion.

The Compassionate Self and Its Benefits

A shame-based identity is not something we usually choose, and it can cause us huge suffering. But supposing we develop an insight into how we became the way we are, and then deliberately choose to cultivate the compassionate potentials within us and make *them* the focus of the self we want to become? Compassion-focused therapy was designed for people who suffer from high levels of shame and self-criticism because developing compassion for ourselves and for others is one of the biggest antidotes to shame.[19] Supposing too we started using our special human abilities for thinking about what other people are thinking and feeling, and for working out what their needs and feelings might be? We have the ability to empathize and imagine what it's like to be another person; so these smart human qualities of our minds—and they are special—can be put at the service of either harming other people or helping them.

Mindful compassion is about recognizing the benefits of deliberately harnessing our caring motives as a way to organize our minds. Compassion, therefore, is not soft or fluffy but is rooted in the fundamental ability in our minds to enlist our smart brains to focus on cultivating motives like compassion, on purpose and with intent (see chapter 4). Without training, our minds can be a chaotic mix of different motives and emotions, but making deliberate choices of what motives and emotions to cultivate can change our minds. This is going to be a principal focus of this book—learning how to cultivate our compassionate self and how to relate to ourselves and others from this standpoint.

The benefits of learning how to cultivate our compassionate selves, which will improve not only our own well-being but also how we relate to others and how we create the societies we live in, is now increasingly backed up by research. Indeed, researchers from all over the world have started to explore the benefits of training our minds for compassion. It turns out that this training is associated with many physiological changes in our brain that are very conducive to our well-being and that help us to form harmonious relationships.[20] Researchers have also shown that if we have compassionate goals (such as genuinely wanting to help others and to avoid harming them) as opposed to ego-centered goals (wanting to get ahead and for others to recognize our good points), we are more likely to have positive relationships with others, be content, and be less depressed, stressed, and anxious.[21] In addition, we often talk about finding a greater sense of connection between ourselves and the world, which arises because compassionate motives are linked to parts of the brain that give rise to feelings of connectedness and meaningfulness.

To understand your own personal mix of motives, shaped by the circumstances and cultures you were born into, consider the following reflections.

Reflection One

Consider how *competitive motives* work within you. Are there times in your life where you are competing against others, be it for a new sexual partner or a new job? Notice how you compare yourself with others and (perhaps) worry about what others might be thinking of you. What fantasies do you have for getting ahead in life? What do you want from achieving success? What happens inside you when you try and fail, and when others do better than you? Are you critical of yourself or can you accept it as part of life? Can you take pleasure in the success of others? What happens to you when you are in conflict with other people and have different points of view? Try not to judge what comes up, but just be curious about how this evolved motive system works in you.

Reflection Two

Consider how *compassionate motives* work within you. What plans or fantasies do you have about becoming more compassionate to yourself and others? What do you think a compassionate self is like? (We explore this in more detail in chapter 10.) Are you worried that being compassionate might make you appear to be weak or soft, or that maybe you do not deserve it (as some people do)? Or do you see it as courageous, wisely authoritative, and at times difficult? When things don't go so well for you, or you make mistakes, can you be compassionate toward yourself? If it's other people who make mistakes, can you be compassionate to them or do you blame them? When people are in conflict with you, are you able to stand back and see their point of view and treat them with respect?

Bringing Our Story Together

This chapter has taken us on a journey into how we became who we are. We have seen that although the brain gives rise to fantastic capacities for science, arts, and cultures, it is a very tricky brain because it also creates problematic loops between our thinking, imagining, and ruminating, on the one hand, and our emotions and motives, on the other. Remember that the zebra will go back to eating soon after escaping from a lion, but a human may well ruminate about a similar experience for days and even be traumatized by it for his or her whole life. This is because of our capacities for thinking, imagining, and ruminating. So our new brain can cause our emotions to be switched on when they *aren't needed* and not be switched off when they *are needed*; in fact, the triggers, frequency, duration, and intensity of our emotions can all be affected by our new brain.

This is where mindfulness comes in because mindfulness is a way of paying attention that interrupts these loops. Rather than being carried away by our thoughts—allowing our thoughts to fuel our emotions and our emotions to fuel our thoughts—we can use this particular kind of *observing awareness*, which is called "mindfulness.' We will explain this in more detail later; what is pertinent here is that mindfulness is a recently evolved human ability. As far as we know, animals (as opposed to humans) cannot deliberately pay attention to the present moment; they cannot observe their own thoughts and know that they are doing so. So mindfulness is a new-brain competency.

In some approaches to mind training, developing mindfulness is seen as a way of developing compassion in itself. However, in both Mahayana

Buddhist and evolutionary approaches, compassion is seen as being rooted in *old-brain* evolutionary systems. Having said this, we should also note that our new-brain competencies for imagining, anticipating, thinking, and reasoning are also fundamental to compassion. These are what enable us to be able to think about and come to understand suffering, the causes of suffering, and the prevention of suffering in much deeper ways than any other animal. Indeed, we know there are areas of the frontal cortex that are very important for capacities like empathy (our ability to think about and understand what's going on in our minds and in the minds of others) that play a key role in compassion. Importantly, these abilities themselves may have evolved because of how they facilitated social bonding, caring, and affiliative relating. This is called the *social brain hypothesis*.[22] The basic story is that developing positive social relationships, such as being cared for by our parents, forming bonds through grooming, developing altruism and cooperative behavior, and the emotions of warmth and friendliness, provides huge evolutionary advantages for humans. Not only do these qualities affect our actual behavior, but we now know that they have a significant impact on our physiological being—our bodies. People who feel part of a supportive network, loved and valued by those around them, have much lower stress levels, better immune systems, and a higher sense of well-being than those who feel isolated and vulnerable to rejection. There is now no doubt at all that affiliative relationships, where you feel friendly toward others, have an interest in the well-being of others, and feel that others are similarly interested in you, are extremely important for our mental and physical health.[23] It is sad that many governments simply don't understand this and are quite happy to maintain and even enhance economic systems that are moving in exactly the opposite direction.

The point is that mindfulness and compassion work together but from different positions. As depicted in figure 2.5, compassion helps us to reorganize our minds by generating particular motives and feelings, while mindfulness helps us to step back and disengage from emotional thinking loops that suck us in, thereby providing the stability and perspective which is the basis for insight. If we start at the lower level of the diagram, we begin with compassion as a basic motive; we commit ourselves to compassion, and this influences our thinking and gives focus and direction to mindfulness. On the upper level of the diagram, we might start with mindfulness, which helps us to stabilize the mind and lay the foundation for the emergence of our compassionate qualities. They work together.

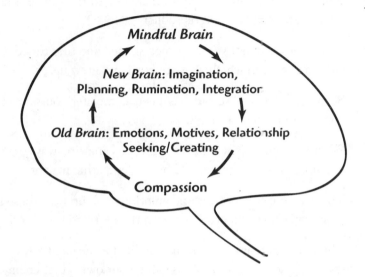

Figure 2.5 Interactions of mindfulness and compassion with old and new brains

Diagrams like this are useful but, obviously, the brain does not actually look like this, with the new brain clicked on top of the old like a Lego brick! Rather, distinguishing between the old and the new brain in this way is simply to help us think about how our minds work. Humans evolved a different kind of mind to other primates over two million years ago, and the differences in our mental abilities are obviously linked to physiological systems in the brain, which are extremely complicated to illustrate in a diagram such as this. What this simple diagram does illustrate, however, is how different *functions* of our minds interact and work together, from which different properties and competencies emerge.

As we noted earlier, compassionate motives are linked to part of the brain that has been associated with parental caring.[24] So compassion may be using old-brain systems, but of course our new-brain systems are vital for it too; for example, the capacity for empathy and the ability to imagine the thoughts and feelings of others are relatively new-brain capacities. The point and central theme of this chapter is that motivational systems organize the mind.

Key Points

- Our brains and minds have been created in the flow of life and are built for survival and reproduction.

- Our values and motives have been shaped and fine-tuned by the circumstances in which we were born and grew up.

- So much of what we are has been completely outside of our control and is not our fault.

- We have a smart new brain that gives us amazing ways of thinking, imagining, planning, and having empathic insight.

- The way that our motives and emotions link up with these new-brain capacities can bring out both the best and the worst in us.

- This calls upon us to take responsibility for the fact that, without training and effort, our minds can be our own worst enemy.

- Standing back and recognizing this gives us an opportunity to cultivate those things within us that will bring us improved physical health, emotional well-being, and better social relationships.

- As recognized thousands of years ago, and percolating through many religions, a mind motivated by compassion can be a source of great wisdom and universal change.

3

EMOTIONAL SYSTEMS

Motives guide us in life but they need emotions to *guide them*. For example, imagine you want to be a famous musician. You will give your energy to practicing regularly. You will experience positive emotions when your practice goes well but may feel frustrated if it doesn't; you will feel good when you get an offer to play a concert but feel bad when you are rejected. Emotions ebb and flow according to what's happening in relation to our motives and goals. Motives, like wanting to be a good parent or musician, can last a lifetime, while emotions, such as anger or excitement, come and go. As we will see, compassion is a motive—not an emotion—but it's linked to emotions in important ways because it also depends upon the ability to feel certain types or combinations of emotions.

Emotions play through the body according to how our motives are going. They give rise to feelings such as anger, anxiety, joy, pleasure, happiness, and lust. Emotions give texture to our lives: we feel love for our children, anxiety if something threatens them; anger at injustice; joy at success; excitement at a new opportunity; and desire for a sexual partner. Think what life would be like without emotions! You would have no feelings if you achieved your goals or if your house was knocked down; you would not be stirred by seeing your children do well or die; nothing would really matter. Life would be meaningless. This little thought experiment helps us see how central emotions are to our lives. We can of course feel more than one emotion in response to the same situation, and our emotions can often conflict with each other. Our emotions are the source of our most meaningful experiences in life, but they can also lie at the root of our deepest problems. Some theorists even think that emotion is the root of consciousness itself.

Our emotions can also have an impact on whether we develop our motives and goals further or whether we give up on them. Many of us know that in order to be successful we have to be able to keep going even when we are tired, experience setbacks, and have feelings of disappointment and frustration. So our motives and life goals will set us on course and our emotions will be like the weather we meet along the way. It matters greatly, therefore, how we come to understand the changing weather of our emotions as we travel through life and the degree to which we allow our emotions to determine how we are in the world.

Even though we have a "smart brain," our emotions can easily hijack it. One reason they can do this is because evolution has designed emotions to make animals behave in certain ways. There is no point in having a threat system that alerts you to a lion if there is not an immediate surge within the body to run like hell when a lion approaches. You don't want your smart-thinking brain slowing you down, weighing up whether the lion is a threat or not, whether it's eaten already, or whether your karate moves would be up to the task of stopping it! This type of thinking needs to be taken "off-line" so that the impulse to action is urgent. So some emotions come with a sense of urgency, and they can knock out the smart brain because they are *designed to take control* in these types of situations.

Problems with Emotions

Although emotions help to give our life meaning, they are not always easy to live with, and we have to learn how to recognize and deal with them as we grow up. For example, as babies, we can't really differentiate much more than between pleasure and pain; but by the time we become adults, we are aware that we can have many different types of emotion such as anxiety, fear, anger, disgust, sadness, joy, excitement, contentment, and happiness. We also recognize that we can have *blends of feelings*, experiencing more than one emotion at the same time; that emotions can conflict with each other (we can be angry about being anxious or anxious about being angry; we can be anxious about getting [over] excited). We can experience emotions when we absolutely don't want to (shaking with anxiety in an important interview or on a date, or getting angry with people we love and then feeling guilty). We can do things to deliberately stimulate our emotions such as watching an exciting film; and then of course some people use drugs and alcohol to try to regulate difficult emotions and feelings as well as to get high. Whereas some people might think it's okay to express anger, sadness, or affection, others can be frightened of expressing certain emotions. And some psychologists have shown that we can have emotions such as anger, anxiety, or even sexual desire that never quite reach our consciousness. We can also use our emotions to justify the way we think, even when our thoughts are quite irrational.[1]

Emotions are also central in our relationships. The emotions we experience when relating to somebody are crucial to how the relationship develops. We tend to find people who exude positive emotions and have what we call a sunny disposition attractive, whereas we might be less keen on people who are rather gloomy and critical. If we get disappointed in a relationship, we might try to do things to affect the emotions of the *other person* (e.g., try to generate more love, guilt, or even fear in them). Finally, many psychologists recognize that the way we think about situations and the interpretations we put on them, which may be linked to our past, play a major role in what emotions get stirred up in us and what we might ruminate on.[2]

So even though evolution has built our brains to be capable of developing and experiencing a range of emotions, it hasn't made life easy for us. This is a very important insight because as we engage with the path of mindful compassion, we are prepared for the fact that engaging with some of our emotions might be very tricky, even painful or frightening, and that's absolutely *not our fault*. Indeed, many mental health problems relate to how people experience and deal with their emotions. Also, if you think about it, many of the horrible things that happen in the world are a result of people just allowing their emotions to rule them.

Mindfulness (see chapter 7) is one of the most important skills in learning to recognize and understand our emotions rather than be carried away by them.[3] For this reason, it makes sense that before we start developing our mindfulness skills, we get to know more about how our emotions are designed and work through us. It's like looking at a map before we set out on a journey so that we will have some idea of what we're likely to encounter. Furthermore, understanding our emotions, where they come from and how they work, contributes to our understanding of compassion, as we will soon see.

Emotional Regulation Systems

Studies looking into how our brain works when it is experiencing emotions have revealed that we have at least *three types of emotion*.[4] Understanding these types of emotion can help us to understand how compassion can regulate and calm some of our more difficult emotions so that we feel more emotionally balanced within ourselves. This in turn helps to create compassionate feelings.

Now, we openly admit that we are simplifying things here a bit and that the neuroscience is less neat and straightforward than we are presenting here,[5] but what is important for the purposes of this book is seeing the overall picture so that we can understand where compassion has its roots and where it can get blocked.

Each type of emotion has evolved to do different things, but of course they interact in very complex ways, as shown in figure 3.1. We are going to refer to them as *emotional systems* because they are groups of emotion that have particular functions.

The three types of emotional systems are as follows:

- Our *threat and self-protection system* helps us detect and respond to threats and harms. It is the source of emotions like fear, anxiety, anger, jealousy, and disgust. When these emotions flush through us, they can direct our attention, thinking, and behavior in particular ways. For example, when we are anxious and our attention is focused on something that might be frightening to us, we might ruminate on this thing, turning it over and over in our mind, and we might behave in ways to try to avoid what we are anxious about, such as applying for a new job or meeting new people.

- Our *drive and resource-seeking system* helps us detect, be interested in, and take pleasure in securing important resources that help us survive and prosper, such as in finding food, sexual partners, friends, money, and careers. It is the source of emotions like excitement and pleasure. Again, when these emotions flush through us, they can direct our attention, thinking, and behavior in particular ways, related to that emotion.

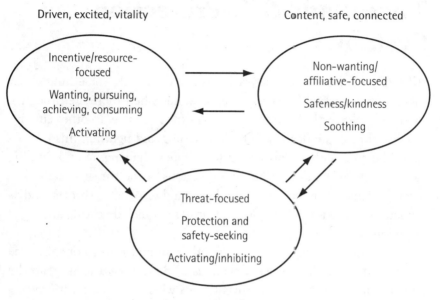

Figure 3.1 Three types of affect-regulation systems
Source: P. Gilbert. 2009. *The Compassionate Mind*. London: Constable & Robinson.

- Our *soothing/affiliation system* is linked to feelings of contentment in situations where we are not threatened or driven to get things we want. It is a source of emotions such as peaceful well-being, contentment, safeness, and feeling connected. These emotions tend to be gentler and slower acting, but when they move through us, they also influence our attention, thinking, and behavior in particular ways, such as opening our attention, softening anxiety, helping us to reason and reflect in more positive, gentler ways, and directing behavior toward slower, calmer actions.

Threat and Self-Protection System

All living beings need to detect threats and then do something about them. Plants curl their leaves to retain water when there are droughts. Insects fly away or burrow. Some animals freeze or flee. In other circumstances, threats are dealt with by threatening and fighting; this is especially the case with social threats (e.g., males challenging and fighting each other). In the flow of life, the functions of the threat system have been fundamental to our ability to detect and respond to threats, and as humans we inherit these old design features of quick detecting and rapid responding.[6]

This system helps us (as it does other animals) avoid or minimize harms and losses. It evolved to alert us to dangers and to gear up the body to take appropriate defensive actions when we need to. It protects us from the suffering we'd experience by becoming a hungry animal's lunch, falling off a cliff, getting beaten up because we've picked a fight with somebody twice our size, getting bitten by things that slither along the ground, or eating something that tastes bitter and makes us sick. That's why it's a *self-protection* system. It's designed to help us spot threats and deal with them quickly. We call it *self*-protection, but it of course extends to people we care about such as kin, friends, and at times the groups we belong to—we can feel anxious if they are threatened too.

Although this system is designed to protect us from suffering, it does so in a way that can actually *create* suffering. Pain is part of the threat system, and it evolved to alert us to damage to the physical body so that we would then protect that part of the body until it heals. People who do not experience pain—for example those with conditions associated with certain genes (a very rare condition of congenital insensitivity to pain)—are very vulnerable to serious injuries. Cases have been recorded of people with major cuts not realizing it and then getting infected, or even walking with broken ankles and bones, and doing themselves great damage in the long term.

So pain is a good example of how a system that has important adaptive features can also become a big liability. Our basic pain system can also give rise to states of agony that we can't do anything about. It makes it possible to be frightened of being in pain and, of course, that opens the avenue for people to deliberately exploit it and inflict pain (as in torture). Sadly, we are evolved to survive and reproduce—being happy or pain free is not part of the equation. Thus many living beings actually die in great pain unless they're lucky enough to have a stroke or heart attack so they die quickly, or are fortunate enough to be treated with anesthetics.

Wired into our threat systems is a range of emotions and action tendencies, such as anger with a desire to act aggressively, anxiety with a desire to run away or avoid, and disgust with a desire to get rid of or destroy. One such emotion is anxiety; it raises an internal alarm and causes us to run away if we are confronted by something or someone that could cause us harm or distress. In this way anxiety helps us to be careful. Let's explore anxiety by doing the following exercise. You might want to have a piece of paper so that you can make some notes as you do it. Try to approach the exercise in a light way and maintain a curious, friendly interest in how anxiety manifests in you.

Anxiety Exercise

Bring to mind a time recently when you felt anxious—perhaps it was when a cyclist wobbled out in front of your car, you put your hand in your pocket and discovered your wallet was gone, or an aggressive-looking drunk took an interest in you as you were walking down the street. Notice how fast anxiety can arise, how it feels in your body, how it affects your attention and focus, and then how it affects your thinking and behavior. Recall how fast your heart rate went up; you might have felt a churning in your stomach, you might have sweated, or your voice might have sounded funny. Your attention becomes narrowed and very focused on the threat and other things that might be of interest are ignored. This is the threat system kicking in.

Next, recall the kinds of thoughts that went through your mind and how they arose, even though you might not have wanted them to. Notice how they might spin around the thing that you're anxious about and how you might be focusing on the worst possible outcome. Just notice how your mind is being controlled by the anxiety. After a few moments, switch your attention to your behavior. What does your body want to do—run away, avoid, melt into the background, apologize, or cry?

Reflect on the fact that the way anxiety takes control of you is *not your fault*; it's what your mind's designed to do, and it will continue to operate in this way until you make efforts to train it and refocus your attention.[7] Even then, because anxiety is such an important part of our emotional system, we might learn how to manage our anxiety rather than stop it altogether.

Another important threat-protection emotion is anger. Anger allows us to respond when we are challenged, thwarted in pursuit of things we want, or need to defend ourselves. Whereas anxiety tends to be an emotion that moves us *away* from the source of threat, anger moves us *toward* it in order to subdue it or damage it in some way, thereby rendering it a lesser threat. Let's do a similar exercise with anger.

Anger Exercise

Bring to mind a time recently when you felt angry—perhaps somebody at work was unfairly critical of you or maybe you were angry at yourself for putting on weight. Notice how fast anger arose. Notice how your attention becomes narrowed and very focused on the things making you angry, while other things that might be of interest are ignored. For example, when we're very angry with our partners, we don't mind how much we might love them, at least not in that moment. Notice and recall how anger felt in your body; maybe you felt your heart racing or tightness in the chest or clenching of the fist. And as these physical experiences were running through you— how did the anger influence your thinking? Next consider the feelings in your body and what anger wants to do; if anger could be in control, what would you do—shout, slam the door, walk out, or something more? Notice how anger can pull your mind into ruminating about the thing you're angry about. Whether it's a rapid surge of anger or slow-burning frustration and irritation, notice how it wanted to take control of your mind. Remember that these things are not your fault; it's what anger is designed to do unless you make the effort to pay attention to it and work with it.[8]

In social situations we can sometimes feel a mixture of anxiety and anger. Anger empowers us to be assertive but also to put our foot down, shout, or even lash out. If it takes control, it will have its own way of reasoning that can seem very plausible at the time. The anxious part of us, though, might be thinking: *I'm going a bit far here; maybe part of the problem is my fault actually; this person will see something in me they won't like and maybe they'll reject me in the future. I don't like myself when I'm in this angry state of mind!* If anxiety and anger are balanced they will help each other, but often they are in conflict, as the next exercise demonstrates.

Anger vs. Anxiety Exercise

Bring to mind a situation in which you felt a mixture of emotions, in particular anger and anxiety. For example, it could be an unwanted argument with a loved one. Once you have got a sense of both the angry and anxious feelings, then think about what your angry self feels *toward* your anxious self. Does the angry self like your anxious self? Probably not much: it is typical for the angry self to be very contemptuous of the anxious self and see it as getting in the way. Do spend a moment breaking off from this book to really think about this in a curious way.

Now switch your attention. What does the anxious self think about the angry self?

It is possibly quite scared of the angry self. The anxious self knows that if left to its own devices, the angry self could be very destructive. It will protect you to the end of its days, it won't let anyone stand in your way, and it won't take nonsense from anyone, but because it's a very basic system in our brain, it's not terribly wise and it doesn't like working with anything that can constrain it. This is how the angry self is designed. Again none of this is our design or fault, but it is important to understand *the relationship* between our emotions—literally what they "think" and "feel" about each other. Mindfulness and compassion will help us recognize and hold these different parts of ourselves in balance. When they get out of balance, and our inner selves become involved in intense conflict, then people can begin to experience mental health problems. Some people can't acknowledge the depth of their rage toward people who they want to be loved by; some people use anger to keep people away and are unable to recognize within themselves a deep sense of sadness and grief, a yearning for love. Aggressive adolescents can often use anger like this because they may have been hurt in the past, so it's a way of defending themselves.

Disgust is another emotion associated with our threat-protection system. It is very useful because it's associated with spitting out and getting rid of toxic substances. If you put something bitter in the mouth of a baby, she will immediately spit it out because she is biologically oriented to do so. Disgust is often associated with bodily excretions or functions, and is designed to prevent contact with things that could contaminate or carry disease. We can have very strong feelings of contamination even when we know it's not logical. For example, would you live in the house of a serial murderer? Disgust emotions can have a very nasty side to them when aroused in certain situations. Disgust is often associated with feelings of badness, contamination, or sometimes even wickedness, and stimulates desires to avoid, cleanse, get rid of, or even exterminate. For example, many tyrants use the language of disgust when talking about their enemies, describing them as "subhuman," "a disease," or "vermin to be eradicated." We saw this during the Rwandan genocide in 1994, when Hutu extremists referred to the Tutsi minority as "cockroaches." Some people justify moral positions using the emotions of disgust, for example in regard to homosexuality.[9] So we have to be very cautious how we use these types of feelings to make moral judgments that guide our behaviors.

Self-disgust is also important because people can feel very bad and want to reject parts of themselves or even self-harm. Some years ago, Paul's research team found that people can actually come to hate themselves and experience strong feelings of disgust toward themselves, and that these feelings can be linked to quite serious mental health difficulties.[10] So, although disgust is an emotion that is often ignored, it is potentially one of the more powerful emotions when it comes to cruelty, both to ourselves and others. This is because it's associated with the desire to cleanse and eradicate—it can really push us into quite cruel behaviors.[11] When some Buddhist practitioners talk about certain kinds of emotions being like "poison," they are using the language and psychology of disgust, which may not be so helpful. We know what they mean—they are actually thinking about the *consequences* of acting on some emotions, such as anger, fear, disgust, or lust, but emotions *themselves* can't be a poison. The key thing with emotions is understanding and transforming them, not trying to cleanse or eradicate them, in part because these emotions are hardwired in our brain—we are designed to experience them—so we cannot simply "get rid of" them.

Disgust Exercise

You can do the same exercise with disgust as you have done with anxiety and anger—thinking about what disgusts you, then noticing how it directs your attention to focus on certain things, how it feels in your body, and how it seeks to control your thinking and behavior. You can be curious whether there are things about yourself, your body, and your feelings that you are rather "disgusted by" in the sense that you feel them to be bad and would like to "get rid of them, or get them out of you"; they may feel like a stain. These kinds of feelings can be common in people who are overweight, for example.

When you do the exercises above, you will gain insight into the fact that the emotions of the threat system can "flush" through us and literally take control of our attention, body, thinking, and behavior. Nobody wakes up and thinks: *I need to practice being more angry today* or *I need to practice being more anxious* or *A bit more self-disgust wouldn't go amiss!* That we still have these emotions is because they are part of our automatic threat-defense system.

This is where training in mindfulness-based compassion is so important because it enables us to notice how these emotions play out and to train our minds not always to fall prey to them. Sadly, we can see many people who simply surrender themselves to anger, and they can behave in ways that are very destructive to themselves and others.

Why the Threat System Gives Us a Hard Time

Although evolved for our protection, the threat self-protection system can give us a very hard time indeed. It is the source of many mental health problems, and even violence. This is because it's not designed for careful thinking; it's designed for fast reaction because that may save your life. If you are a rabbit munching away in a field and you hear a sound in the bushes, the best thing to do is to run away. Nine times out of ten, it is likely to be a false alarm—but that doesn't matter. So it's better to be oversensitive to threat and make mistakes that overestimate danger than to be the other way round, because sooner or later the tenth occasion will arrive, with the sound being a real predator this time. We call this "better safe than sorry" thinking.

Now your threat system was designed over millions of years in these conditions of high threat where predators were common and, if you got injured, there was no modern medicine to help you. There are very fast-acting pathways in your brain that, with the first flush of threat, bypass your frontal cortex and rational thinking.[12] So it's very important to realize that in fact your brain is actually *designed to make mistakes in certain contexts*.[13] It will overestimate danger for you; our ancestors who acted out of "better safe than sorry" survived, as did their offspring. Unfortunately, this tendency to overestimate threat is one of the reasons we have so many problems with anxiety—it's just very easy for our minds to go into anxiety mode. If we are prone to anxiety, it is not our fault, but likely to be a combination of the way our brains are and the things that have happened to us in our lives. This means that we will need to work to overcome these tendencies—as we will see in the practice section of this book.

Another way our threat system gives us a hard time is that it directs our attention in such a way that it blocks out positives. For example, going back to the little rabbit munching on one of the sweetest lettuces it could find and maybe eyeing Miss Bunny close by, if a signal indicating "possible predator" appears on his radar, he needs to lose interest in the lettuce and Miss Bunny immediately and run. The threat system immediately turns off any interest in anything else. If you watch birds feeding on your lawn you will see that most of their time is spent looking around anxiously and gingerly approaching the food rather than actually eating it, often flying away before they do. And as we saw before, more problems arise when we get stuck in those old-brain/new-brain loops where threat emotions are fueling our thinking and then those thoughts fuel our emotions, which continue to flush through us—even when the threat is long gone. The result is that not only can we continue to feel bad long after a threat has gone, but we will also continue to block out positive experiences.

Here's another example that indicates how our threat system can block compassionate awareness. Imagine you're out Christmas shopping and you go into ten shops. In nine of the shops, the assistants are extremely pleasant and actually help you buy presents for less money than you were planning to spend. You're really pleased. But then you go into one shop where the assistant is chatting to a friend, has very little interest in you, appears bored and at times rude, and, on top of it all, tries to sell you something that's of inferior quality but at a higher price than you are willing to pay. When you go home with your presents, who do you talk to your partner about? Will you say, "I love Christmas because it reminds me that 90 percent of the people I run into are so helpful, kind, and imbued with the festive spirit"? Unlikely—the threat system will make you focus on the one person who was unhelpful, and you may end up speaking to your partner throughout dinner about how rude sales-people are these days!

Gaining insight into how our threat emotions work and often con-flict with each other lays the basis for learning to relate to them mind-fully and compassionately. It's important that we are not harsh or critical of how our emotions operate, because they're all built into us by evolution—they are not our design and not our fault. When we give up blaming and shaming ourselves, we can step back and genuinely take responsibility to work with them as best we can. This is a key component of training in mindful compassion.

Drive and Resource-Seeking System

We have seen that threat emotions help us avoid harms and losses. However, we are also motivated to acquire things: to find food, shelter, sexual partners, and to get on in the world. Here positive emotions are very important for gearing us up to get on with these life tasks. However, when it comes to positive emotions, it is crucially important to distin-guish between two very different types of positive emotion.[14]

The first positive emotion system is the one that most people are very familiar with, namely the *excitement and drive system*. It's the one that our society focuses on a great deal. It is linked to achievement and acquiring and consuming things. The second type of positive emotion is very different because it doesn't create that hyped-up sense of drive; rather it is associated with a more peaceful sense of well-being, content-ment, and connection to the people and world around us. This *soothing system* has an important role in helping us regulate and calm down some of our threat-based emotions and keep our excessive drive-based emotions in check. We will look at this positive emotional system shortly— but for now, we will focus on the excitement and drive-based emotions associated with seeking, getting, achieving, and acquiring.

As we noted, the drive- and resource-seeking system evolved to motivate us to go out and achieve the things that are important for our survival and reproduction. So when we encounter things that could be helpful to us, we are motivated to pursue them, and if we acquire them, we get a buzz of pleasure. This buzz means that we're likely to try to do the same thing again. Psychologists call it *positive reinforcement*, but the important thing to identify is what gives us the feeling of the "positiveness." It turns out that it's linked to a brain chemical called dopamine and to an increase in the activating system in the body called the *sympathetic nervous system*. The sympathetic nervous system has effects on our muscles and hearts because it gears us up for action. It can be activated when we are under threat as well as when we are excited because it is a sort of "let's go" system. In contrast, the *parasympathetic* system does the opposite; it slows us down and helps us to feel calmer and quieter so we're not activated to take actions, or *to do* things.

Now imagine that you win $100 million in the lottery. What do you think will happen in your body? You are likely to become very excited and even agitated; you will have a rapid (sympathetic-driven) heart rate and a cascade of racing thoughts; you may become quite giggly; and you may have a lot of trouble sleeping for a night or two because of your elevated dopamine and sympathetic arousal. When really good things happen to us, we get a big buzz from the excitement and drive system. Passing an exam that is important to us or going on a date with someone new can give us a buzz of pleasure. We can also get something of a buzz from *anticipating* good things happening. This is where our new, smart brain comes in: just as we can ruminate on worries and fears, so too we can focus on hoped-for outcomes and imagine how we will feel if we pass an exam or win a competition. We can also spend a lot of time ruminating and thinking about how to achieve these goals because they are associated with good feelings.

Of course the more we live in the daydreams of success and the more unrealistic we allow our fantasies to become, the harder the comedown will be when we encounter our everyday reality and things don't go quite so well; also, of course, the threat system will then be activated all the more as we fail to live up to our dreams. And then there are some people who don't bother with all the effort of achieving things to feel good and look for shortcuts to these feelings. They take drugs such as cocaine and amphetamines as a way of getting that energized, positive feeling. Unfortunately, these drugs are highly addictive and the comedown is pretty horrible.

There have been many concerns that Western societies and competitive businesses are overfocused on elevating the excitement- and drive-based emotions associated with pride in accomplishment, owning, and controlling. This striving, getting, having, achieving, and owning is almost like an addiction—partly because we are constantly overstimulating our dopamine and sympathetic nervous systems.[15] The constant pursuit of material possessions or money, status, or sexual relationships, and so on, can be problematic. Indeed, some people can *only* feel good if they're constantly achieving or satisfying certain drives. Spend some time watching television advertisements over the next few days and notice how many of them appeal to excitement states: excited, smiling people getting hyped up for all kinds of reasons related to the goods and services on offer. This is particularly true for advertisements aimed at younger people, and it creates a climate in which people believe that this is what good feelings or the good life are all about—simply getting hyped up, having a good time, and so on. So while the drive system is important to achieve certain things, we have to be careful that it doesn't get out of balance so that we become overly focused on achieving and feel frustrated and depressed when we do not succeed.

One consequence of materialistic self-focus is that it undermines our interests and efforts to build, be part of, and contribute to, our social communities. Indeed, some people can become so work-focused that they hardly get to know their neighbors. This materialistic and competitive striving and needing "to have and own" has been linked to deteriorating mental health, especially in young people.[16] In addition, we can feel under increasing pressure to strive to achieve, to keep up, to prove ourselves, to do more for less; we may fear not being able to keep up. Paul's research team has shown that fearful striving to avoid being seen as inferior or not up to the job is actually linked to mental health difficulties, especially depression, anxiety, and stress.[17] There is increasing worry about the rates of liver disease and alcohol-related problems because middle-class and older people are drinking more. But if you talk to them, what you find is that their busy lives are so stressful and exhausting that when they come home, all they want to do is open a bottle of wine to unwind and relax. It is very important that medical agencies understand the link between our lifestyles, stress, and drinking and not simply think that the solution is to raise the price of alcohol. So once again, it's a question of balance and direction, and again the Western mind seems very out of balance when it comes to competitive psychology—and we haven't touched on the fact that it's our excitement and drive system, our competitive psychology, that will gobble the Earth's resources if allowed to, leaving polluted environments in its wake.

Perhaps one of the most serious consequences of an out-of-control excitement and drive system is that when opportunities arise for acquiring large amounts of resources, we can be driven to become deeply immoral and corrupt. Much has been written on the banking crisis, the excitement of bankers doing deals and getting carried away with opportunities to make masses of money—and all of us can get caught up in that. The problem is that individuals get locked into the drive system and simply do not pay attention to the potential damage they can do. Social psychology tells us that this is not because people are evil; it's because this is what happens in certain social groups if they are allowed to do these corrupt and immoral things, because the social group creates the values and contexts for people's behavior. This is why governments are so important for compassionate regulations. These need to be put in place, perhaps by organizations like the government to encourage people to behave in more morally and socially aware ways. Without them, people can behave destructively. Harnessed, drives are helpful and essential, but unregulated, they can be extremely damaging. Excessive drive leads to excessive self-focus, as well as immoral and corrupt practices because of the enticements of such practices, as has been shown in various investigations into top businesses that have fallen from grace. And of course countries have been ruined because of corruption, with their populations left destitute and in fear because the people who are supposed to protect them are involved in the corruption too. Frankly, without regulation either from the outside or within our own moral codes, drives can lead to the worst types of greed and corrupt immoralities, which people will even try to justify.

So while all too human, unregulated drives grossly distort our sense of our common humanity, where some individuals are worth billions, justifying it and believing they are "worth it," while others just down the street may not have enough to eat. In our hearts we know this is simply wrong. Pandering to our collective drive system has led to it being out of control in modern society, as exemplified by the current, widely held belief in the value of unregulated competition, and it's difficult to know how to restrain it. Unregulated drive can promote callousness and indifference toward those who suffer.

The issue for us is to recognize how our economics, politics, business models, media, entertainment, and education systems are constantly stimulating the competitive mind and excitement- and drive-based emotions and how this will have consequences for how we think about ourselves, get to "know ourselves," and relate to each other. The problem is not just with us as individuals; it's the way social systems work and how our minds both generate these systems and then become trapped by them. We end up feeding the very systems that are causing us problems, and this is because we've lost control of the systems we've created. Lacking both mindfulness and compassion, we simply go along with it because this is what our drive emotions push us into—constantly striving for states of pleasure. So if we keep in mind the Four Noble Truths, and if suffering is really the focus of our attention, then mindful compassion is not just "training our own minds or meditating for personal benefit" but about really opening our eyes to these drive-linked realities. This brings us back to the Buddha's concept of the Middle Way.

Compassion enables us to understand the importance of regulation and the rule of law—it is not just an appeal for everybody to be kind, but the recognition that it is our social context that can bring out the best as well as the worst in us. As we have said before, if we the authors had grown up in violent drug gangs, we would not be writing a book like this! So we will need to find ways in which we recognize the limits of our individuality, that we are all partly socially constructed and need new political ways of thinking that understand this in a deep way (beyond the small differences between political left and right), and begin courageously to build the kind of society that we want our children and our grandchildren to grow up in.

Now it might seem that we are giving drive emotions a very bad name. But just like the threat emotions, they have an important role when understood and wisely approached. Drive and excitement emotions are important in affiliation—the joys and pleasures we get out of being with others and sharing with others. In this respect, it is useful to keep in mind that compassion can also harness drive and excitement emotions to help a person become highly motivated, enthusiastic, and determined in pursuing compassionate goals, such as finding a cure for cancer or working for a just society. What is so important, then, is the motive underlying what we are driven to do. What do you become *excited* about and what gives you *energy*? Is it making money, killing your enemies, scanning the Internet for pornography, shopping, going clubbing with friends, or working for a compassionate cause? Of course at different times an answer might be "all of these," but then the question comes—which do you really want to focus on and make more prominent in your life? Emotions can attach themselves to very different motives, and for this reason, motives are crucial. In the context of mindful compassion training, this means that we become increasingly aware of our motives and desires, for example, to excel in a career, make money, impress other people, be accepted and not rejected, avoid shame, and help others as best we can. What we place at the center of what we want and seek in the world will determine the direction in which our drive-based emotions will take us.

Drive Emotions and Our Social Relationships

For the majority of us, the most important things associated with drives are our relationships. Imagine winning a $100 million lottery jackpot, but then being told that you will have to live the rest of your life on a desert island. The island will have everything you want: a wonderful home, comfortable beds, swimming pools, saunas, fancy sports cars to drive around on hundreds of miles of empty roads, wonderful scenery, boats to sail the crystal-blue seas, the best food in the world, and a perfect climate—it is a place where every physical desire can be satisfied! However, the catch is that you will never see another human being again, you will never know affection and love, and you will never be able to talk and be intimate with anyone. Would you make that trade-off? Or would you prefer to stay where you are, relatively poor perhaps but socially connected?

This is extraordinary when you think about it because it brings home to us just how important relationships are, even though we live in a world that constantly promotes the fact that material things are what bring us happiness and that we must constantly strive for that competitive edge.[18] In fact, from the day that we're born, our positive emotions are constantly being stimulated by our interactions with others who smile, laugh, and play with us. Relationships are really the lifeblood of our positive emotions and drives—just as they can be a source of our greatest threats, sadness, anxiety, rages, and cruelty.

Consider too that we have enormous socially focused drives to be approved of, valued, esteemed, desired, wanted, and loved; and, on the other side, to avoid being criticized, shamed, rejected, or forgotten.[19] For most of us, *social drives and needs* are at the core of our sense of self and what motivates us, even if people take them for granted. But we then just have to consider what it would be like to be completely alone for the rest of our lives on a desert island with every physical comfort met, and it soon becomes obvious that these kinds of pleasures become meaningless in a world of loneliness and social disconnection.

Finally, consider that we love doing things together, to become a "we" and not just a "me," be it by playing on a football team or in an orchestra, working together to land somebody on the moon, or as part of a charity. Forming groups and feeling a part of a group because of shared interests and values can be very important for our sense of identity and security. So we can experience joy from doing things together. Of course there is also a downside in that groups can be very competitive with other groups and even aggressive to people they do not see as members of their own groups. As we well know, rival football fans often get into fights. So this tendency to easily form into groups and then be aggressive to "nongroup" people is something that can be a serious bias in us. Evolution has designed our brains, like those of other animals, to be very sensitive to who we see as part of our group and "one of us" and those who we don't see that way. However, the key question is, are we happy just to do what our brains seem to push us into? Once we recognize this, as mindfulness will help us to do, we can choose to work against that bias and genuinely follow a more spiritual view that all of us are on this journey together as part of the same flow of life and common humanity.

The Soothing/Affiliation System

If, in Western society, the drive system is overdeveloped, overvalued, too much directed at material wealth, and focused on achieving individual rather than collective goals, then the one system that seems sadly *undervalued* is the one that gives us a sense of contentment and peaceful well-being. This is the one that also speaks very much to our need for social connectedness. If you have spiritual beliefs, it's also the one that is more likely to connect you to a spiritual sense of well-being. We can call this the *soothing/affiliation* system. It too evolved under certain conditions and has specific functions.[20] Importantly, this system, which enables calming and soothing, became adapted for creating attachments with others and the care of offspring. Soon we will look at this in more detail because it helps us to understand how and why *feeling cared for* can be innately calming for us and is associated with a sense of well-being.

When animals aren't defending themselves against threats and don't need to achieve anything because they have enough, they can be content. Contentment is "being happy with the way things are," feeling safe and neither striving nor wanting.[21] It is characterized by an inner peacefulness that is a very different feeling from the hyped-up excitement or "striving and succeeding" feelings associated with the drive system.[22] As noted above, whereas activating emotions are linked to what is called the *sympathetic nervous system*, slowing down and being at peace is linked to what is called the *parasympathetic nervous system* (sometimes referred to as the "rest and digest" system). When people practice meditation and sit quietly, these are the feelings they describe: not wanting or striving, but feeling calmer, slower, and more at peace with themselves, and more connected to others and the natural world. The sympathetic and parasympathetic nervous systems come more into balance.

Now it's important to recognize that this meditative state is not just a relaxed state, because it can involve a heightened state of awareness and openness of attention; so, for example, you are more likely to appreciate a walk in the country, noticing the smells and colors, feeling chilled out, neither wanting to achieve anything nor worried about anything; the thinking mind is "off" and you are engaged directly with your sensory world. These feelings seem linked not only to a particular balance between the sympathetic and parasympathetic nervous systems but also to an important chemical in the brain called an *endorphin*, which interestingly is also a chemical that tones down feelings of pain. People who take heroin sometimes report similar feelings because heroin tends to stimulate the endorphin system—the flip side is that there can be some very nasty comedowns of course, and it is highly addictive.

It's useful to experiment with taking time out from our competitive and pleasure-seeking drive system by going somewhere quiet, perhaps in a beautiful part of nature, to spend time just *being there*, and to allow ourselves *to slow down* and engage with our senses: feel the earth beneath our feet, listen to the sounds of nature around us, and appreciate the ever-changing sky. In so doing you might get a glimpse of that sense of feeling peaceful, content, and connected to the world around you. The *slowing down* is very important. In our everyday world, we have to *deliberately* do this because our senses are constantly being stimulated by neon lights, cars, televisions, computer games, and so on; not to mention the stresses we all experience in trying to get so many things done in the day. Even if we go shopping or to a restaurant for lunch, we can't get away from distracting music and bright lights. In fact, very few places exist where it is possible to be silent and still. When we go to bed, there may still be a constant hum of traffic outside. And if we can't sleep many of us turn on the TV or log on to social networking sites, thereby stimulating ourselves yet again.

The point is that the extraordinarily high rates of sensory stimulation in our world make it very difficult to access the (parasympathetic-linked) soothing system. And it is not uncommon that when some people do deliberately try to slow down, they become fidgety and agitated, almost as if they're suffering from a kind of withdrawal. In contrast, if you ask people on a mindfulness retreat how they feel at the end of it, they typically report a feeling of slowing down and becoming more peaceful within themselves. Unfortunately, sometimes it doesn't last that long because within a few days of being back in their normal environment and the hustle-bustle of life, their drive systems are ramped up again, meeting deadlines and rushing here and there. So we become more aware of the fact that the world is in sensory overdrive, with all the TV channels, enticing advertisements, bright lights, stimulating music in every shop, traffic, and sheer noise. This has a major impact on how our brains work. When higher-arousal states of drive are being constantly stimulated, with the desire to acquire more and go faster, this greatly accentuates the problems of greed, frustration, stress, depression, and even immoral behavior.[23] Of course, these are not new messages, and we also need to remember that all over the world, in charities and many professions, people are working for the benefit of others. In fact, although we can be "mindlessly" greedy and self-focused, we also have the capacity for enormous goodwill to each other. Mindfulness and compassion training are ways to tap into and cultivate these basic human qualities, which can soften our economically driven "drive system."

Soothing and Relationships

In chapter 7, we will describe ways to slow down your breathing and connect with your body as a way of consciously accessing and developing your soothing system. Right now, however, we are going to explore something that is extremely important in understanding how and why the soothing system regulates the threat and drive systems.

When babies are in a state of distress and their threat systems are aroused, what is it that calms them down and makes them contented? It's normally the caring, loving actions of another person (usually their mother, but not always, of course). Even as adults, if we are stressed and upset, we usually find that the understanding and kindness of others really helps; this is partly because our brains are set up to be *calmed down in the face of kindness.*

Indeed, experiencing kindness can reduce our heart rate and blood pressure, thereby slowing down our body. This is the very opposite of what happens when we feel threatened, are rushing about, or are excited.

How did it come about that the caring and affection of other people can soothe our threat system? The story goes like this. For many millions of years, living beings did not get looked after. For example, turtles hatch from their nests with hundreds of other brothers and sisters, and have to dash to the sea as quickly as they can. Sadly, many die on that very first day and are eaten by predators that are lying in wait for them. It is estimated that 98 percent of them do not make it to adulthood.

Around 120 million years ago, however, an adaptation occurred with mammalian mothers taking care of their infants.[24] The effect was fewer births so that the mother (usually) could invest in her young, look after them, provide them with food and warmth, be attentive to their distress calls, and try to relieve that distress. Now a number of things are happening here. There have to be changes in the brain and nervous system so that the infant doesn't try to get away from the parent or protect itself (as turtles might try to do). The mammalian infant in contrast *turns toward* the parent and seeks closeness. So there need to be mechanisms in the brain that guide the infant to seek closeness and feel safeness when the parent is close; and become alarmed if the parent becomes too distant. And of course, there need to be evolved mechanisms that motivate the parents to take care of their offspring.[25] For humans, these basic motivations—"to take care of; look after; prevent harm, feed, and see flourish"—are the foundations of compassion. Indeed, as we saw in the previous chapter, the work of Simon-Thomas and her colleagues has shown that compassion tends to work through similar mechanisms associated with parental caring.

Early Life, Attachment, and Soothing

Let's stand back and reflect on how the evolution of caring and affiliative relationships affects the organization and development of our emotional systems. Some years ago, the British psychiatrist John Bowlby studied how parents interact and develop relationships with their babies and how these affect the baby's development. Evolution, he argued, created systems in the mammalian brain that make infants seek closeness to their carers, and their carers respond to the needs of their infants. He called this the *attachment system*. He argued that how we experience our early attachment relationships will have a major effect on how we experience and come to regulate our emotions, views of ourselves, and abilities to relate to others.[26] In his day, this was a revolutionary idea because most developmental thinkers tended to focus on simple rewards and punishments as the focus for development. He went further and argued that it's the *availability* and *basic affection* of the parent that is key to a child's development because the child's brain, which is laying down many hundreds of thousands of connections a day as he or she is growing and developing, is highly influenced by those early life experiences— something that today has been shown to be absolutely correct.[27] The parent, he argued, creates a safe place/base, and this is fundamental to regulating the child's experience of threat in the world. The parent is always somebody the child can turn to in order to be calmed down and soothed when upset, as well as for stimulation. So when a child is distressed and the parent picks the child up to be cuddled, this reduces the child's distress. In other words, *the parent stimulates the baby's soothing system, which then calms down the threat system.*[28] Ideally, this goes on throughout childhood with the parent acting as a source of comfort to the child when he or she is distressed. However, at times the parent must also act as a stimulator of the drive system (as in play and joyful interactions) and engagement with threat; that is to help develop the child's *courage*. Indeed, we call it en*courage*ment. This happens by providing a safe base for children to go out and explore things that they might otherwise be anxious about. In this way, the child develops an experience of her- or himself and others as *being in an affectionate, supporting, and "encouraging of independence" relationship.*

These qualities of affection, kindness, and encouragement from others also help soothe us as adults when we're distressed. When we feel soothed, we feel safe in our everyday lives. These feelings of soothing and safeness work through brain systems similar to those that produce peaceful feelings associated with fulfillment and contentment.[29] In fact, interestingly and importantly, there seem to have been changes to the parasympathetic system (the system associated with slowing down and feeling calm and contented) that were especially important for the development of affiliation and especially attachment. So, in a way, the soothing parent is able to activate an aspect of the infant's parasympathetic nervous system. This work is especially developed by the researcher Stephen Porges.[30] The bottom line is that kindness and feeling connected to people will help balance your sympathetic and parasympathetic nervous systems—and this can be the case whether the kindness and affiliation come from yourself or from those around you.

One research study[31] found that if you ask people to imagine making their favorite sandwich, which stimulates the drive system, this slightly shifts people toward more sympathetic arousal, as one would expect because it's activating. If you ask them to imagine another person being kind to them, this seems to increase parasympathetic activity and produces greater balance between the sympathetic and parasympathetic nervous systems. It can also reduce cortisol (a chemical in the brain), which is linked to the threat system. So this suggests that even just *imagining* compassion and kindness is enough to start to activate the soothing/

affiliation system and tone down the threat system. Thus, again, evidence informs us that kindness brings the sympathetic and parasympathetic nervous systems into balance as well as reducing threat processing. The one problem with this, though, is that it is not the case for everybody because people who are self-critical actually can appear to become *more* threatened by imagining kindness. The reasons for this are explored in chapter 6.

Substances in our brain called endorphins, which link to feelings of calmness and peaceful well-being, are also released when we feel kindness. In monkeys, grooming behavior like holding and stroking is associated with releases of endorphins. Indeed, endorphins are fundamental to social interactions and how safe we feel in our environment and relationships.[32] It is possible that when we are being kind and helpful to ourselves, experience kindness for others, and focus on loving-kindness, we might also be releasing endorphins.

There is also a hormone called *oxytocin* that links to our feelings of social safeness and affiliation. Oxytocin is very important for mammals' attachment; if you eliminate it, animals don't form attachments to their offspring. Oxytocin has been linked to trust, liking people, and feeling safe and supported.[33] Paul's research team has also found that oxytocin seems to enhance feelings associated with imagining receiving compassion from another person, indicating that compassion might be linked to oxytocin systems.[34] But once again, it turns out that some people, especially those who are self-critical or self-disliking, can experience feelings of kindness toward *themselves* less positively. They might actually feel more lonely when given oxytocin! We think this is partly because oxytocin opens up affiliation systems in our minds, but if we have difficult memories, of, say, feeling alone, it can remind us of those things. This is related to how our memories work. For example, for most of us, going on holiday is a cause of excitement, but suppose on one occasion something terrible happened? You may get over it then, but much later somebody does something that makes you think about holidays again, and what will come back to you may not be the pleasure and excitement of that holiday but the horrible memory and feeling. It may be the same for self-critical people, that if we stimulate the affiliative system, it puts them in touch with a loneliness, linked to the kindness they wanted (perhaps as a child) but didn't get. Now this is something we are going to talk about in chapters 5 and 6 too, because fear of the feelings associated with compassion and kindness can obviously be a major block to becoming compassionate.

Taken together, then, we now know that the mammalian (particularly the human) brain is designed to be highly responsive to signals of affection and care that emanate from others. There is a whole range of specialized systems that have evolved in our bodies and brains to respond to kindness and affection, help our bodies function optimally, and create feelings of peacefulness, safeness, and well-being. Indeed, we now know that even *genes* can be turned on and off in a baby's brain, depending on the amount of and type of affection the child receives early in life.[35] Sadly, children who are abused or severely neglected can show quite severe changes to their brains, and are different than those who are loved and cared for while they were growing up.

John Bowlby also pointed out that children develop ideas, expectations, and beliefs about other people and how they are going to relate to them. So children who receive love and affection in early life tend to see other people in relatively benign terms and can turn to them when they need to.[36] In addition, experiencing love and affection regularly will constantly stimulate important areas of the brain, enabling them to develop and grow. So it's not just that we develop positive beliefs about others, but that our brains are geared toward openness and expectation of others as being friendly and helpful. In contrast, when things go wrong in early childhood, children can develop beliefs, expectations, and feelings about others and see them as less benevolent; they may see others as easily rejecting, criticizing, or hurting.

Distinguishing Safeness and Safety Seeking

It's clear, of course, that the feelings of safeness in this context also go with feelings of freedom, openness, and even exploration. To some extent, these are drive-linked experiences in that we can actively seek them out or try to create them. So all the time we have to keep in mind this issue of *balancing the three emotion-regulation systems*. Indeed, part of life is learning to feel safe enough to be in control of what we are doing, despite facing challenges; we feel safe enough to take that driving test and face up to the challenges. In events like the Olympics, many athletes will thank their family, friends, and trainers for all their support and love. They demonstrate with absolute clarity that feeling safe, supported, and encouraged by others can help us take on major challenges.

We can contrast safeness with safety seeking where people are motivated to try to avoid bad things happening or to escape. If we are in flight mode, we try to get away. This is really safety seeking and part of the threat system because our attention is highly focused and our body is experiencing some kind of anxiety. We might feel relief if we manage to get away from the perceived threat. Safeness, however, has an open attention and explorative orientation to the world that allows us to be more integrated in our thinking. In general, when we feel safe, our emotions are neither excessively excited nor threat focused. When we feel safe, we are more likely to be relaxed and we *can play*. This also can create joyful relationships.[37]

The Importance of Affiliation

The parts of our brain that support and enable attachment are also linked to more general feelings of affiliation, empathy, and friendship.[38] And so it is the case that when we move out of our home environment, we may experience school as being a pleasant environment and our peers as a source of connection and support; or alternatively, we may find the environment to be unpleasant and one in which we get bullied. This too will have a major impact on how we develop our inner sense of safeness and our ability to be open to friendship and to deal with conflicts. This is the basis of affiliation.[39]

Equally important, the way we have experienced other people relating to us can have a major impact on how we relate to ourselves. You probably won't be surprised to learn that individuals who come from loving and caring backgrounds tend to like themselves and feel worthy of being loved. In contrast, people who come from more difficult backgrounds may find it hard to open up to the love of others and can be very self-critical and even self-loathing. The problem with being critical or disliking oneself is that it constantly stimulates the threat system, which creates stress in our body and mind. Consequently, if the soothing/affiliation system is not stimulated or developed, then our capacity for being compassionate can become dormant. Practicing mindful compassion, however, is specifically designed to stimulate those brain systems that foster a sense of peacefulness, safeness, and contentment; and these qualities are so important for offsetting tendencies toward self-criticism, anger, and self-loathing.

We will come back to this later in this book, but the key point here is that our brains are influenced in so many ways by kindness and compassion. From the day we are born until the day we die, the friendliness and kindness of others will have a huge impact on our brains and states of mind. There is absolutely no getting away from the fact that humans are biologically designed to respond to kindness; we have specific brain systems that are designed for giving and receiving kindness. Although there are, of course, conditional factors, in that we tend to feel more affection and kindness for those we are genetically related to or part of our group, this shouldn't detract from this fundamental design feature.

Affiliation is closely connected to a sense of community. In Buddhist teaching, the three jewels of refuge are taking refuge in the Buddha; taking refuge in the teaching; and taking refuge in the community. The concept of community is therefore vital to our sense of safeness and calmness. In any work environment, people are happiest when they have a sense of belonging and of feeling supported, validated, valued, and appreciated by those around them. If you look at people who take time off work due to stress (for example, in the UK, especially those in the National Health Service), this is usually because these qualities have been absent. Mindful compassion therefore is not about isolating yourself in meditative practice but recognizing the importance of being part of a community. Keep in mind, as we said above, that competitive materialistic approaches to Western life, which are on the increase, seem to disrupt and fragment people's sense of community. This is a serious problem because it has major implications for how our brains work and the degree to which we are able to function optimally.[40]

There is another key element to affiliation, and this is that it *builds courage*. Just as the attachment relationship between parent and child can encourage the child to engage in things they might be fearful of, so can affiliative relationships help us to face things that threaten us. Many people who have anxiety problems and avoid doing things often "feel alone" *when anxious*, as if the two fuse together. So if we ask someone who is having an anxiety attack, "Do you feel alone right now or do you have a sense of connectedness and sharing with others?", they will typically respond, "I feel alone and separated from other people." It is this sense of aloneness that can seem fused with anxiety and can make anxiety so difficult to face. But suppose people do not feel alone. If you think about people in, say, a war situation, they will do extraordinarily courageous and heroic things because they feel part of a team or that other people need them; they don't feel alone. When we feel supported and understood, this really helps us build courage. This is important because *compassion provides the courage to face the things that we may not want to face.* For example, by becoming more self-compassionate, a person who is agoraphobic may develop the courage to go out; or a shy person may develop the courage to go to a party. So we develop courage often in the context of affiliation, and feeling the connection with others really helps us to cope with our fear.

In summary, there are a number of things we can say about the importance of affiliative relationships:

- They are the source of some of our greatest joys and feelings of contentment but also the source of some of our fears and sense of loneliness.

- They involve both drive (taking pleasure and joy in relationships) and soothing systems (feeling contentment in relationships).

- They form the basis for feeling safe and have the power to calm us when we are stressed and feeling threatened.

- They stimulate the development of kind and benevolent feelings toward ourselves and others.

- They enable us to feel safe enough to use our abilities to begin to think about our own minds and the minds of others; that is, they are the basis for empathy and the capacity for both inward and outward reflection.

- They give meaning to life, and, indeed, working with and to help others is one of the most meaningful activities that humans pursue.

- Learning to focus on how to access, stimulate, and utilize these very important affiliative brain systems, which have been evolving for millions of years, is one of the keys to emotional well-being and social harmony.

- Stimulating the affiliation system helps us to build courage and engage in the things we find difficult.

- Cultivating these brain systems is the basis for developing compassion.

Consequently, compassion needs to be understood within the context of this long, evolved process by which affiliative relationships have come to be so important for the regulation of our minds and for our relationships in the world. If the systems in our brain that regulate the experience of contentment and affiliation are compromised, or we become frightened or dismissive of the feelings associated with them, then we can get seriously out of balance. In effect, we then lose the ability to use one of the most important emotional regulation systems that evolution has bestowed upon us.

Exercise: Three Circles

Let's take this knowledge and turn it into personal insight. We will stand back and reflect on how these three emotional systems are actually working within us. Remember that all these exercises are intended to be done with a sense of friendliness and curiosity, so if you find yourself getting distressed by the exercise for any reason, then take a break.

Find a large piece of paper—a loose sheet or a notebook especially for this purpose will do—and consider the three circles shown in figure 3.1, in chapter 3. Focus on each one for a moment, reflecting where you spend most of your time and energy, and then draw circles for yourself accordingly. So if most of your time is spent worrying and ruminating, then draw a big circle for your threat system; and if you spend very little time feeling safe and contented, then draw a small circle for the soothing system. Once you have done this, we can move on to the second part of the exercise.

Let's begin with the threat system. Think about the things in your daily life right now that can trigger your threat system. It may be small things such as needing to get to work on time or concerns about the traffic or completing a piece of work; or it might be something more serious such as facing a divorce or a worrying health problem. Write these things down in your circle. Think about how much of your time is spent in this emotional system and how often these worries and concerns ripple through you. Over the next few days, more things might occur to you, so you can write them down too. Note how thoughts and feelings from this system can just pop into your mind.

Now pause for a bit and then focus on the things in your life that give you a sense of pleasure and enjoyment: things you feel excited about and look forward to, positive things that make you want get out of bed each day. This could be something you want to achieve or it might be the thought of going on a holiday; it might be looking forward to coming home to a nice meal, going to the movies, or doing a good piece of work. The key thing is the experience of being energized by whatever it is you think of. How preoccupied are you by things that excite you and give you a sense of purpose and direction? We could call these _energizers_. Keep in mind, though, that some energizers can be threat focused: for example, wanting to achieve things not for enjoyment of the thing in itself, but because you are frightened that if you do not, then people might reject you. So, strictly speaking, they fall into the threat-system rather than the drive-system circle. In your notebook or on your piece of paper, make a note of how much time you spend in the drive system.

Now pause for a bit and then focus on the things in your life that give you a sense of slowing down, chilling out, and being content, and allow you to feel a sense of well-being, of not wanting to achieve anything or go anywhere because you are content with the way things are right now. What things, activities, or relationships in your life foster this sense of feeling safe, connected, and content? How much time do you spend in the soothing/affiliation system?

When you have completed this task, stand back and think about which system you spend most of your time in. Which system would you wish to cultivate more? It's not unusual for people to realize that they spend more time than they want to in the threat and/or drive system, feeling stressed out, worrying, or rushing. Some people even start to feel a bit anxious if they spend too much time in the soothing system! It's as if the drive system kicks in and makes them feel guilty about not doing or achieving something.

Another way you can do this exercise is simply to focus on specific parts of your life. You could do it for your life at work or at home and notice how different places influence these three systems differently.

It's not that one system is intrinsically good and the other bad. Rather, it is all about *finding balance and seeing how they work together*. For example, David was feeling a little unwell and went to his doctor only to discover that he had very high blood pressure. That's a major threat. The consequence of this was a recognition that he needed to de-stress and spend more time "slowing down and chilling out." So he became motivated to find ways to do that, for example, by spending more time in his garden and learning to be more present in the moment.

When Karen got depressed, she became aware that she spent most of her time in the threat system ruminating, worrying, and being self-critical. Even the things that she had previously enjoyed, such as going out with friends, became a threat because they now made her feel anxious, so she tried to avoid doing them. And she devoted no time at all to slowing down and focusing on things she found she could enjoy. She certainly did not focus on how to generate kind feelings for herself and others and she was highly self-critical. So Karen was very out of balance. What helped her shift her focus was to understand how her thoughts and behaviors were maintaining the threat system and how doing little things that gave her pleasure helped her activate the other emotional systems. Through gradually learning to shift the focus of her energies and address the sources of the stress, she recovered.

The point of these stories is to show how it is not always easy to bring our minds into balance in the culture we live in but that through learning to apply the skills of mindful compassion (in part II), we can gradually bring them back into balance.

All Want Love and to Be Loving

Buddhist texts argue that we are all the same to the extent that we all want happiness and none of us want pain and suffering (see chapter 11). Research has shown, however, that there is more going on than just seeking happiness—that we also all deeply want to be loved and to be loving. We know this because researchers have looked at what happens in people's brains when they focus on feeling loved, and on feeling loving toward others. This work has shown that there are specific systems in our brain that respond to receiving love and kindness and to being loving toward others. Moreover, we see that our mental health; our immune system; the maturation of the frontal cortex; and our capacities for empathy, creativity, and lower stress—indeed, almost all facets of our being—function best under conditions of feeling loved and being loving, in contrast to feeling unloved and feeling anxious or angry.[41] In these conditions, we feel safe and can be open. Even for people who have mental health problems and who can be quite aggressive and destructive, this often settles down when they begin to feel valued, respected, and loved—once they have overcome their fears of these affiliative feelings, which can themselves be intense.

So although we can be incredibly destructive and cruel, selfish, materialistic, greedy, and grasping—as the last few thousand years have sadly shown—if we keep in mind how evolution has actually created our mind to work at its most optimal, it's our affiliative capacities that shine through. This gives us real hope for creating a better and fairer world. Learning more about how to stimulate, promote, and work with affiliative relationships that excite us and give us joy, as well as soothe and create a sense of safeness, is the challenge of the future.

Key Points

- Emotions texture and color our minds. If we didn't experience emotions, life would be very gray. However, emotions are also the source of some of our greatest difficulties because they can so easily to take control of our minds.

- We have different types of emotion that have evolved for different purposes: to cope with threat, to go out in the world and achieve things, and to be content and form nurturing relationships.

- The way our emotions develop and how they link to our sense of self is very much influenced by our genes and our early life experiences.

- From the day that we are born until the day we die, our relationships play a fundamental role in our mental well-being, and they do so because they give us access to the soothing/affiliation system.

- If this soothing system is not accessible to us, then balancing our emotions can be very difficult. Indeed, many people with mental health problems experience their emotions being out of balance and playing out powerfully in their everyday experience.

- An important role of the soothing/affiliation system is to regulate threat-based emotions and bring us back into balance. Becoming kind and loving toward ourselves and others is a way of stimulating this emotional system and regulating our difficult emotions.

- When we practice mindful compassion, we are therefore learning how to balance our minds and make the soothing system more accessible.

4

EMERGENCE OF COMPASSION

One of the ideas conveyed in chapter 2 is that our motives help to organize our minds. If we deliberately choose a motive like compassion to be the guiding principle of our lives, this is going to organize what we pay attention to, and how we think and behave. We have referred to this as a *social mentality* because compassion, like other motives, can organize a variety of psychological abilities and capacities, such as attention, feelings, and the way we think about ourselves and others to achieve particular social outcomes and relationships.

So our basic motives, life goals, and the kind of person we want to become are all hugely important in guiding and thus shaping our lives in very significant ways. When we consciously place compassionate motives such as caring, helping, encouraging, and supporting other people and ourselves at the center of our lives, this can have far-reaching impact on how we relate to ourselves, other people, and the world we are living in. This insight has been around for thousands of years and is common to many religions. In the Mahayana Buddhist tradition, compassion is seen as the fundamental agent of transformation that allows us to shift from a life centered on self-focused concerns to one focused on service to others. This is expressed in the classic Mahayana aspiration and heartfelt desire for all beings to be free from suffering and the causes of suffering, and in making the commitment to do whatever we can to bring this about.[1] This aspiration and commitment is referred to as *bodhicitta*.[2]

The Buddhist scholar Geshe Tashi Tsering speaks about the meaning of *bodhicitta* in the following way:

> *Bodhicitta* is the essence of all of Buddhist practice. The word "bodhicitta" itself explains so much: *bodhi* is Sanskrit for "awake," or "awakening" and *chitta* for "mind." As enlightenment is the state of "being fully awakened," the precious "mind" of *bodhicitta* is the mind that is starting to become completely awakened in order to benefit all other beings. There are two aspects to this mind: the aspiration to benefit others and the wish to obtain complete enlightenment in order to do that most skillfully.[3]

The recognition that we need to "enlighten ourselves" in order to help others is very important. For example, if someone falls into a fast-flowing river, you may well be tempted to jump in to save them. But if you can't swim yourself, then two people may end up dead. And of course there are many areas of life where we recognize we need *to train ourselves*, for example as doctors and nurses, in order to be able to help others—desire itself is not enough. These motives, of wanting to develop our own skills of mind because that's how we will eventually help ourselves and others, are the life blood that flows through the various Buddhist practices and enables them to come alive. In traditional Buddhist texts it is said that if one practices meditation without *bodhicitta*, it simply does not work and is tantamount to building castles of sand in the wind.

So, according to the Buddhist tradition, the best possible way to serve other living beings is to become enlightened ourselves. This means fully cultivating our own inner capacity for wisdom and compassion. With the clarity that comes from wise self-awareness, and the warmth and expansiveness that come from compassion, our limiting barriers of focusing just on ourselves and grasping to achieve more, have more, and hold on tightly to what we have, naturally relax and subside. As we become more enlightened by developing our capacity for compassion, we gain more clarity and effectiveness to help others become freer from suffering and happier too.

A key function of *bodhicitta* motivation is to organize the mind in a particular way. It is the central axis around which all of the other meditation practices and teachings turn. So every time Mahayana practitioners sit down to perform a meditation practice, they make a specific aspiration and commitment to invoke the compassionate mind. What this does is orient the mind in a particular way so that there is a sense of *guiding intention for their practice.* This lends power and energy to what they do because it is framed by an intention of compassion that is greater than one's narrow self-preoccupations.

In this respect we can see then that mindfulness alone—even with a loving-kindness focus—may not awaken this profound transformational process because *bodhicitta* is operating deep in the motivational and emotional brain (chapter 3). We can see too how powerful compassion is and how far-reaching its effects are. This is something we will now explore in more detail.

What Is Compassion?

Fossils show that about one million years ago our ancestors evolved into a species that looked after their old and diseased, as well as their young. This means that they were using caring motives in thoughtful and reflective ways, which is key to skillful compassion.[4] However, the word "compassion" comes originally from the Latin word *compati*, which means "to suffer with." As we will see, this is *not* such a helpful definition because the key to compassion as we think of it today is not just suffering or even "suffering with," but the motivation to relieve it and acquire the skills to do so. When we begin to look at the key qualities of compassion, science reveals a very hazy picture here.

In an effort to clarify the meaning of compassion, the American psychologist Jennifer Goetz[5] and her colleagues recently attempted a major review of the meaning of the term "compassion" and its evolutionary origins and functions.[6] Mostly, compassion is associated with words like "sympathy," "empathy," and "kindness." Compassion has also been linked (quite incorrectly) to pity in some English dictionaries (and in some other languages as well), but compassion has nothing to do with pity, as this involves a sense of feeling sorry for and looking down on another person. So the word itself is tricky.

In the Mahayana Buddhist tradition, sadness can awaken compassion. In some texts it is said that when the Buddha first emerged from his golden palace and saw the suffering of the world, he was overcome by sadness and it was this that created his commitment to try to do something about it. There are many stories about how different *bodhisattvas* of compassion turn back to see and hear the cries of the world and then are so moved by the cries of suffering that they reenter the world of suffering again, to try to do something about it. It is actually quite easy for us to connect with this inner sadness we carry. For example, try this exercise for contacting your inner sadness. Of course, *don't* do it to the point of feeling overwhelmed, but rather just until you start to feel touched by something that will awaken your own inner *bodhicitta*.

Exercise

Sit quietly and bring to mind some of the images you've seen on television. Remember that right now many thousands of children are dying from lack of food and water, mothers are in despair, many people are in pain or dying because of human violence and cruelty, and many are dying in pain because of diseases.

It doesn't take very long to let those images come to mind and to realize that although our world has beauty in the sunsets, the snow-covered mountains against blue skies, the forests, and the new flowers of spring, it's also a world of immense suffering. We should not be so dazzled by beauty that we forget suffering. However, if we only hold onto those images, then eventually they can be draining and depressing.

Now sit for a moment but this time focus on all the wonderful charity work going on around the world. Bring to mind images of people building wells for clean water, schools, and hospitals, and developing new treatments for painful conditions. Imagine the joy that is created when these come to fruition. Create in your mind images of individuals acting with each other to relieve suffering and the pleasure that flows from doing that. Did you feel what happened in you?

As Matthieu Ricard points out, while it's important for us to open our minds to suffering and not to hide away in our golden bubbles of personal satisfactions, it is also important we generate positive feelings linked to loving-kindness (or more accurately, friendly-kindness) and genuine wishes for the happiness of self and others—that suffering and the sources of suffering cease (personal communication, 2013). Compassion stimulates important motives and actions; it is *not* about being sucked into the mud of suffering and then becoming stuck there.

It is not about being overwhelmed by our inner sadness or wallowing in it. This is not sadness as a sense of pity or sentimentality, but the sadness that accompanies clear insight into the human condition; seeing things as they really are. In addition to what is actually happening around us, we can also see how we all go round and round making the same mistakes and creating suffering for ourselves without necessarily meaning to. We can see how we are all caught in the flow of life without exception, playing out the dramas of the brains that have been designed for us, that give rise to the experiences of pain and loss. There is also a close link between sadness and sympathy (one of the attributes of compassion described below). By being open and attentive, we become emotionally attuned to pain, loss, and suffering (you can develop a sympathetic connection with it). So this aspect of compassion requires us to open our hearts and be touched by the pain of life, and with this often comes sadness. The important point is that if we just keep it personal, this can result in "poor me" syndrome, but if we see how others are in a similar or perhaps even a worse situation, this connects us to others, and is a powerful basis from which compassion can arise. It is what Kristin Neff calls our "common humanity."[7]

In psychotherapy, we also know that sometimes people are angry in order to avoid being sad—some people find anger is easier than sadness, but it's recognizing and engaging with our sadness, then processing it so that transformation can take place, that is important; strange as it may seem, sadness can be very transforming and inspiring. It is sometimes said that it is our tears that can water and give birth to the lotus of compassion from the mud of suffering.

Healing: Definition of Compassion

There is no universally agreed-upon definition of compassion, so it is useful to look at a few.

In Wikipedia, compassion is defined as: "A virtue—one in which the emotional capacities of empathy and sympathy (for the suffering of others) are regarded as a part of love itself, and a cornerstone of greater social interconnection and humanism—foundational to the highest principles in philosophy, society, and personhood." This definition rests more on Christian and Western concepts of virtue (see also the next section, "Compassion, Kindness, and Love").

The simplest definition that emerges from traditional Buddhist thinking is compassion as "sensitivity to suffering in ourselves and others with a deep motivation and commitment to alleviate and prevent it."[8]

Two major thinkers in the area of compassion, Christina Feldman and Willem Kuyken, take into account Buddhist concepts of compassion as well as recent evolutionary thinking on compassion:

> Compassion is the acknowledgment that not all pain can be "fixed" or "solved" but all suffering is made more approachable in a landscape of compassion.
>
> Compassion is a *multitextured response* to pain, sorrow, and anguish. It includes kindness, empathy, generosity, and acceptance. The strands of courage, tolerance, and equanimity are equally woven into the cloth of compassion. Above all compassion is the capacity to be open to the reality of suffering and to aspire to its healing.[9]

They then go on:

> Compassion is an orientation of mind that recognizes pain and the universality of pain in human experience and the capacity to meet that pain with kindness, empathy, equanimity, and patience. While self-compassion orients to our own experience, compassion extends this orientation to others' experience.[10]

In teaching the importance of developing compassion in a therapy context, and to get across the idea that compassion is not about being soft, weak, or simply "nice," we suggest that compassion is a way to, as Paul often notes in his lectures, develop the kindness, support, and encouragement to promote the courage we need—to take the actions we need—in order to promote the flourishing and well-being of ourselves and others.

What is important about these definitions is that, while they acknowledge suffering, it's the alleviation and prevention of suffering and the idea of flourishing and well-being that are central to compassion.

As Matthieu Ricard has noted many times, compassion can also be seen as a form of altruistic love and is made up of a whole range of subattributes, abilities, and skills including sympathy, empathy, and motivation.[11] Indeed, he suggests that, at its heart, compassion is a *deep-felt wish* for others to be free of suffering and the causes of suffering and to flourish and find happiness. That motivation arises because we see clearly the suffering all around us. In a meditation practice Paul recently attended, the Buddhist scholar Geshe Tashi Tsering suggested that, rather than dwelling on the awfulness of suffering, our focus should also be on *the joy* we would feel to actually see others relieved of suffering.[12] Matthieu Ricard makes the same point: to be in touch with suffering is more like empathy, which is a key component of compassion, but compassion itself is a much more complex and larger process focused *on the release from suffering* and its causes (personal communication 2013). In this respect loving/friendly-kindness is the emotional tone needed for the harnessing and cultivating of compassion, focusing less on the pain and more on the wish for the ending of suffering and the joy we would experience if we could bring this about. Loving/friendly-kindness is the emotional texture that helps soften suffering.

Compassion, Kindness, and Love

Kindness and compassion are often overlapping concepts. It is important to recognize that some schools of Western philosophy, and of course Christianity, have placed kindness, charity, generosity, and compassion as central to the important qualities humans should cultivate. In their recent book *On Kindness*, Adam Phillips and Barbara Taylor point out that kindness can encompass a variety of sentiments, such as

> …sympathy, generosity, altruism, benevolence, humanity, compassion, pity, empathy—and that in the past were known by other terms as well, noticeably *philanthropia* (love of mankind) and *caritas* (neighborly or brotherly love). The precise meanings of these words vary, but basically they all denote what the Victorians called "open heartedness," the sympathetic expansiveness linking self to other.[13]

They go on to point out, "For most of Western history the dominant tradition of kindness has been Christianity, which sacralizes people's generous instincts and makes them the basis of a universalist faith."[14] The edicts of "love thy neighbor as thyself" and "turn the other cheek," and the story of the "good Samaritan," are central to the Christian life. So Christianity was first and foremost based on an appeal to kindness and compassion.

In addition, the last few thousand years have seen repeated philosophical and spiritual appeals to recognize the importance of our interconnectedness and that compassion is at the heart of a meaningful and happy life.[15] When kindness and compassion influence social and political discourse, the results can be dramatic as shown in the nineteenth century. As Adam Phillips and Barbara Taylor point out, this was a time when there was a major wave of humanitarian activism in Britain and America. Many of the horrors of child neglect, slavery, and cruelty to animals were openly debated and addressed, whereas before they had been accepted as normal ways of life.[16] The desire to "create a better life for all" was the sentiment in the rebuilding, post–Second World War years. Though close to bankruptcy, and with very little infrastructure, within fifteen years Britain had built the National Health Service that was the envy of the world and many other educational (such as school and university buildings) and support services for the elderly and poor. The post-war politics of the time were to some degree based on a "sensitivity to suffering and the desire to relieve it." The suffering the Second World War created was immense. However, such compassion has arguably been gradually eroded by the politics of individualism, competitiveness, and materialism. So now kindness is more likely to be seen as "nice but for losers" and not affordable in the cut and thrust of competitive life.[17]

Such ideas have been taken up by the psychotherapists John Ballatt and Penelope Campling in their important and fascinating book *Intelligent Kindness*, which looks at kindness and health care provision.[18] They offer a different insight into kindness by pointing out that the word "kindness" is linked to "kinship" (one of a kind) and that it grows particularly from a sense of interconnectedness and interdependence with others. These concepts of kindness capture many overlapping features with compassion. Whereas in Buddhism, loving-kindness (or, more accurately, friendly-kindness) is bracketed together and relates to the sense of feeling, the Western approach to kindness is more encompassing than that.

Yet another approach to defining compassion and, specifically, self-compassion, has been developed by Kristin Neff.[19] She focuses on three major dimensions:

- *Kindness*—Understanding one's difficulties and being kind and warm in the face of failure or setbacks rather than harshly judgmental and self-critical

- *Common humanity*—Seeing one's experiences as part of the human condition rather than as personal, isolating, and shaming

- *Mindful acceptance*—Awareness and acceptance of painful thoughts and feelings rather than overidentification with them

Here again we see the concepts of kindness and interconnectedness as central in our understanding of compassion. We should be careful to not simplify compassion into a single concept because, for hundreds of years and in different traditions, compassion has long been associated with kindness, sympathy, and, as Matthieu Ricard points out in books like *Happiness* (2003), the idea of altruistic love.

We can see, then, that the concept of compassion rests on slightly shifting sands, and many people are working on trying to understand the processes that are involved in compassion and the nature of the compassionate mind. Personally, we prefer this slightly open-ended definition, which allows us to have a feel for what we are talking about, rather than a concrete definition and process. The other important issue that is very noticeable is how most thinkers now don't try to define compassion in terms of a single motive or emotion, but recognize that it's more like (as we would say) a social mentality—in other words, a coordination and integration of different elements of the mind (e.g., motivation, attention, sympathy, empathy, action). When we present our model and approach to compassion below, we will see the same basic thinking—namely that compassion needs to be understood as consisting of *multiple* attributes and skills—and yet we will hold to the fact that at its core is motivation: the desire for all living things to be free of suffering and the causes of suffering.

Compassion and the Importance of Nurturance

Interestingly, in Buddhist texts, compassion is often compared to the love a mother has for her child, but the concept of "nurturance"—the act of offering warm and affectionate physical and emotional support and care—is not commonly used when referring to compassion, though it is perhaps implied. However, the psychology of nurturance may well have something important to teach us about compassion. To give you some understanding of how Paul came to the model of compassion that we will present below, and why the concept of nurturance is important to it, we will mention something of its history. Back in the 1980s when Paul was working on social mentality theory[20] (see "Motives Coordinate the Mind"), he was very influenced by the work of Alan Fogel, Gail Melson, and Jane Mistry,[21] and in particular, their ideas about the nature of caring and nurturing. They suggested that nurturance involves

- *motivation* to nurture;

- *awareness* of the need to be nurturing;

- *expression* of nurturing feelings;

- *understanding* what is needed to be nurturing;

- *matching* what is given with what is required to meet some developmental goal;

- *feedback* as the ability to change and adapt what is given according to how the target of care is responding.

Nurturing, then, needs to be skillfully carried out. Paul also suggested that these aspects can be self-directed as well as directed toward external people or objects. The concept of self-nurturance preceded the concepts of compassion.[22] So, our approach to compassion is influenced by Western psychological concepts of compassion as well as Buddhist ones.

Compassion as a Social Mentality: Its Multidimensional Nature

A further source of insight for the model we present has come from a number of years of working with people who struggle with being able to nurture, be kind to, or have compassion for themselves or others. These are *blocks to the flow of compassion*, between self and others and within oneself (self-compassion). The idea of overcoming blocks to the flow of compassion is also central to the Mahayana Buddhist practices. It has become clear that people struggle with compassion for different reasons. For example, some people are simply not motivated to be caring, perhaps because they are too caught up in, say, anger or fear, or because they are convinced that compassion is soft and weak. When it comes to being open to compassion from others or self-compassionate, although some people realize it would be helpful to them, they feel they don't deserve it or that it's simply beyond their ability to develop.[23] Some people are very motivated to be caring and helpful, but they are not very empathic. They rush into things rather than being thoughtful and reflective, and they tend to be rescuers rather than helping the other person develop the qualities *they need*; or they may become too distressed when they engage with other people's distress and end up tuning out.

Thus, the compassion circles were developed (1) by taking guidance from the original Mahayana Buddhist traditions and teachings and the works in this tradition; (2) through reference to current research on nurturance and altruism, caring, and helping; and (3) by working with people who struggle with compassion (especially self-compassion), and trying to identify where their difficulties in developing compassion lie.[24] We present compassion as two circles to reflect that the various attributes and skills of compassion overlap, work together, and enhance one another; it is not a linear process. Compassion is a complex and multifaceted social mentality, and if any of its attributes or skills are not working so well, then compassion as a whole can falter.

The Two Psychologies of Compassion

Compassion is of course more than just the alleviation of suffering and involves prevention of suffering and desire for the *well-being* of others. The focus on prevention is obvious because it's about removing the causes of suffering. So the point of spending effort training our minds is not just to relieve suffering when we see it but also to prevent it arising. This is true with all training; we train to get physically fit or eat a healthy diet to prevent health problems. In other words, we seek to remove or alleviate the conditions from which suffering arises.

Alleviation and prevention in this context does not imply a "fix it" approach to suffering like you might fix a car that has engine trouble, nor does it imply something has gone wrong. Our minds can get into all kinds of difficulties not because anything "has gone wrong" but because of the way they are. Alleviation and prevention are therefore about creating the conditions for clear insight and change, and that often means facing and accepting what is painful and difficult rather than turning away from it.

It is also clear that when we focus on compassion, and engage in various meditations and mantras, such as "may you/I be free of suffering," there is also added the mantra of "may you/I be happy" (see exercise 10). Freedom from suffering is accompanied by the desire for well-being and happiness, as Matthieu Ricard has outlined many times.[25] So we can see compassion as a kind of diamond process, as presented in figure 4.1. We turn toward, not away, from suffering (engagement); we have skills for the alleviation of suffering (know what to do); we seek to remove the causes of suffering (prevention), and create the conditions for well-being and happiness to arise. As one aspect improves, so the others become more accessible too—so they are interdependent.

As with all these kinds of summaries and diagrams, it should not be seen as some hard-and-fast rule, and there are different ways this could be presented. Note also that these are interacting processes so that as, say, our well-being increases, this may also increase our preparedness to engage with suffering. And as our skills for alleviating suffering improve, so does our preparedness to engage with suffering. It is of course partly about confidence, as with most things in life, so as our experience and confidence in our abilities increase, the more we are prepared to engage with more and more difficult things.

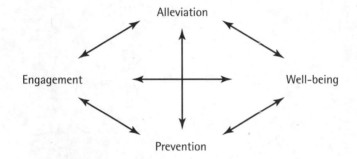

Figure 4.1 The compassion diamond

We now come back to the basic building blocks of compassion. These revolve around the actual attributes that are necessary to help us engage with pain and suffering, as well as the skills for the alleviation and prevention of suffering. Both the attributes and skills are usually infused with warmth as opposed to cold detachment. Combined, these attributes and skills constitute what we refer to as the *compassionate mind.*[26]

We can represent the compassionate mind with two interacting circles of attributes (for engagement) and skills (for alleviation and prevention) (see figure 4.2). We have two circles because there are *two different psychologies* involved with compassion. If we go back to the simplest definition of compassion as "a sensitivity to the suffering of oneself and others combined with a commitment to do something about it," then we can see that *engagement* (the ability to turn toward and engage with suffering as opposed to avoiding or trying to deny and suppress it) and *alleviation* (the ability to soften and help alleviate sources of suffering) are different. So the inner circle of attributes allows us to engage: to be motivated to engage with suffering, to understand it, to be moved by it, but also to tolerate it.

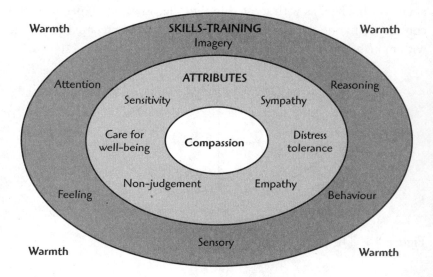

Figure 4.2 Attributes and skills of compassion
Source: P. Gilbert. 2009. *The Compassionate Mind*. London: Constable & Robinson.

The outer circle of skills, however, is related to the process by which we try to alleviate suffering—the wisdom we bring to bear on what will be helpful and effective in alleviating suffering.

The Attributes of Compassion: Engagement

Motivation

The first attribute of compassion is motivation; this is central to the Mahayana Buddhist position and also our evolved caring systems. It is the deep desire for ourselves and all living things to be free from suffering and the causes of suffering; and to be free from the causes of suffering means we have to be motivated to discover the causes and then antici-pate and prevent suffering. Care-focused motivation is the fundamental motive that coordinates and choreographs the other attributes. For example, empathy without a desire to be caring could be used for exploitation (see the "Sympathy" section later, for examples of empathy). Or why open your attention to suffering unless you are motivated to do something about it? So the motivational system provides the focus, the purpose and point of the other attributes. In addition, we need wisdom and insight. Wisdom ensures that compassion is not adopted as a "should or an ought," or just trying to be a nice person so that we are liked. In the Buddhist tradition, compassion is something that emerges together with wisdom: first, we see and understand how things are (Four Noble Truths, or the flow of life), which is the wisdom aspect, and then we are moved to do something about it, which is the compassion aspect.

Our motivation can be stimulated by role models; that is, we can see in others' qualities that we would like to develop in ourselves. People become examples that we aspire to. For example, many young men want to be like their football heroes so regularly practice their football skills, or women try to look like the fashion models in their magazines. Having people who demonstrate traits that we admire can become a source of inspiration to us—we may wish to be like them, learn from them, and have a sense of belonging to their group; for example, a young man following a football star and wanting to play for the same club, or a student being inspired by a teacher to take up the same area of study. This fosters a powerful source of self-identity. In Buddhist traditions, the compassion heroes we identify with are embodied in the *bodhisattva* ideal—they are people who have gained some wisdom and who are then motivated to respond to and alleviate suffering; they could be famous doctors, charity workers, or spiritual leaders, or even someone you know personally whom you deeply admire.

It's no different really than if you want to be a skilled piano player or football star. You identify your motivation, you identify who can help, you learn and train from those you respect and admire, and later maybe you teach the next generation.

So then we have to turn inward and train our minds to become more like this kind of person from all the possible selves that could emerge and flow through us. In Buddhist traditions, identification and aspiration, which are often focused on a teacher or guru, organize the mind in a particular way and shape how we think, speak, and act. In this way, identification with a *bodhisattva*, a person dedicated to bringing compassion into the world (see "The Self We Might Choose"), stimulates our inner motives, self-identities, and social mentalities that organize and shape how we respond to the world, and this in turn influences our attention, thinking, feeling, and behavior.[27] In some Buddhist traditions, Christ is seen as a *bodhisattva* because of what he inspires us to develop within ourselves.

As we become more mindful, we become more aware of compassionate experiences and the things that block compassion; we begin to notice how our compassionate motives of caring, encouraging, and being supportive of self and others can become blocked as we become angry or anxious, or more materialistic and self-focused. As we become more mindful, we also recognize that we can be very motivated to achieve certain goals, such as losing weight or getting fit, but we may not put the necessary effort into making these things happen. So motivation needs to be accompanied by effort; it is more than just a desire for something. This is why we emphasize the importance of training and practice in part II.

Sensitivity

This attribute is a capacity to be sensitive with *open attention*. Developing sensitivity of attention means that we are in touch with the moment-by-moment flow of our experience and we are less likely to turn a blind eye or use denial or justification to avoid engaging with things we find painful. Perhaps we have to become open to sadness to begin with. In later chapters we will focus on developing openness of attention and the ability to allow ourselves to become tuned in to suffering. We will see how mindfulness is core to this aspect of sensitivity (see chapter 7). With mindfulness we train to become more and more tuned in to the inner and outer flow of experience and the connections between our sensations, feelings, thoughts, and actions.

Some individuals really struggle to notice triggers to emotions linked to suffering. This could be because their minds are distracted and all over the place, or it may be linked to more specific causes. So even if we keep to the motivation of the wish to relieve suffering and the causes of suffering, we still need to work quite hard to be attentive enough to notice the triggers and causes of our reactions. This is where insights from modern psychotherapy can help because there are many models now to help us understand how our *emotional memories* can set us up for suffering and then play out in various unhelpful ways. We can start avoiding painful things in an effort not to notice and not to suffer. Mindfulness practice can benefit us enormously here by helping us pay attention to our bodies and what is going through our minds, because changes in the body can indicate that certain emotions are present.

Some people, however, are not so good at recognizing emotions in themselves or others; they simply are not tuned in to emotional states (this is called *alexithymia*). So no matter how motivated we are to face our difficulties, if we struggle to tune in to our feelings, compassion can get tricky. As we saw in chapter 3, one of the reasons for this can be that our emotions and motives are in such conflict that we feel overwhelmed. For example, some people who have had very difficult backgrounds might experience intense rage, but accepting those feelings seems to run against the kind of person they want to be, so they can feel enormous shame and fear of that rage; and for this reason, it gets blocked out. When they start to become more mindful, they get glimmers of unprocessed rage or sadness or yearning which then confuse or overwhelm them, so they then become defensive and avoid their own internal experience. Some therapists believe this even results in people becoming unconscious of these conflicts. When people's emotions are very blocked in this way, they often require professional help. But even so, the process of noticing enables people to develop wisdom that enables them to recognize that they need help, and through compassion, they can open themselves to being helped by others without feeling shame.

Sympathy

Sympathy is the emotional ability to be moved by distress in ourselves and others. Interestingly, in Christianity, sympathy is a core attribute of compassion and kindness; the ability to feel in tune with, and be moved by, the emotions of another, as in the story of the good Samaritan. Psychotherapists Phillips and Taylor noted how the eighteenth-century Scottish philosopher David Hume saw sympathy as core to our humanity and compared the transmission of feelings between people to the vibration of violin strings, with each individual resonating with the pains and pleasures of others as if they were his or her own.[23] We are "taken out of ourselves" into the emotional worlds of others, Hume wrote; or, as Adam Smith put it in his *Theory of Moral Sentiments* (1759), "we become in some measure the same person. ...This is the source of our fellow feeling."

Although empathy as a way of understanding other people, in contrast to simply feeling what they are feeling, is a later concept that was introduced into English in 1909 by the British psychologist Edward Titchener, sympathy and empathy are often confused. So to clarify how *we* use these two different concepts, here is a simple table to help you think about the differences as we are discussing them.[29]

Table 4.1 Differences Between Sympathy and Empathy

Sympathy	Empathy
Sympathy involves a heightened awareness of the suffering or needs of another person as something to be alleviated. The focus is on the other person's well-being.	Empathy involves a heightened, focused awareness of the experience of another person (not necessarily suffering) as something to be understood.
Sympathy is relatively automatic and effortless.	Empathy is effortful and depends on abilities to imagine being the other, to "walk in their shoes."
Behavior is on immediate actions to alleviate—it may or may not be what is needed.	Behavior is on listening, engaging, finding out, knowing, conceptualizing, and understanding—the basis for thoughtful/skilled actions.
In sympathy, the self is moved by the other.	
The other is the vehicle for understanding, and some loss of identity can arise.	In empathy, the self reaches out for the other.
	The self is a vehicle for understanding and never loses its identity.

Source: Adapted from P. Gilbert. 1989. *Human Nature and Suffering*. Hove: Psychology Press. Used with permission.

Although there are debates about such distinctions, sympathy can be taken to be our immediate emotional reaction, without conscious thought and reflection. For example, a friend phones you up and tells you that her child has been killed in a car crash or has a terrible illness. You're immediately flushed with feelings without thinking. Or, when you see a child playing happily and then he falls over and hurts himself, you feel an immediate emotional wince at his sudden cry or scream, which "hits" you in the stomach. We don't need to think or reason to feel an immediate sympathetic connection—it's there straight away. But, like many other aspects of compassion, sympathy is not necessarily helpful by itself because sometimes we are simply overwhelmed by our feelings and we can't quite distinguish them from those going on in the other person. In this case, we can lose a sense of perspective and rush in without thinking in a desperate effort to turn off distress or even turn away from it because we can't tolerate it; we have too much personal distress.

Blocks to Sympathy

Other problems with sympathy can arise because it gets blocked in certain ways. For example, studies show that sympathy can be extremely painful and takes its toll when it involves, for example, connecting to someone we love or feel responsible for who is in pain and/or mentally ill.[30] Another type of block arises when we try to be emotionally attuned to suffering in an environment that's excessively demanding, for example, if we work somewhere that is short staffed, punitive, bureaucratic, and nonsupportive. There have been various reports about compassion failures in the National Health Service in the UK as a result of these processes.[31] Yet a different reason for dulling our capacity for emotional attunement can be that we are brought up with a news media that constantly focuses on death, disease, dying, humiliation, and shame but leaves us feeling powerless to do anything about it—so we get angry, shrug, and switch off. Add this to an entertainment industry that is constantly encouraging us to take pleasure in seeing the bad guys get injured, mutilated, or killed, and it would seem that we are constantly invited to turn off sympathy and be emotionally *unmoved* by suffering.

Sympathy and Guilt

It's also important that we are able to develop some degree of sympathy for the pain *we ourselves cause* others (that is, we are emotionally moved by it) because this is the basis of guilt, which, unlike shame, gives us feelings of sorrow and regret (see chapter 6). So if we shout at somebody and are critical of them, we are able to recognize that we have upset them and then our sympathy for the pain they are experiencing may alert us to try to rectify the pain we've caused. If we are very egocentric, however, we might even become angry with them for getting distressed about our criticism; we might see their pain but then think, "Oh, they are weak. Why don't they toughen up?" or "Well, life is tough—they've just got to get on with it." The point is, there are many things, both inside us and in our cultures, that can deaden our sympathy and disconnect us. Without sympathy, we have very few emotional bridges to connect us to the feelings of others.

Distress Tolerance

Many researchers in this area recognize that connecting to pain within ourselves and others can actually stimulate much *personal distress.* How we deal with that can have a huge influence on whether we go forth with compassion for engaging or avoidance, or whether we try to help people in distress because we want to turn off our own distress.[32] So the fourth quality of compassion is distress tolerance, which enables us to stay with the experience of being emotionally tuned in to suffering.[33] People who feel overwhelmed by distress in themselves and others tend to turn away from it. Some may reach for all kinds of medications to remove anxiety and depression, and while sometimes that is a compassionate thing to do (if this suffering stems from treatable diseases and conditions), at other times it may not be so helpful. Being able to bear and cope with distress allows us to actively listen and work out what is helpful. However, distress tolerance is not intended to foster some macho endurance, but is based on a caring motive that facilitates long-term recovery or development. If you put your hand next to the fire, it is simply crazy to leave it there in the false belief that you have to learn how to tolerate or accept it—sometimes it's important to learn when we don't need to tolerate distress.

Distress tolerance arises from motivation again, which is a *willingness* to engage. Much psychotherapy today focuses on the importance of developing acceptance and willingness—that is, motivation to engage with difficult experiences and feelings rather than close down to them.[34] What is important, though, is recognizing that the more supportive and kind we are, the more we will be able to tolerate difficult things and therefore be willing to try to engage with them. In contrast, if we are self-critical, then there is less tolerance. In Buddhist and Western traditions, distress tolerance also involves cultivating patience. Patience is an essential antidote to acting out frustration. Now while some people seem more naturally patient, "laid back," or easygoing than others, it can also be helpful for us to recognize what undermines our ability to develop patience (e.g., having too many things to do—too much drive system) and seek to address those causes of impatience.

Learning how to tolerate distress is the basis of *courage*—for example, thinking about the Four Noble Truths (how everything is impermanent and how suffering pervades all of life) and becoming aware of the flow of life. This could be quite a downer and rather difficult to bear. So we might just turn away from it, get out the red wine, and enjoy life for ourselves as best we can. But when we engage the compassionate wish to prevent and alleviate suffering as best we can, that changes our orientation.

Empathy

As noted above, philosophers, neuroscientists, and psychotherapists tend to have slightly different views about empathy and sympathy, so here we are going to follow the more psychotherapeutic view. Wikipedia gives a huge range of different definitions for empathy. So we will try to clarify our use of the term. It has been said that empathy is one of the most important attributes that evolved in humans. It is what makes us distinctive as humans and separates us from other animals.[35] Human empathy is different than sympathy because it involves our ability for *awareness and intuitive understanding.* Whereas sympathy is an automatic resonance with the feelings of others, empathy is much more about insight and understanding. It is our ability *to understand* not just that someone suffers but also why, to see into the causes. More complex is empathy that enables us to work out how to communicate and act in order *to help the other person understand* what is in *our mind*. In fact, without some deep capacity to understand each other, it is unlikely that civilization would have developed to the extent that it has.[36]

We can start our exploration of empathy by noting that one of the major evolutionary adaptations to the human cognitive system is what is called *theory of mind*. This is a technical term for explaining that we relate to other people differently to how we relate to our car or a food mixer! Cars and food mixers don't have motives, intentions, and emotions, and they don't suffer or feel joy in the way that living beings do—you don't need to impress them nor can you shame them. Of course, if they go wrong—say the food mixer sprays cake mix all over you, or the car decides not to start when you have to go for an important interview—you might hit them! In contrast, when it comes to other animals, and particularly humans, we understand that they have minds with feelings and intentions. Empathy is our ability to understand and emotionally recognize the feelings, motivations, and intentions of another human being.

There is a huge amount of academic literature on empathy and its use in psychotherapy stretching back over sixty years to the humanistic psychotherapist Carl Rogers.[37] He suggested that people can find ways to change and grow if you treat them with positive regard, genuineness, and empathy. He defined empathy as the ability to *imagine* oneself in the minds of other people, *walking in their shoes*. So, for example, seeing somebody in tears allows us to understand that they may have experienced a loss of some kind. Whereas with sympathy we are emotionally moved by the distress of someone in tears but do not necessarily understand its source, with empathy we try to understand *why* this person is feeling distressed.[38] As noted in table 4.1, this is not automatic like sympathy but requires us to imagine what is happening for them; we imagine what is going on *from their point of view* and step into their shoes. Maguiles talks about the "wonder of empathy"—the way in which we have to be open, curious, and fascinated by "the other" in order to connect to them.[39] Being curious is an important way to develop empathy.

These days the clinical use of empathy has become a major focus for understanding the process and effectiveness of therapeutic work. We now know that empathy is a cycle of communication whereby a therapist tries to understand what's going on in the patient's mind (without empathy, this would be impossible), then relays this *back to* the patient so that the patient feels understood and validated; and then the patient behaves in such a way as to show he or she has been understood. Our understanding of empathy is *interpersonal*; in other words, it grows out of how we relate to other people and how other people relate to us.[40] As for compassion, if we have no idea of the source of suffering, then clearly we may have no idea of how to respond to suffering.

Empathy and Emotional Containment

Empathy allows us to contain our own emotions. In this respect, it is connected to distress tolerance. For example, imagine you are going to Jane's fiftieth birthday party. Just before you go, you hear that a mutual friend Sally has been diagnosed with cancer, and this greatly upsets you. If you have a capacity for compassionate empathic containment, then you would still go to Jane's party but you would refrain from telling Jane what has happened to Sally because you know that it would ruin her party and it might be best for her to learn the bad news the following day. Your empathy has predicted that for Jane to hear the news would destroy the joy of her party, and your caring motivation prevents you from doing this. Here is another example: You have had a very stressful day at work and want to talk to your partner when you get home. Before even finding out what kind of day your partner has had, you simply dump all your woes on him or her. People who struggle to contain their emotions often share things with people when sometimes it's not always helpful to do so; they are not really able to recognize the impact of their behavior on others. Compassion training really helps here because it teaches us to slow down, pause, and, with empathy, reflect on how our behavior impacts on others.

Empathy vs. Projection

Empathy is sometimes contrasted with projection. A classic case of projection is when we can feel sad about taking a beloved car (we have an affectionate attachment to it) to the scrap-yard—we can almost feel guilty at leaving it there to be broken up—as if we are doing something bad and the car will feel abandoned by us! Projection is also when we think that other people think and feel the same way we do. For example, it's your birthday and you would love a new guitar. Your wife understands this and buys you one. You're delighted. Next month is your wife's birthday so you think to yourself, "What would I like? Hmm, I really enjoyed getting a new guitar—ah, ha! I have the perfect present then—a new guitar!" But the problem is, she doesn't play the guitar. So if we only use our own preferences, desires, and wishes to make judgments about other people, we can get things wrong.

The curious thing about empathy is that, on the one hand, we have to use our own feelings, intentions, and desires as the basis for understanding others or else people would be like aliens to us. However, we also have to be able to recognize the *differences between us*: that I know things that others may not, that I have desires others may not, that I can do things easily that others cannot.[41] True empathy means that we try to imagine what it's like to be other people, to walk in their shoes, and not simply to see them as carbon copies of ourselves. When you hear people saying, "I really can't understand him or her; after all, *if I was him or her* I would do this and not that…," this is an issue of lack of empathy because understanding that *someone is different from you* is the first step to trying to work out what it is they are really feeling and *how* they are different from you.

One of the big debates about our human tendencies to project our own thoughts and feelings into the minds of others is religion and belief in God. Humans tend to create gods with very humanlike motivations and emotions (such as being loving and caring or vengeful) just like a human mind. Using our own minds to think about the mind of God allows us to have some kind of relationship and to wonder what would cause God's love or anger for oneself.[42] Males used to sacrifice virgins to the gods because they assumed gods were like them—easily persuaded by a few virgins! Although our emotions were honed on the fields of evolution, we assume God has a mind like ours. If not, it would be impossible to form a relationship because the mind of God could be totally alien.

Unhelpful Empathy

One question we are often asked is, Isn't empathy the same as compassion; or isn't empathy always compassionate? We hope by now you see that the answer is definitely *no*—empathy is a very important attribute of compassion, but compassion is much more than just empathy. Not only that, but empathy can be used in all kinds of noncompassionate ways. The worst torturer to have is an empathic one. The nonempathic one puts the gun to your head, but the empathic one puts it to your child's head. Empathic advertisers know exactly how to stimulate you to eat more than is healthy for you, and they care little about putting your life at risk through obesity. Indeed, there is so much in the commercialization and competitiveness of our modern world that is very empathic but very destructive too. For example, politicians are constantly working out how to get people to support them by relying on complex research that studies how our brains react to certain messages.[43] Consequently, without a caring motive, empathy is of little use by itself and may even be very destructive. Time and time again, then, we come back to the issue of motivation and how we orient ourselves to become a certain kind of person, which requires us to train our minds and not take compassion for granted.

Blocking Our Empathy

Sadly we are an incredibly tribal species, and a major block to empathy comes from our tendency to form groups very easily and then become aggressive or contemptuous of other groups. Once we have identified the attributes that define our group, it becomes very tempting to think that members of other groups are "not like us" and then to show very little interest in understanding how and why they are actually fellow human beings like us. Moreover, when conflicts arise between opposing groups, leaders often deliberately undermine empathic connection between rival groups even to the point of denigrating the others as vermin, a disease, a corruption, or a danger to our way of life. Tribalism is probably one of the most tragic causes of blocking empathy and compassion; we don't want to pause to think of our enemies as fellow human beings, who want to be free of suffering, to be happy, to love their children and see them grow and flourish; we block from trying to see the world through their eyes. Tragically, one way empathy could be recruited is when we try to work out how to really make them suffer!

Empathy blocks can also arise because we cling to our own tightly defined and socially constructed self-identity. Consider the fact that 2,500 years ago, at the time the Buddha was teaching the Four Noble Truths, just a few thousand miles away many people in Rome were enjoying watching people butcher each other in gladiatorial contests. It can be difficult for us to imagine being like our Roman ancestors because we want to reject those passions in ourselves. But those screaming in delight over the spurting of blood were not aliens; they were simply human beings like you and me. It is just that they were part of a very different culture and inhabited minds that were socially influenced in different ways. By being empathic we can understand this; we can become much clearer in our minds about how cultures shape us and what we need to do if we want to live in a genuinely compassionate culture. This would almost certainly mean rejecting our addictions to competition, individualism, and materialism, and finding more balanced ways of living.

The main point is that while we might have empathy for someone who is similar to us, the more different they are, the more difficult it becomes. So empathy for an anxious person might be easy, or even for an angry person, but what about empathy for a callously violent or sexually abusive person? What happens to our empathy when we are confronted by someone we do not like or someone who has seriously upset us? Empathy can require a decision to move into places that are difficult. For example, when your boss is being unpleasant to you, can you try to imagine what is going on for him or her, or do you just hate him or her?

With this example, bear in mind that compassion is not the same as submissive acceptance. While it is important to develop empathy rather than avoidance or fear, the courage of compassion may mean we have to be assertive and stand up to our bosses. Similarly, we can understand that violent people often come from violent backgrounds, so we try to treat them compassionately, but that does not mean that we just let them carry on being violent, because this is neither wise nor compassionate. So we can be compassionate to the person and empathize with their struggles, and have a heartfelt wish that the causes of their destructive behavior disappear, yet still take appropriately tough action against their negative behaviors.

Matthieu Ricard points out that empathy is not a precondition for the arising of compassion. Although empathy helps greatly because we are able to step into the shoes of another and sense what they are going through, in certain circumstances it comes about directly through wisdom. In a personal communication Matthieu Ricard suggested

Empathy can be an important trigger to compassion, when it triggers an emotional resonance with the suffering of others and alerts us to their needs and to their suffering. But empathic resonance is not always necessary, since the wisdom aspect of compassion, which is to recognize the deep causes of suffering (the third of the three kinds of suffering according to Buddhism, the all-pervading suffering due to ignorance) and wish that beings might be free from that basic ignorance that is at the root of all suffering, is a cognitive state, not an emotional or empathic state.

Nonjudgment

Compassion involves being nonjudgmental in the sense of being noncondemning. In both Buddhism and Christianity, not acting out on others or not seeking to harm people out of anger or vengeance are seen as important parts of kindness and compassion (e.g., let he who is without sin cast the first stone). Now clearly the brain is making judgments all the time, and we are unaware of many of them. The issue here, however, is not acting on our automatic judgments but being more reflective so that our actions are based on compassion, wisdom, and choices. If we just become critical and angry about things, this can interfere with compassion. We end up being caught up in the threat-processing system, and this system lacks wisdom. Nonetheless, anger at the suffering around us can sometimes be the first step to compassion.

Nonjudgment and acceptance is not "doing nothing." For example, we learn not to judge ourselves for being depressed but at the same time do what we can to overcome it; we do not allow a violent person to continue to be violent. So the key to nonjudgment is as a mindfulness skill that allows the flow of the mind to reveal itself without fighting with it. This gives us the ability to clearly discern what is happening and make choices about how to act wisely.

Compassionate nonjudgment is not necessarily based on liking. For example, we might never like a psychopath who has beaten up people and is cruel to animals. But through empathy, we can try to understand what her mind is like and, moreover, we can have a sense of enormous *gratitude* that we don't have a mind like that. On the basis of this understanding and gratitude, we can open up to the possibility of being nonjudgmental toward this person, but again, this doesn't mean that we allow her to continue to be harmful; and if we didn't, say, put her in prison, we might be failing in our efforts to prevent harm to others—an important moral issue. Compassion is aimed at the wish for the processes that create cruelty within the psychopath to stop, and it is based on the understanding that she, like us, just finds herself here, with a brain designed by genes and social conditioning (with that spark of consciousness) she did not choose. Cultivating hateful feelings toward the psychopath is only going to stimulate the threat systems in our brain, and then, before we know it, we will start to tread the path of the person we loathe.

Nonjudgment doesn't mean nonpreference; it doesn't mean not working for things that you believe are important. In fact it is exactly the opposite. For example, the Dalai Lama and other spiritual leaders spend a lot of their time traveling around spreading compassionate values. This is something that is very important and dear to them. So nonjudgment doesn't mean not having values, aspirations, or ambitions. It means that when things are not as we want them to be, we don't fight with them; we learn to ride them out. We will look at this skill in more detail when we learn to practice mindfulness in chapter 7.

Bringing the Attributes Together and the Emergence of Compassion

People with different approaches suggest different qualities and attributes for compassion. For us, these attributes we have discussed above are the crucial ones, and if you remove any of them, compassion will begin to struggle. For instance, if you take out the motivation to be caring, the whole compassionate endeavor starts to collapse, but it will also falter if you lose sensitivity and don't pay attention to suffering because you simply don't see it; or if you see it but you can't tolerate it, so you turn away from it; or even if you do see it and turn toward it, but you can't understand it and are not sure what to do because your empathy is struggling.

There are ways in which we can focus on each of these attributes, but what's interesting is that because these are part and parcel of the compassion process (what we call a social mentality), when we do certain mindfulness and compassion exercises *these attributes tend to co-arise*— that is, they tend also to build and support each other. As we build empathic awareness, this helps distress tolerance; and as we become more tolerant, and able to stay with, contain, and explore our emotions and those of others, we become more empathic and open. It might be worth recalling how we discussed the importance of emergence (see chapter 1, "Emergence and Interconnectedness") and the way in which patterns are created through the interaction of their components above. In this case you can see how compassion gradually emerges in the mind through the cultivation of these interacting attributes of compassion.

In chapter 8, we will work with these attributes in an experiential way and show how they can be applied to the moment-by-moment working of our minds in such a way that we engage fully and honestly with our experience as it unfolds.

Skills of Compassion: Alleviation and Prevention

We will now discuss the outer circle of figure 4.2. In the Mahayana Buddhist tradition, meditation has two aspects: first, there is familiarization with the workings of the mind, which is what is commonly developed through mindfulness; and, second, on the basis of becoming familiar, there is the cultivation of certain qualities and potentials, which is what is understood as compassion training. In other words, there is insight based on observation that leads to wise discernment of what to do. The compassion circles are similar. The inner circle focuses on tuning in to suffering so we can understand and tolerate it, while the outer circle focuses on what to do about it, namely using our skills for alleviating suffering. In the Buddhist tradition, there is talk about *skillful means*, which is learning to skillfully relate to suffering once we have become aware of it. Knowing *how to be* helpful is part of compassion and wisdom. Of course this is one of the reasons people train in medicine or therapy, or will spend years doing mindfulness practice, so that they can learn to become skillful helpers and work to prevent suffering.

Compassionate Attention

As we will see when we explore attention training in part II of this book, our attention can be focused on anything we like—from our left foot to our right foot to the ice cream we are about to eat to the TV program we're watching. And when you focus your attention on something in particular like this, other things fade in the field of your awareness. We will do an exercise on this a little later (see chapter 7). Compassionate attention is simply recognizing how you can voluntarily direct your attention to themes that are helpful to you and others.

To illustrate the difference in attention focus between the inner circle of attributes and the outer circle of skills, imagine a doctor coming to see an injured patient. First, the doctor's attention must be on the injury in order to make an accurate diagnosis. The doctor will listen carefully to the story of what happened, investigate the symptoms, and maybe prod here and feel there. The doctor will become familiar with the pattern of symptoms and pains that are being presented. This requires skillful attention and mindful engagement. However, once this is done, the doctor does not stay focused on the injury but switches attention and brings to mind what is needed to heal the person. At that moment, the doctor's attention changes and so do his or her feelings. So we need one type of attention to become aware of the injury and then a different type of attention to focus on its alleviation.

Here's another example of these two types of attention. Remember the ten shops we went into when we were doing our Christmas shopping where nine people were kind to us and one person was unkind? Mindfulness enables us to see how our attention is focused on the one unkind salesperson and how we don't see the other nine who were kind; it enables us to become familiar with this fact. This opens up the possibility for compassionate attention in which we now deliberately choose to bring to mind and focus our attention on the nine salespeople who were helpful; we remember their facial expressions and what they said, and we remember our joy as we left the shop with a nice present.

Now compassionate attention is not always about simply being accurate. Aaron Beck, the originator of cognitive behavioral therapy, for example, once pointed out that if you are on the third floor of a burning house and have to climb down the drain pipe, it may be true that if you slip you could die. This is a perfectly accurate thought, but it's not very helpful to focus on it in this context! What is more helpful is to focus on your grip and on your footing as you climb down. So what we focus on can be extremely important, and it's not always about being accurate, but being mindful of what is helpful in that moment.

Compassionate Imagery

Imagery is now used in a number of therapeutic approaches.[44] It is regarded as a more powerful means of producing psychological and physiological change than verbal exchanges alone. Imagery is central to many types of Buddhist meditation that are designed to help people get in touch with inner processes, feelings, and motivations.[45] In chapters 9–11, we explore compassionate imagery in some detail, including the fact that many people misunderstand imagery, thinking it's just about trying to create pictures in the mind. Images sometimes arise spontaneously because of the state of mind we are in, but we can also deliberately create images that can then influence the hormones cascading through our body. This is important because when we engage in compassionate imagery, we are stimulating key emotional and physiological systems in our brain and body. If we do this on a regular basis, it will start to forge different tendencies within us that will begin to organize our minds in different ways, in effect laying the foundation for the emergence of the compassionate mind.

Compassionate Feelings

In the inner circle of attributes, compassionate feelings arise through our sympathy for pain and our sense of feeling connected to it. In regard to the outer circle of skills, however, our feelings are focused on the alleviation of suffering, and we approach suffering with *friendliness and kindness*—sometimes called *metta*. As we have seen, kindness has a particular meaning in Western philosophy linked to the sense of interconnectedness.[46] What is important here is the heartfelt wish for suffering to be alleviated and the joy and excitement of this happening.[47] Matthieu Ricard has frequently talked about the importance of the *heartfelt wish* as being at the root of compassionate feeling.[48] So we can think of compassionate feeling also as a two-stage process: first, mindful attention makes us aware of the reality of suffering and sympathy engages it with mirror-like feelings; second, the skills of compassion recruit the positive feelings of kindness and friendliness and, with enthusiasm, try to alleviate suffering.

Important too is recognition of voice tone; that is, when we are thinking about ourselves or other people, we *deliberately try to create an inner, kind, and warm voice tone* as opposed to a neutral, harsh, aggressive, or critical one.

Compassionate feelings are also linked to other important Buddhist elements, patience and tolerance—different but linked to distress tolerance above—which support the ability to wait and allow rather than force and hurry. So patience is the ability to stay calm even when things are not moving in the way that you would ideally like. We will have more to say about compassionate feelings later.

Compassionate Thinking

As we have said many times, our human new brain has the ability to think, reflect, analyze, predict, imagine, anticipate, and plan. These are extraordinary feats. The key question, though, is how do we use our powers of reasoning and thinking? What motives do we pursue with these new brain skills? Do we let our reasoning be dictated by whatever culture we find ourselves in, and so, in our modern competitive culture, simply go along with how to get the competitive edge and not worry about anybody else? Compassionate thinking is making the decision, to the best of our ability, to reason compassionately. This involves first mindfully standing back, slowing down, and observing what is going on in our minds, and, second, thinking compassionately in a range of ways.[49] In fact, a whole approach to psychotherapy called cognitive behavioral therapy focuses on ways of helpful thinking: how to keep things in perspective, treat yourself like you would a friend, and check out the evidence for a particular worry or concern. We can gently *ask ourselves questions* about how we would see this if we were in a different state of mind, if we were at our most caring and compassionate, our wisest and calmest. In our approach to compassion, these are very helpful indeed.[50]

Compassionate thinking has to work against our natural biases in thinking. We know that when we are threatened or when we are in high drive states, our thinking and reasoning can become very biased. For example, when we have an argument with somebody, our angry self can come up with all the reasons why we should be critical or attack the other person. If we are experiencing anxiety, our thoughts can make us even more anxious: "Oh my gosh, what happens if I have a heart attack or this person rejects me or I make a mistake?... I will never get over it. It will be a disaster," and so on. The way we think, reason, and ruminate about things can have a big impact on whether we pour gasoline on the fires of our threat system or learn to calm it down. Indeed, certain types of rumination are well known to lock us into stress and suffering. Compassionate thinking is an antidote to this.

Compassionate Sensory Focusing

Compassionate sensory focusing is where we learn to focus on the sensory qualities of compassion. In the practice section (part II), we look at how to breathe (called *soothing breathing rhythm*) in such a way that we may stimulate the parasympathetic nervous system, which then provides a firm platform for compassionate work (see exercise 3). We also look at compassionate postures, facial expressions, and voice tones, and use images to imagine ourselves as compassionate beings.

Compassionate Behavior
Compassionate Courage

Compassionate behavior relates to the inner and outer circles in different ways. One of the most important qualities of compassionate behavior is *courage* because without it, no matter how empathic or motivated we are, it could be difficult to follow through with a course of action. For example, the fireman who rushes into the burning house and risks his life to save a baby is showing compassionate courage. Another example might be the thousands of people who put themselves and their families at risk to save Jewish people during the Second World War.[51] What is interesting here is that some of these individuals were not necessarily overly kind or tender, and some may have been quite autocratic, yet their behavior could be seen as little other than compassionate because it was based on the motivation to alleviate and prevent suffering.

So the outer circle is different from the inner circle in that you can get different elements operating independently—compassionate behavior without compassionate feeling, for example. This is important because both Buddhist practice and modern psychology suggest that behavior often comes first. If we learn to behave in a way that will help ourselves and others flourish, then even if we don't have a deeply compassionate feeling about this, it is still a very important path to compassion and gradually feelings may follow.

When it comes to helping people develop courage we use the term "en-couragement" and this requires a degree of empathy. For example, there are times when we would rather avoid difficult things, but the encouragement of others—and sometimes *even the pressure they put on us*—helps us jump over an obstacle. So we can recognize then that compassionate behavior can take different forms. In the case of an agoraphobic, compassionate behavior might involve going to the front door with her and then seeing how far she can get, while learning to be kind, supportive, and validating with every step forward when anxiety starts to kick in. Compassionate behavior isn't soothing yourself by sitting on the couch eating chocolates and watching TV; it's not about having a relaxing warm bath. Compassionate behavior is focused with intention and purpose. A compassionate therapist may even be quite "pushy" when trying to help the patient overcome his reluctance to face, experience, and learn to tolerate his anxiety or other avoided things. With children too we sometimes have to help them face their fears even when they don't want to. Compassion is not the same as never upsetting anybody or being "nice" all the time. Sometimes people might not like you when you encourage them to face things.

The Christian story is ultimately one of courage. Whether or not you believe Jesus was the son of God, the idea of dying in that way to save humanity can only be seen as extraordinary courage—and indeed it is the call to courage, to stand up for the poor, the sick, and the suffering, which is at the heart of Christian compassionate values. Sadly, some politicians can turn that on its head, with rather little interest in providing for the sick or the poor and with more interest in personal advancement, and claim the latter as Christian ethics.[52] In the Mahayana Buddhist tradition, too, courage, or fierce compassion, is one of the key attributes of the *bodhisattva*, or spiritual warrior, who embodies the compassionate ideal, able to tolerate his or her own fear in order to face the pain and difficulties of life, and who may put his or her own safety at risk in order to alleviate the suffering of others.

Compassionate Kindness

Kindness has had a checkered but very important history.[53] It can be seen as an emotion, motive, or action. Doing kind things that bring happiness to others has long been recognized as being helpful to ourselves too. Indeed, some recent approaches to happiness involve doing random acts of kindness for somebody each day. Kindness may not require any courage at all, and it can be pleasurable to do (such as buying someone a birthday present or going next door to cut an elderly neighbor's lawn). It can be associated with feeling good about ourselves, and for this reason many psychologists recommend it precisely because it has positive effects on our own moods and emotions. In this sense it can be seen as having a selfish component. In fact, the Dalai Lama often says that the best form of selfishness (i.e., the one that brings the highest dividend to oneself) is being kind to others. Simply put, if you spread sunshine to others, it can brighten you up too.

The idea that somehow our compassionate behavior should give us no positive feedback is simply wrong. Not only do we experience other people's gratitude, but more importantly we are stimulating brain systems that can be good for us. Even if we dismiss gratitude, we can't ignore the fact that acting compassionately affects our brain. On the other hand, if we engage in compassion *only* because we want to be liked and be seen as nice, or if we are acting out of submissiveness, then our *motivation* is not really compassionate and therefore it may not have the same impact. Paul is currently researching this.

So, what determines compassionate behavior in any given situation can sometimes be tricky, and for this we need wisdom to recognize that many of our motives and behaviors are actually mixes and blends—some will be conscious to us, others will not. Nonetheless, we can still spend time openly reflecting on what compassionate behavior in any particular situation might be and we can pose ourselves the question: "What is the compassionate thing to do in this situation?" By slowing down and reflecting, we can access our inner wisdom. The problem is that people simply don't stop and ask themselves the question! Sometimes compassionate behavior will require courage, other times kindness, and often both.

The Two Psychologies of Compassion: Bringing Them Together

In conclusion, there are two distinct but interdependent psychologies that make up compassion: the psychology that enables us to be motivated to engage with suffering, to stay with it, and understand its causes in a nonjudgmental way; and a second psychology that enables us to work skillfully toward the alleviation and prevention of suffering and its causes. This whole process is contextualized in a mind that is mindful, observant, and familiar with its own workings. Indeed this process would be very limited without such mindful awareness.[54]

We can use a concrete example to bring this together. A friend tells you that he has cancer. *Motivation* is wanting to help; *sensitivity* is the attentiveness to his experience; *sympathy* is being moved by his pain and fear; *distress tolerance* is being able to stay with that pain and fear, neither turning away nor trying to superficially rescue; *empathy* is imagining what it might be like being him and what he may require of you; and *nonjudgment* is accepting without fighting or raging about this tragedy. For the outer circle, *attention* is focusing on things that would be helpful; *thinking* about what would be helpful and how to act skillfully; *behavior* may be going with your friend for hospital appointments and holding his hand; *feeling* is holding to your heartfelt wish that he can either recover or his pain be eased; *sensory focusing* is awareness of your body and the emotions flowing through you.

A simple depiction of the interaction of these psychologies is given in figure 4.3.

We suggest that this interaction supports both wisdom and courage. We also suggest that wisdom and courage are key to the continuing development of our abilities to engage with, alleviate, and prevent suffering. The emotion regulation system that will be especially helpful for developing these two psychologies of compassion is the soothing/affiliation system. It is this system that gives us feelings of caring and enables us to take an interest in the well-being of others. It is the basis for our ability to experience affiliative and "kind" emotion. Remember that animals without attachment or affiliation systems have no interest in the well-being of others of their kind. They don't have the systems and the brains for it. So, as we showed in the previous chapter, these feelings emanate (mostly) from the soothing/affiliation system. If this system is compromised in some way, so that people struggle with these feelings or do not value them, then compassion itself can begin to falter.

Compassionate Process

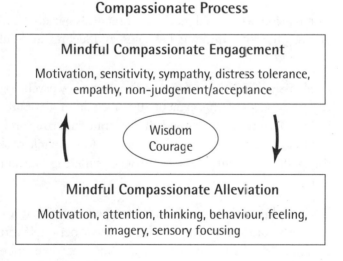

Figure 4.3 Building the compassionate mind for engaging in the suffering and the causes of suffering

We will look at some of these blocks to compassion in chapter 6. But, once rooted in the soothing/affiliation system, the qualities for engaging with suffering can spring forth from appropriate soil and so too feelings of joy at the prospect of alleviating suffering.

So these two psychologies support each other and are underpinned by the important emotional systems we discussed in chapter 3.

Key Points

- Compassion arises from deep insight into *how things really are*. In Buddhism, this is the Four Noble Truths. In the evolutionary model, it is seeing how we all just find ourselves here, created from our genes and social conditioning, with an evolved brain that has all kinds of problems.

- Insight into the nature of suffering and being in contact with it stimulates motivation to do something about it.

- Compassionate motivation stimulates and recruits multifaceted processes involving specific attributes and skills.

- Compassion, as a social mentality, organizes our minds in terms of our attention, thinking, behavior, and feeling, and cultivates our self-identity.

- Compassion "as lived and enacted" has two key psychologies: (1) the psychology of engagement (inner circle of attributes)—the ability to open to, understand, and tolerate suffering; and (2) the psychology of alleviation and prevention (outer circle of skills)—the skills of knowing how to alleviate suffering and uproot its causes.

- The Buddhist monk Matthieu Ricard points out that if we only stay with our experience of suffering (the inner-circle attributes, especially sympathy and empathy), it can become unbearable. What is necessary is to focus on the path of alleviation and prevention of suffering, which are the skills of compassion.

- Buddhist approaches also link the ending of suffering with a desire for happiness, that all beings have happiness and well-being. Hence compassion has a positive motivational focus as well.

- Being loved and being loving is one of the surest ways to happiness.

- So we draw on the inner qualities of compassion, as embodied in the compassionate self (see chapter 10), then focus on suffering, and generate positive feelings of kindness, understanding, and care, and a keen and enthusiastic wish that it comes to an end and happiness emerges.

5

THE CHALLENGE OF MINDFULNESS PRACTICE

The previous chapters explored why coping with our minds can be so difficult. In chapter 1, we saw how the Four Noble Truths inform us of the impermanence of all things, yet we have a brain that is biologically designed to grasp after permanence, solidity, and continuity. It responds with anxiety, anger, grief, and pain to losses and threats. In chapters 2 and 3, we saw that the flow of life has created a brain that has a number of glitches: we are saddled with an old brain that has very powerful motives and emotions, and a new brain that is capable of thinking, imagining, planning, and anticipating. While these two types of brain are the source of so much that we value as humans, such as science and culture, they can also be the source of great suffering. In chapters 3 and 4, we saw the enormous importance of the mammalian evolution of brains that are capable of caring, affiliation, and affection. Science has shown us that these qualities affect how our brain grows and develops and even how our genes are expressed; they influence our capacity to regulate our emotions (e.g., via our frontal cortex) and develop a particular type of self. And since motives organize our minds, one of the most important Buddhist teachings, and indeed one taught in most spiritual traditions, is that we need to cultivate compassionate motives because these will organize our minds in such a way as to foster individual well-being and social harmony. Left to their own devices, our minds can follow some very destructive motives if the environment stimulates them.

To cultivate anything requires us to understand why and what we're trying to achieve and also to have the tools to do it. In the practice section of this book (part II), we develop these tools in detail—in particular mindfulness, acceptance, and a range of compassion-focused exercises such as cultivating the compassionate self. However, this chapter and the next prepare you with something of a warning: both mindfulness and compassion practice can become unintentionally undermined. Keeping this in mind will allow you to be suitably prepared and will provide you with a context of understanding should this arise for you.

The Role of Mindfulness

We have spoken a great deal about the cultivation of the motives and attributes of compassion, but before we can cultivate anything, we need to be aware of where our mind habitually goes and learn to direct our faculty of attention in ways that serve us. This is the role of mindfulness in the context of compassion training, and it is the first tool we will be working with in the practice section.

Definitions

We need to say from the outset that mindfulness is not an area without controversy, and there are now important and fascinating debates in this area. We look at the practice of mindfulness in the next chapter, but here we can briefly note that there are different definitions of mindfulness. In fact, the whole history of mindfulness over hundreds of years is itself not without debate and controversy.[1] One of the Western world's most renowned mindfulness teachers, Jon Kabat-Zinn, defines mindfulness as "the awareness that emerges through paying attention on purpose in the present moment, and nonjudgmentally, to the unfolding of experience moment-by-moment."[2] Another mindfulness teacher, Ronald Siegel, has a somewhat simpler definition of mindfulness as "awareness of present experience with acceptance,"[3] while Rob Nairn says, "Mindfulness is knowing what is happening while it is happening no matter what it is."[4]

The theme of nonjudgment is important to all definitions because judging as good or bad can set us into loops between the old-brain and the new-brain processes (see chapter 2)—we start trying to push "that" thought or feeling away, or make "this" thought or feeling happen more. Mindfulness helps us cultivate a particular type of attention and awareness and to become a skillful observer of what's going on in this tricky mind of ours. In this way we are less likely to get caught up in three types of problem: (1) *attention hopping*—where our mind wanders all over the place like a butterfly, alighting on whatever object of the senses it happens to find; (2) *rumination and brooding*—where our mind gets stuck in a loop, going round and round specific themes that are often negative and a source of depression and anxiety; (3) *emotional avoidance*—where we try to block out of conscious awareness the things that are very painful or don't fit with how we see ourselves.

Present-Moment Awareness

People often get into mindfulness because they are trying to cope with some personal distress or even mental health difficulties; but importantly, Jon Kabat-Zinn tells us that mindfulness is not just a technique—*it is a way of being.* For this reason a key element of mindfulness is *to remember* to be mindful. It's to remember to be fully present in our lives as we live them, as well as during a formal daily practice.

One of the Buddha's great insights was that in becoming more aware of how our mind bobs about like a cork on a stormy sea, we can begin to settle it and learn to rest in present-moment awareness. We get a sense of how distracted our attention is when we start mindfulness practice (see chapter 7). At first, holding our attention on the breath can seem as tricky as grasping for the soap in a bath. Many of us will also be familiar with our lack of mindful attention to what we are actually doing because we have had experiences of driving home and not really remembering the drive because we were thinking about 101 other things.

However, reflect on this key issue: *Where do you actually exist?* It can only be in this *present moment.* Although we only exist right here and right now (neither in the moment to come nor in the moment just gone), our attention and focus are seldom *here*. Most of the time our mind is off planning, anticipating, ruminating, problem-solving, regretting, hoping, or just daydreaming, that is, caught up in new-brain hustle and bustle!

Mindfulness brings us back to the present moment and to a simple awareness of our physical senses.[5] At a deeper level it helps us begin to separate the mind that is "simply aware" from the contents of experience that are constantly flowing through it. In his lectures and at retreats Matthieu Ricard likes to say that consciousness is like water. It can contain a poison or medicine but it is not the poison or medicine; it is pure unto itself. A mirror can reflect many things but is not the things it reflects. Similarly, our mind can be filled with many different emotions and thoughts that pass through it moment by moment, but none of them affect the quality of this "right now and only now" awareness that remains changeless and pure. Many clouds pass across the sky but the sky itself remains constant. At its deepest level, mindfulness is a way of becoming more aware of the passing clouds and learning to rest in a sky-like awareness.

Not Our Fault

In our way of approaching mindfulness, a key attitude is the recognition that the reasons why our mind gets so easily pulled away from the present moment is *absolutely not our fault*. It has to do with the evolution of our new brain that enables us to dwell, worry, anticipate, imagine, and plan, in effect, reliving past events or anticipating future events and then weaving a "story" around them. As we noted in chapter 2, unlike the zebra who is chased by the lion but manages to escape and then very quickly returns to grazing on the savannah, humans have the capacity to relive the incident endlessly: "What if the lion had caught me? I would have been done for"; images of being ripped to pieces or eaten alive might pop into our mind—all very scary and traumatic. Humans are also constantly thinking: "What if...and suppose that..." for good and for bad. Mindfulness helps us *witness* the constant chatter, plans, and inner dramas going on in the movies of the mind. It helps us step back and pay attention, "observing from the balcony" so to speak. In this way, we become keen observers of the inner workings of the mind; and as the Buddha discovered, the mind becomes our greatest teacher of all.

Default-Mode Network

Interestingly, research has shown that we have what is called a *default-mode network* in our brain. This network is active when we have a "wandering mind" as opposed to a focused mind. It seems to be the part of the brain that keeps us on our toes and is constantly seeking out things we should be attending to—a bit of threat here, a bit of action there. It's linked to our capacity for thinking, planning, and anticipating, which can be so helpful to us humans. The problem is that this default mode can do its own thing and constantly be toning up different circuits in the brain. So if we wander off into threat-focused thinking (becoming angry or anxious), then we're going to stimulate the threat system, as we saw in chapter 2. What meditation does for us—and this is very important—is that it may make our default-mode network settle down. Researchers have found that experienced meditators show much less activation in this brain network when they are meditating.[6] This allows the mind, with its magnifying glass of attention, to settle and stop stimulating circuits that can be difficult for us. When we stop stimulating threat and drive circuits, we may be naturally settling into the soothing/affiliation system that can then give us a novel experience of just "being." Indeed, in a very important contribution to the mindfulness literature, Daniel Siegel outlines how mindfulness seems to affect brain circuits that are deeply involved in affiliation and kindness, namely the soothing/affiliation system that we explored in chapter 3.[7]

Origins of Mindfulness

As we saw in chapter 1, mindfulness derives from the teachings of the Buddha and was taught as part of the Fourth Noble Truth—the truth of the path. Within it, he set out four foundations of mindfulness, which are the four main areas of focus in mindfulness practice:[8]

1. *Mindfulness of the body*—This refers to mindfulness of our bodies, physical activities, and our sensory experiences of hearing, tasting, touching, seeing, and smelling. In some practices, we learn to become mindful of the body in action—in walking, eating, or breathing.

2. *Mindfulness of feelings*—This refers to the feelings that arise in response to the sensory activities of hearing, tasting, and so on. The Buddha identified three main feelings: unpleasant, pleasant, and neutral. In mindfulness practice, we become aware of how we can be addicted to pleasant feelings and constantly trying to avoid negative feelings. This can drive our thoughts and actions.

3. *Mindfulness of mind*—This refers to the thoughts, images, and mental associations that arise in response to feelings, in particular the thoughts of "me" and "mine." In practice, we become aware of thoughts and mental activity. In Western psychology this is called *metacognition* and sometimes *mentalizing,* and it is the ability to be aware that "I am having the thought that...."

4. *Mindfulness of the dharma*—This refers to mindfulness of the very nature of things, or the underlying processes and relationship between things. In this way, mindfulness helps us to see more deeply into the nature of the life process itself.

We explore these four foundations in an experiential way when we look at acceptance in chapter 8.

What is important to bear in mind is that the Buddha taught mindfulness in a particular context. In the Theravada tradition, mindfulness has always been seen as an *integral part* of what is called the noble eightfold path. This applies to how we build our intentions, think, speak, behave, and so forth. It does not stand alone. It rests on a firm ground of ethics that revolve around nonharming, and it is oriented toward meditative stability (*samadhi*) and wisdom (*prajna*). In the Mahayana Buddhist tradition, mindfulness is what keeps the *bodhisattva* on track and guards against falling prey to the conflicting emotions; in this respect it is a protector of the awakening mind of wisdom and compassion, called *bodhicitta*. Again, it is closely allied to a system of ethics and values, and it is informed by a body of wisdom. In this respect, Ken Holmes, director of Buddhist studies at Samye Ling Tibetan Center in Scotland, says

Mindfulness itself, unlike awareness, is charged with ethical values. It is about setting up the intelligence needed for taking one's life in hand and shaping it into what one would like it to be. In Buddhism, how one would like it to be is naturally rooted firmly in Buddhist values.... Mindfulness could be taken very literally as the mind being full of, i.e., not forgetting, its purpose. In Buddhism, mindfulness is synonymous with remembering or, more precisely, not forgetting. The general outline is: being very aware of what is happening in the moment, one remembers wise counsel, because one cares deeply about the outcome.[9]

Secular Mindfulness

Over the last forty years there has been growing interest in the West in the benefits and effectiveness of mindfulness, especially in relation to physical and mental health problems. What is interesting is that an entire discipline is emerging around the practice of mindfulness that is secular and somewhat divorced from its Buddhist roots.[10] There is no doubt that this emerging tradition has been hugely beneficial to many people because it has offered a set of tools for working with the mind in a very direct and immediate way.

A prominent pioneer in this respect is Jon Kabat-Zinn, whose application of mindfulness in dealing with chronic pain has evolved into a highly successful eight-week program called Mindfulness-Based Stress Reduction (MBSR). This program has been well researched, and there is now a good evidence base for its efficacy in dealing with stress, boosting our immune system,[11] and even influencing how our brains work.[12] An application of mindfulness for preventing relapse in depression called Mindfulness-Based Cognitive Therapy (MBCT) also has well-established benefits.[13] So mindfulness practice is making increasing contributions to education, therapy, and health care throughout the West.

However, we need to bear in mind where mindfulness comes from and the fact that it has always been charged with ethical values and linked to a higher vision of wisdom and compassion. And so, in applying the ancient wisdom of Buddhism for the West, we need to be careful not to lose this basic foundation. This is a theme we explore now and return to in the next chapter.

Problems That Can Arise with Mindfulness

As we mentioned earlier in this chapter, the practice of mindfulness is not without controversy.[14] So we also need to be mindful (no pun intended!) of the ways in which mindfulness can get subverted from its core purpose. There are obvious reasons why mindfulness meditation can become difficult for people: some people might have difficulties with paying attention in particular ways or be in states of high distress or excitement. Apart from these cases, there are many other ways in which mindfulness can be misunderstood and then misapplied.

Mindfulness and Motives

Mindfulness is primarily a skill of how we pay attention, and therefore it can be linked to a variety of different motives. Many of the martial arts have mindfulness as a major training component. Some top athletes, who have a ruthless desire to win, have learned mindfulness skills. Musicians are now being trained in mindfulness. This is possible because mindfulness involves training a faculty of attention that could potentially link up with any motivational system. There are therapists now teaching mindful sex and mindful eating (not at the same time though!). This kind of mindfulness is somewhat stripped of its deeply transforming potential. As Ken Holmes says

> Simply being very aware is not necessarily virtuous in itself. One could be vividly aware yet doing horrible things and enjoying them. Therefore, the essential characteristic of this Buddhist awareness is to be aware of whether or not one is being *mindful of noble purpose*. Put another way, it is helping us to live to our highest ethical standards and not "turn a blind eye" to the more negative habits....[15]

Mindfulness and Compassion

Although mindfulness does seem to stimulate brain circuits associated with affiliation and calming, mindfulness and compassion should be seen as separate processes that need to be *explicitly cultivated in their own ways*. This is because mindfulness can easily be seen as only learning how to pay attention in a particular way—learning how to create inner motives and emotions that tap into specific old-brain systems that enable us to engage with suffering and alleviate it (see chapter 4). Only when they work together can they bring about lasting change and transformation in our lives. This is indeed the approach that we are taking in this book. We are also beginning to discover that mindfulness and compassion might have overlapping but also quite different effects on the brain.[16]

With some notable exceptions,[17] the secular mindfulness tradition has not worked with the cultivation of compassion *in an explicit way*, nor has it explored the problems in doing so (see chapter 6); rather it has included compassion implicitly through the way in which mindfulness practices are led by a compassionate teacher or by introducing specific loving-kindness practices that engender feelings of compassion for ourselves and others.

From our respective disciplines of meditation and clinical psychology, we have come to the conclusion that framing mindfulness training within a compassionate orientation is very important. In Choden's experience (of the Mahayana Buddhist tradition), compassion is what anchors us in the ground level of our experience; it helps us hold and contain the difficulties, raging, and turmoil of the "inner mud" of our life experience—something we look at in detail in the next chapter. It holds the motivation to engage with pain and suffering with the heartfelt wish to alleviate suffering and remove the causes of suffering—something that always brings us back down to earth. Without the anchoring of compassion, there is the risk that mindfulness practice can become a subtle way of avoiding difficulties by trying to keep one's mind in an "observing" or "breath-focusing" mode and not engaged with painful things. In fact, many people come to mindfulness meditation in order to resolve complex emotional difficulties and deal with psychological pain,[18] but it's almost impossible to engage with this material without some kind of compassionate focus. Consider what psychiatrist Edel Maex, a long-time Buddhist practitioner, says:

> It can happen that I sit on my meditation cushion in the evening and suddenly remember something really stupid that I did, a blunder I made, something ridiculous.… I was so busy during the day that I totally forgot it. Then in the evening I remember it on the cushion and there is no escape. It would be cruel to become aware of my own stupidity without kindness. We need kindness to make it possible and bearable to have open, receptive attention. I have to let go of judging myself, and reproaching myself for my thoughts and feelings. The act of being cognitively aware is impossible without a compassionate attitude.[19]

This important statement directs our attention to the central issue of shame that can so haunt and destroy humans, as we'll see shortly. So there needs to be clear development of compassionate motives and clarity as to *why* we are engaging in mindfulness practices, for example, by engendering the commitment of *bodhicitta*, which is the commitment to understand one's own mind with compassion in order to be helpful to others.

Mindfulness and the Threat System

Some people are very resistant and even fearful of experiencing mindfulness and compassion and the deeper levels of connectedness that this can involve. The reasons for this are complex. Many of us carry emotional wounds in our minds and bodies that originated in our relationships with others—maybe as far back as childhood. The problem is that mindfulness meditation can begin to lift the lid on painful and unprocessed emotions (see Choden's own experience in the chapter 6 section "Descent: Choden's Personal Journey"). If there is little ability to experience or tolerate affiliative, soothing emotions that can soften our threat system (see chapter 3), there may be little ability to contain our emerging inner experiences in compassionate, warm, and receptive ways. If we are living in an inner world of self-criticism and self-dislike, mindfulness can become very tricky indeed.[20] What becomes helpful in this instance is to develop the compassion circles (chapter 4); this builds the capacity to contain and transform what mindfulness brings forth. Therefore, we can see how mindfulness practice can be undermined if people become too overwhelmed with threats and losses—some of which may be rooted in their unprocessed past emotions—because the soothing/affiliation system is inaccessible to them or is itself associated with painful feelings.

Mindfulness and Shame

We should certainly be aware that mindfulness meditation can take us to high-intensity areas of threat in ourselves that lie at the root of what we fear disconnects us from ourselves, our humanity, and our relationships with others. The big monster that can start to emerge as we become familiar with our minds is called *shame*. Remember how in chapter 2 we talked about the importance of identity and our sense of a separate self? Nowhere does this sense of a separate self created by our brains cause us more problems than with shame. Shame is that self we do not want to feel and do not want to be in touch with. It comes with a feeling that there is something not quite right or indeed very wrong with us, that if people knew what was going on in our minds, they would not like us very much and might even be repelled by us. That is why shame can be so difficult to talk about or open up to.

We can feel shamed by our fantasies, secret desires, and lusts; the strength or destructiveness of our emotions; or our cowardliness. We can feel shame about the shape and size of our bodies or how they are functioning; this can become a source of disgust and loss of dignity. We can feel shame about things that happened in the past, or feel haunted by memories of abuse or bullying or just the sense of feeling unwanted. Well, you name it, and we can be ashamed of it. It can be subtle or it can be profound, but the sense of being unacceptable at some level can affect all of us very deeply, and especially so in the West. It can sometimes be quite useful to sit quietly and in a nonjudgmental way observe the kind of things you might feel ashamed of. Just touch the shame, rather than going deeply into it. What thoughts arise? What is that condemning voice of shame like? What are its textures, tones, and emotions? How does it capture you and carry you away? How does it convince you to listen to it? Have you ever asked it, "Do you have my best interests at heart? Do you take joy in my progress and development?" Usually the voice of shame does not; it's only interested in condemning.

The problem with shame is that it puts us into hiding not only from others, but also from ourselves. It can be one of the main sources of what is called *emotional avoidance*; we just don't want to look at the stuff that makes us feel so awful about ourselves. Mindfulness meditation can begin to lift the lid on all this. Shame nags at us as we sit there meditating, "You are not so lovable really; if people really knew you or what goes on in your mind, they would not like you; you're no good at this; you call yourself a compassionate person but look at how unkind you were to Jane!" These may not arise as clear verbal thoughts but more as a feeling or sense that hangs over us like a dark cloud or seeps into us unawares. And, of course, lying behind shame is the blocked soothing/affiliation system—that yearning for connectedness, to be valued, to be wanted, to love, to be loved, and be lovable. Shame is that finger that wags at us and says, "But not for you."

Interestingly, too, we found that when some people begin to touch the need for kindness and closeness, they can feel rather awkward and even embarrassed and ashamed; sometimes they can feel tearful as becoming mindful can stimulate a sense of being out of control or feeling empty, and so they turn away from it. Sometimes they can be frightened that the feelings invoked might overwhelm them with sadness and reopen painful early life memories.[21] So the question that arises is whether mindfulness practice on its own can contain or work through shame.

It is the compassionate mind that awakens the emotions of kindness, affiliation, and caring that heal shame.

Mindfulness and Acceptance

Things can get even more tricky. Part of the mindfulness process is acceptance and nonjudgment of the present moment; to "simply accept" what comes up.[22] So we might well try to "accept" what is going on within us, and yet it might become another strategy of our subliminal preference and judging system. We might say to ourselves, "Okay, let's try another route; let's try to acknowledge the difficult feelings that are arising; let's allow them to be there and notice where we feel them in the body."

However, we don't really appreciate how complex and entangled these feelings can be with their mixture of anger, anxiety, sadness, and doubt all fused together (see chapter 3). And so in the back of our mind there is the secret hope that if we "accept" these difficult feelings of shame, loss, and yearning, they will go away and we will be at peace again; we will become lovable, and then we can practice the *real* mindfulness. Without a compassionate holding, however, acceptance becomes tough. Shame is one of the biggest impediments to acceptance because we want change, to find a way of feeling acceptable, lovable, and connected. However, the sense of not being okay and not acceptable remains firmly in place because we have not attended to the real issue, which is the wounding of our soothing/affiliation system and our deep yearning to feel loved and connected to others.[23]

Mindfulness and Aloneness

Mindfulness meditation may not resonate with the overwhelmed, frightened, or shamed self that feels isolated and alone in the world without its having built compassionate capacity. This is especially the case if mindfulness is used to perpetuate the idea that we can "go it alone." Choden's experience is that one sometimes encounters this view with people who go on long meditation retreats. There can be an underlying sense that you can sit there on your meditation cushion and "work through" all these things on your own. It is as if you are trying to be a personal hero, confronting painful material within oneself, but alone. But what arises often calls for something different, and in many cases, the process of sitting there alone and working through your "stuff" may not address the issue. For many people what surfaces is the *deep wounding of their soothing/affiliation system* and awareness that the very emotional fabric of their being is crying out for relationship, connection, and love (see "Emergence and Interconnectedness" in chapter 1). While some people can have "breakthroughs" (where they begin to see through the nature of reality and consciousness) by simply holding to a very strict meditative orientation, this is not the case for others. Sadly, for some people it becomes so painful that they find themselves falling apart and having to leave, and then maybe seeking out psychotherapy of some kind.

So what is needed is something different. It is mindful compassion that opens up connectedness, heals the feelings of shame and disconnection, and allows us to be touched by another. This is where the power of compassion really helps. Compassion is as much about reaching out to others for help as it is about reaching inside ourselves—it's not just about going it alone. For thousands of years, meditation was practiced in communities and monasteries and it was only the very experienced practitioners who chose to spend time meditating for long periods alone in caves and remote places. Similarly, Western science teaches us that it is through relationships that we change and grow just as much as by working alone on our own minds.[24]

Remember that there are three sources of refuge (or support) in Buddhism: Buddha (our inner enlightened potential, symbolized by the historical Buddha); Dharma (the teachings and practices); and Sangha (the community of spiritual practitioners). The Sangha is perhaps the one that needs the most attention in the West. This is where people really struggle, and this is why we need to pay more attention to thinking about how to build compassionate communities instilled with the values of genuine sharing and support.

Mindfulness as a Way of Controlling the Mind

Despite the huge interest in mindfulness meditation in the West, many people misunderstand meditation in fundamental ways and run into problems.[25] Mindfulness meditation actually means *becoming familiar* with and *getting to know* the mind, and the way we do this is through open attention and observation. This point cannot be overemphasized. One of Choden's Tibetan teachers described how many people sit there thinking "I am meditating," but this thought just gets in the way, stops meditation from happening, and ends up becoming a subtle form of control. Given the very subjective nature of the practice, it is often not so easy to identify when someone is going off track. If someone works as an apprentice carpenter, for example, the master craftsman can watch the apprentice closely and see exactly what the apprentice is doing; but this is not so easy with meditation, which is highly subjective inner work.

Mindfulness and Avoidance

An issue closely related to control is that of avoidance. There is now strong evidence that a lot of unhappiness and mental health difficulties are linked to what is called *emotional avoidance*: avoiding or suppressing feelings, fantasies, or memories because when they come into our field of awareness, they trigger bodily feelings that can be overwhelming.[26] Indeed, for all kinds of reasons, our present-moment experience can be so painful and conflicted that *we don't want to be there*. We feel that if we stay there too long, collapse, implosion, or emotional eruption might occur. This might not be the case in the beginning. When we start meditation practice and have our first experience of stepping back from the repetitive storylines that continually run through our minds to just watch them float by, there can be a feeling of joy and release as we see firsthand how we do not always have to be carried away by our thoughts.

But this can be a honeymoon period. In Choden's experience of mindfulness training, it is when we start running into the deeper levels of emotional resistance that mindfulness practice risks sliding into a process of thought management in which we subtly promote certain ways of thinking and feeling and reject others. It is like having a nice, tidy desk with everything in its rightful place, and constantly rearranging it so you have a sense of maintaining control. Very quickly meditation can be hijacked by this process—certain things are allowed in but others are not. You can tell this when people say, "I've been practicing mindfulness for eight weeks now, but I still can't stop feeling anxious or getting irritable," indicating that right from the outset, mindfulness was understood as a way of *getting rid* of painful emotions rather than being more fully present with them and learning how to hold them with compassion and thus to tolerate and accept them. Behavior therapy works in exactly the same way. For example, you would take an agoraphobic out into the streets so that they can experience anxiety *more fully*, learn to tolerate and work with it, and so be less frightened of it. In the case of the agoraphobic, avoidance is obvious, but for the mindfulness practitioner, it can be far more subtle.

According to Rob Nairn,[27] one of Choden's mindfulness teachers, this process of avoidance and suppression happens subliminally, and before we are even consciously aware of it, we may find that we have *already* bought into attitudes of identification and avoidance—almost as if some shadowy doorkeeper to our subliminal world says that "this" is permitted entry but "that" is not. And then an even more subtle voice of authority follows quickly behind and says, "This is the way it must be."

As an instructor of mindfulness, Choden sees this as a very real dilemma we can encounter with the practice of meditation. It can unwittingly assist the process of suppression of emotional pain, grief, and trauma held in the body. We can spend years keeping the lid shut, subtly suppressing all our painful and unprocessed emotional experience as our system of preferences—what we like to experience and what we certainly do not want to experience—gradually infiltrates and takes over the practice of mindfulness. And, this process of infiltration can happen at an unseen, subliminal level, just below the threshold of consciousness, like the hands of a puppeteer moving the puppets on a stage in such a way that nobody sees what is happening. This is recognized by people working both in mindfulness and therapy.[28]

For some people, meditation practice can follow a different route. Instead of shutting the lid down on our deeply buried hurts, emotional memories and wounds, the practice can open these up, sometimes in sudden ways, while at other times a crack can open in the closed chambers of our emotional memories. When this happens our immediate instinct can be, "I don't want to go there; I don't want to feel this.... This is too much. I thought this mindfulness was supposed to help me feel better!" We do recognize that this can be terribly frightening, and it's no surprise that people want to move away from it. So although the basic instruction is to practice bare attention of whatever arises, allowing ourselves to feel our experience as it is, we might instead find ourselves freaking out: "Oh no, this is not what I signed up for; I thought this was about gaining mastery of my thought process so I am not prey to random, distracting thoughts. I thought it would help me feel better. I did not bargain on this...."

On the one hand, then, we are training to be present, while, on the other hand, deeply held resistances arise with a strong command: "I do not like this. I do not want to feel this. This is not okay." At these moments it is as if the puppeteer of the threat system pops his head over the backdrop and exclaims, "This is too dangerous—game over." In this way our preference, monitoring, and threat system lays down the law that was perhaps written when we were young children—when it might have been appropriate to close down and react in the way we are now doing, but which might be entirely inappropriate this time around. Now this is much more likely when we haven't built compassionate capacity because it is compassionate capacity that gives us the emotional environment to hold some of this difficult and painful emotion.

Mindfulness of the Chaotic Mind, Not Just the Still Mind

Getting closer to the "still mind" is often the subtle gold we think we are looking for, and we may find ourselves monitoring our practice closely to see if we are approaching our benchmark. We can sense this subtle process of striving happening when people talk about having a "good" meditation as opposed to a "bad" one, even though the key instruction is to be aware of the flow of our thoughts and emotions in a nonjudgmental way. Someone might say, "That practice session was awful—my mind was all over the place" or "My mind was really centered today—my practice seems to be going well." So what we find happening is that the practice of mindfulness can gradually be undermined by our threat and drive systems that are monitoring our practice and making judgments like "This is good or that is bad."

We might not even realize that we have fallen under the power of these brain systems, but the effect is that they can take us away from the open quality of being that is associated with the soothing/affiliation system.

The key issue here is that monitoring our practice according to whether it is a "good practice" or results in a "still mind" automatically generates resistance to those experiences that fall into the other extreme and threaten to overturn the apple cart. It is like a boatman who sails his boat around the harbor relishing the calm water and admiring the gentleness of the breeze but is terrified to venture into the deep seas for fear of capsizing and drowning. This is understandable for those of us who have experienced abuse, neglect, feelings of rejection, or major losses because staying present with these experiences can be very tough indeed; and this is especially the case if they're not contained in a compassionate way or if we are trying to go it alone. But the deep sea can be flat and beautiful as well as stormy and treacherous, and our ability to sail safely through storms can greatly extend the range of what we can explore and come to know.

In this way, the practice of mindfulness meditation can become a way of seeking calmness and stillness rather than familiarity, understanding, and insight. While our boatman rather likes the calm waters of the harbor, in fact, what he needs is to learn to sail on the open seas. This is the dilemma that is central to the integration of compassion with mindfulness. Compassion enables us to stay afloat on the turbulence of the open sea, while mindfulness is the way in which we skillfully navigate the sea.

Mindfulness and Relationships

Consequently, without "care," mindfulness meditation can lead us headlong into a brick wall of our deeply held resistances or expectations of how things should be. And, furthermore, because we are frightened of some of the things that go on in our minds, we can stay in hiding. As we have seen, this may be because of shame or fear of what might happen if the disowned parts of ourselves emerged in conscious awareness. This is a serious issue because hiding can prevent us from understanding some fundamental things about ourselves like the tricky, evolved brains that we have in common with all other human beings; and it can also prevent us from healing painful inner wounds.

This is precisely the time when we are called upon to trust others and reach out for help. We are a deeply social species who, from the first days of our lives, are engaged in the process of co-creating our life experiences with each other. In her book on self-compassion, Kristin Neff, a pioneer of self-compassion, honestly addresses a sexual difficulty she had when she would become very childlike and tearful in the bedroom and not understand why.[29] However, it was through her openness to this experience and the acceptance and love of her husband that, *together*, they were able to work through this issue.

It is a mistake to believe that growth, insight, and change come *only* from sitting there on our cushion and going it alone. Monasteries were never set up like this but were always community based. In addition, Western psychotherapy actually shows the importance of relationships in the process of changing and growth: that we move from a position of dependency toward independence as our inner abilities for reflection, empathy, and emotional regulation are developed in and through our relationships. In the Buddhist tradition, an important source of help and support comes from one's spiritual friend or guru, who will have spent many years practicing. In the West, support might come from someone who actively listens, reflects, and helps us gradually work through things we are frightened of; or this support may come about in a group context. Indeed, many mindfulness teachers have acknowledged that *being together*, sharing together, and witnessing what others go through is crucial in bringing about insight and healing in mindfulness groups. Certainly, in the research that Paul and his colleagues are now doing on compassion and mindfulness, this sharing quality comes up time and time again as one of the most important factors that facilitates growth and healing.

A foundation for all sharing that heals is the awareness that no matter what we feel, all of our experiences are part of a common human mind—*common humanity.* We are not alone in what we go through because so many others will go through something similar too. This is the compassionate wisdom that can "de-shame" us. What is crucial here are relationships. Self-help books like this one can be helpful but cannot replace building genuine relationships based on mutual connection and support. Rather, they can help us develop the courage to build supportive and encouraging relationships with other people. Perhaps the ideal of the Buddhist hermit meditating alone in a cave is not one that we should aim for in the West. Instead, what might be more appropriate to our time is becoming more mindful and compassionate while *in relationship with others.*

Key Points

- Mindfulness is a skill that involves paying attention to the present moment on purpose and without judgment.

- However, mindfulness is not just a technique; it is a way of being, an orientation that we take to life itself. A key element of mindfulness is to remember to be fully present in our lives as we live them.

- What our attention focuses on will stimulate very different brain systems and emotions.

- It is not our fault that our minds get pulled away from the present moment in the ways they do. This is to do with the evolution of our new-brain capacities and how our minds have developed from our life experiences.

- Historically, mindfulness has always been based on ethical values and allied to a body of wisdom; it has not stood alone as a skill in its own right.

- It is important to frame mindfulness training within a compassionate orientation. When unaddressed issues begin to surface, such as feelings of grief, shame, self-criticism, or self-loathing, compassion enables us to hold these feelings with kindness and understanding.

- Compassion training provides a context for working "mindfully" with our tendencies to avoid or suppress our emotions. Mindful Compassion helps us heal the wounds to our soothing/affiliation system and offers a sense of connectedness.

6

THE LOTUS IN THE MUD

While mindfulness has been shown to have great benefits in helping people with personal distress and suffering,[1] the Mahayana Buddhist tradition has always seen mindfulness as the *servant* of the awakening heart and compassion as the key transforming agent of the mind. It is the force of compassionate motivation that reorganizes the mind and brings about lasting change, but mindfulness has an important role in alerting us when we are doing things that are harmful to ourselves and others.[2]

Compassionate motivation has many levels. At its most simple level, it is the wish to be kind and helpful to ourselves and others. But at a deeper level, it is connected to wisdom. This arises out of an emerging understanding of how tough life is and how we are really "up against it" in its flow: everything is impermanent; living beings arise, flourish, decay, and die, sometimes very painfully; our bodies are fragile, easily injured, and vulnerable to thousands of diseases; our brains are easily tipped toward cruelty and horrendous violence. All of this comes with the package of being alive. The Dalai Lama says: "When we lack an understanding of the suffering nature of existence, our attachment to life increases. If we cultivate our insight into the miserable nature of life, we overcome our attachment."[3]

Moreover, as stated before (see chapter 2), we are socially constructed, and have limited choice about the kind of person we become. To return to our favorite example, if we (the authors) had been snatched as babies and brought up in violent drug gangs, our sense of who we are, our values, the wiring of our brains, and even the expression of our genes would have taken a completely different turn. We would be extremely unlikely to be in a position to write this book or even be interested in writing books. The chances are we might be violent, have poor control over our emotions, or be dead. Our brains are very plastic, and the social circumstances of our lives literally build different brains and therefore entirely different selves.

This insight can cause us to "tune out" and focus instead on fancy cars, fast food, sex, drugs, and rock 'n' roll; or it can plunge us into the depths of despair. But following the Middle Way of the Buddha that we explored in chapter 1, we can work on cultivating a different kind of life: one where we are not prepared to stand by and be indifferent, but instead are motivated to do whatever we can to reach out to suffering. This requires us to stand back and observe the way life really is—that we inhabit a mind and a brain that to a large extent was built for us by evolution, on the one hand, and the environments we grew up in, on the other.

This insight also makes it possible to engage with our life struggles and pains without overly personalizing them and without feeling ashamed. Healing shame begins with the process of recognizing that it's not our fault that we are the way we are, while at the same time taking full responsibility to do the best we can to repair the harm we might have done others, and then working on developing the qualities of the person we want to become. It's much the same as when you buy a new house and want a lovely garden, but find that the plot is covered in mounds of rubble. You don't just leave it like this. You begin to clear the rubble, bring in new soil, and then start to cultivate it.

In following this approach, we are aspiring to tread in the footsteps of the *bodhisattvas* of old. They engendered *bodhicitta*, the awakening heart of compassion, and their primary concern was to do whatever they could to free living beings from suffering and the causes of suffering. In the language of modern experience, however, they would first aspire to understand the flow of life: how we just find ourselves in situations that have been shaped for us, how socially constructed we all are, and how this life is so transitory and impermanent. This is the basis of wisdom.

When the practice of mindfulness is accompanied by compassionate motivation and grounded in wisdom, there is a depth and a power to the path we follow and the practices we do. In fact, the *bodhisattva* commitment goes further and includes the sincere wish to awaken from the sleep of illusion so that we can wake up others too (see "The Self We Might Choose," in the Introduction). Within Buddhism this is referred to as "enlightenment," but this term might be a bit misleading. Lama Yeshe Rinpoche, one of Choden's teachers, once said a more accurate term is "self-liberation"—freeing the mind from its limiting concepts of self and recognizing the unbounded awareness that is its true nature. It is like being imprisoned in a small, dusty room for your whole life and not realizing that the door has been unlocked all along, and all you need do is push it open and walk outside—but getting to this point might take a long time!

In this book our focus is on how we get trapped, how this is no fault of our own, and how we can begin to take gradual steps to spotting that door, and so begin to feel some release from the limiting loops of our minds. A big part of this process is to acknowledge our connection with everything that lives—how we are interconnected and part of the flow of life. In this way, through awakening our inner capacities of wisdom and compassion, we gradually begin to emerge from the prison of emotional avoidance, self-criticism, and shame.

When we approach the conflicts and struggles of our lives from this orientation, there is the potential for deep transformation. The *bodhisattva* is a spiritual warrior who follows the heroic archetypal story—someone who is willing to step outside the prevailing paradigms of her time, who is prepared to open up to the pain of life, lift the lid on the hidden chambers of her being, and allow a process to unfold even though she does not know where it will lead. This is a life of surrender in which we allow ourselves to become templates to work through the pain and struggles that mark our age so that we can find a path that others can follow. When we approach mindfulness with this kind of motive, it becomes a transformed process. It is animated with a vision that raises it to another level. It becomes infused with the vibrancy and aliveness of our deep connection and affiliation with one another.

Understanding How Compassion Can Be Undermined

This all sounds well and good, but in practice, it might not be so straightforward. Just as we looked at how *mindfulness* can be undermined, we are now going to look at how *compassion* can be undermined too—mostly through problems in the emotional systems that underpin it, and through misunderstanding of what compassion is and what it can do.

Compassion calls upon us to engage with suffering by being sensitive and open to it (inner circle of attributes [see chapter 3]), while also generating the feelings of kindness, affiliative connection, and warmth (outer circle of skills [see chapter 3]) that can soothe and alleviate suffering. For many people, however, engaging with suffering might feel overwhelming and distressing, and generating these compassionate feelings might be very hard too. It might be easy to acknowledge that we all want happiness and we don't want suffering, but the problem is that the psychology behind this is not so straightforward. If you understand this, it may help you recognize some of the issues that could come up for you and how you might begin to work with them. This is something we explore in detail in the following section.

Compromised Soothing/ Affiliation System

One of the main reasons that some people struggle with compassion is because the soothing/affiliation systems is not working very well. Now there are many reasons for this, and one of them might be biological. For example, it seems that psychopaths are not emotionally responsive to suffering or motivated to care. Also, if people are in severe states of distress or depression, their soothing systems can be almost impossible for them to access or feel. In other cases, people struggle with soothing themselves because they simply don't have connections with other people; for whatever reason, they have become isolated, and there is no one they can form relationships with to talk to or feel understood or soothed by. As we keep stressing, affiliation and connection are crucial for activating the emotional systems that underpin compassion so that we do not see people as disconnected social beings who should be able to "sort their heads out" all by themselves.[4]

Misunderstandings About the Nature of Compassion

In addition to these underlying emotional issues, compassion is easily misunderstood. These misunderstandings can create resistances within us that block us off from feeling compassion for ourselves and opening up to compassionate relationships with others. Men are especially tricky! When we mention the word "compassion" to some people, especially men, there can be a slightly embarrassed look as if compassion is "kind of fluffy"—a good thing but not really "tough" or what we need in a crisis. A colleague of ours, Dr. Christopher Germer, working at Boston University and author of the book *The Mindful Path to Self-Compassion* (2009), has noticed a very interesting thing about compassion. When he runs retreats and courses on mindfulness, he has about 50 percent men and 50 percent women turning up. But when he runs a compassion retreat, it's more like 90 percent women and only 10 percent or fewer men. So we have a problem in the West with men misunderstanding compassion and not taking it seriously.

Paul has also met resistance from fellow psychotherapists who fundamentally misunderstand what compassion is about and think it's just about being "nice" to patients. Compassion is okay, they say, and of course all therapists have to be compassionate, but the real purpose of therapy is to get involved with people's pain, rage, anxiety, and depression (like conscious and unconscious processes, core beliefs, abuse memories, and so forth). We agree, of course, but as we hope we've made clear, this is the job of compassion; and indeed, without compassion, therapy can be a very painful and lonely journey. In this respect, some therapists lack insight into the complexity and different psychologies of compassion (see chapter 4).

Fears of and Resistances to Compassion

We now explore the resistances to and fears of compassion because they can throw us off course very early on in the process of developing a mindful and compassionate mind. However, the more we become aware of how these fears and resistances arise and how they are part and parcel of the human condition, the less likely we are to take them personally or to blame ourselves for them, and the more workable they will then become.

For some people, efforts to generate compassion toward oneself and others actually stimulate difficult emotions rather than pleasant ones.

Research has found that some people can have deep fears about developing compassion even if they see the value of it. Gerard Pauley and Susan McPherson looked at the meaning and value of self-compassion in a depressed group. They found that while depressed people viewed self-compassion as potentially very helpful to them, they also saw it as being very difficult to develop, in part due to the impact of their illness. They noted that "an interesting related finding was that many participants reported that it was not just that they found it difficult to be self-compassionate, but also that they experienced the exact opposite of self-compassion, when depressed or anxious."[5] They experienced shame and self-criticism instead.

For a few years, Paul's research team has been exploring a variety of fears associated with compassion.[6] Now of course any therapist will tell you that if people come from traumatic backgrounds where they have been abused, bullied, or neglected, it is only natural that anything that begins to stimulate a feeling of "connectedness" is going to be problematic. Nonetheless, we have looked at three types of fear of compassion: fear of being compassionate to others, fear of receiving compassion from others, and fear of being compassionate to and for oneself. We measured these by giving people a series of statements and then, to explore these fears, we asked them to rate how much they agreed with each statement:

- *For the fear of being compassionate to others, we gave statements such as:* "People will take advantage of me if I am too compassionate"; "If I'm too compassionate, others will become too dependent on me"; "I can't tolerate others' distress."

- *For the fear of receiving compassion from others, we gave statements such as:* "I fear that if I need other people to be kind, they won't be"; "I worry that people are only kind and compassionate if they want something from me"; "If I think someone is being kind and caring toward me, I put up a barrier."

- *For the fear of being compassionate to oneself, we gave people statements such as:* "I fear that if I develop compassion for myself, I will become someone I don't want to be"; "I fear that if I am more self-compassionate, I will become a weak person"; "I fear that if I start to feel compassion for myself, I will be overcome with loss/grief"; "I feel that I don't deserve to be kind and forgiving to myself."

So what did we find? First, there was a tendency for people fearful of one form of compassion to be fearful of others. Second, if people were frightened about other people being compassionate to them, they also had difficulties with being compassionate to themselves. Now just reflect for a moment about living in a world where we find it very difficult to let in love and compassion from people around us and where we are not compassionate or kind to ourselves at all. If we dislike or even hate parts of our self due to shame (see "The Shamed Self" in chapter 2), think about what's going on in our minds on a day-by-day basis. The soothing/affiliation system is going to have very little stimulation, while the threat system will have lots. Yet if we don't stimulate the soothing/affiliation system, then how will it function in our brains when we need it to? Research has shown repeatedly that we need to stimulate different brain systems to help them develop.

If we cut ourselves off from compassion, we're going to starve our soothing/affiliation system, and it won't be available to us when we need it. Indeed, our research shows that fears of compassion make us much more vulnerable to depression, anxiety, and stress. In addition, people who have these fears also tend to be self-critical—and you can see why. They can't afford to make mistakes because they don't have any way of calming and soothing themselves if they do but typically feel frightened or angry and launch into self-criticism instead.[7] Effectively, they live on a knife edge.

Fear of Happiness

We also know that some people are anxious about having any positive feelings at all and even fear being happy. There can be a puritan taboo surrounding pleasure that derives from feelings of fear and guilt. Many books now focus on how to be happy, but few of us have really thought about the fact that many people are surprisingly frightened of happiness. Once again, it is Paul's patients who have been his best teachers, and he simply turned some of the fears of happiness they talked about into questions to see how common these fears are and how they relate to states like depression. In the course of the research previously mentioned, we asked people how much they agreed with statements like "I am frightened to let myself become too happy"; "I worry that if I feel good, something bad may happen"; "I feel I don't deserve to be happy."

When we did the study with students, we were surprised to find that this fear was *very* highly associated with depression, anxiety, and stress. In other words, people who are vulnerable to depression may well have fears of happiness; they struggle *to allow themselves* to feel happiness, and when they do feel it, they can become anxious. One of Paul's patients noted that "It's when I feel happy and think things are going well that ideas come into my mind about what would happen if my husband or one of my children died or something went wrong. When I am depressed, I don't think about these things so much." Happiness reminded her of life's fragilities.

Feeling undeserving of happiness can be common to and can arise in families where a parent is ill. Karen's mother was divorced and had a number of physical conditions, which meant she couldn't get out much. When Karen was a teenager she recalls "never really feeling okay with going out and having fun because I would always be worrying if Mum was okay and feeling guilty that I was out having fun and had left her at home alone."

Mindful compassion allows us to acknowledge these thoughts without blaming and shaming, to see them as understandable and often linked to social backgrounds in which life was difficult and happiness fairly short lived. In these cases we are living with the programming of our pasts. It's not surprising then that people stay depressed if they are constantly blocking off their ability to experience positive feelings, and it's not surprising that eventually their positive feeling systems will take a nose dive.

Emotional Memory

One of the reasons people can run into fears and unpleasant experiences when they try to be compassionate is because when they begin to touch these emotions, they trigger their emotional memory. How does it work? At one level it's very simple. For example, imagine that when you were young, you were bitten by a black dog. Later in life you're walking home and out jumps a black dog. Your body memory causes your body to be flushed with anxiety—there is no thought, just that the moment you see it, your body's memory activates the anxiety system. So all of us know we physiologically react to things that have had meaning for us in the past. Interestingly, though, nice feelings can be turned into unpleasant ones. Imagine this: you love cheesecakes, and when you see them, you get a warm feeling of anticipation and imagine how lovely they are going to taste when you eat them. But then one day you have a cheesecake, and it makes you seriously ill. Okay, so what happens to those lovely warm feelings toward cheesecakes when you next smell one? They've gone, and in their place are feelings of nausea and dread. Even if you still want to enjoy eating cheesecakes, your body will remember how you got sick. You can't help how you feel—you have been *conditioned*. And those feelings of nausea will override your conscious wishes and thoughts—that's the key point. In time, you might desensitize these aversive feelings and get back to your love of cheesecakes, but not immediately; and this will definitely not happen if you now avoid the aversive feelings.

So our emotions can be linked and conditioned to other emotions—positive feelings can become triggers for negative feelings. Here's another example: Sally's mother was agoraphobic, often depressed, and at times volatile. Sally could remember many times when she looked forward to going out, and one time in particular she was excited about going to see Santa Claus. Sadly, at the last moment her mother had a panic attack, collapsed into tears, and said she couldn't go. And to make matters worse, her father was in the house and became really annoyed with his wife, and the atmosphere "turned horrible." Sally described how, if she ever felt excited about something, it often turned out badly like this. So now she tries not to feel too good about things, because in the back of her mind—her emotional memory—there is always the feeling that something bad will happen or something will go wrong. In fact, she notices that when times with the possibility of having fun come around, like Christmas, she becomes uneasy. You can see how that's understandably rooted in her emotional memory system. You can see too how different types of emotion are fused together here, such as anger and sadness.

Affiliation and Emotional Memory

We can think about this from the perspective of attachment and affiliation too. We are biologically set up to want to form loving relationships and attachments, initially with our parents, and to be calmed and soothed by them.[8] However, what happens if this system is activated, but then the people who are supposed to provide you with love and support don't, or, even worse, they actually harm or threaten you? Now of course there are always conflicts, arguments, and disagreements in all relationships; so we are not talking about the everyday situations here. It's when these forms of neglect become regular, persistent, or intense that our body memory is coded with the idea that "getting close to people will hurt me." So when we begin to experience those natural feelings of wanting to be close to others and to feel loved, our memories remind us of what happened in the past, and we then feel very uncomfortable. In a way this is no different from the cheesecake example where something that you would normally want and enjoy becomes something that you find extremely unpleasant and avoid. It is called *emotional conditioning*, and it's a very important factor in understanding why our soothing/affiliation systems can become blocked. Feelings that are normally pleasurable, such as closeness and affiliation, can become contaminated by experiences of threat or hurt, and it's those feelings that now show up when you stimulate the soothing/affiliative system.

Even more tricky and complex are blockages to the soothing/affiliation system that arise in people who come from emotionally disruptive, harsh, critical, or affectionless backgrounds. This may be more common than we think. Some people say that their parents cared for them and made sure they had enough food and material possessions, but they had very few memories of physical affection or feeling that they were regarded *with joy* in the minds of others. Maybe their parents were too busy with work or were fatigued, or simply not comfortable with sharing affectionate feelings; or maybe these people felt they had to constantly compete for affection or perform and be successful to get attention—something that's becoming sadly more common in our competitive society. People from these types of abusive, affectionless, and/or competitive backgrounds tend to be especially self-critical, partly because they are driving themselves too hard, are desperate to be successful or near perfect (to be valued), and are alarmed by mistakes and failure. For these people, the notion of accepting themselves "warts and all" is frightening—so too are feelings of affiliation and self-compassion. Sometimes they may even be contemptuous of these feelings and distrusting of people, and so keep them at a distance. The issue here is not so much having negative ideas about compassion, but that the actual experience of compassion is problematic.

Our soothing/affiliation system can be likened to a computer, in that it can "shut down" if it gets hurt. The problem is that when we start to rekindle it—for example, by doing compassion practices—it can open at the place where it originally shut down. So, if we experienced our early life attachments as being threatening and painful, when the soothing/affiliation system comes back online, we are likely to have negative feelings rather than positive ones. Now, this is tragic, but it's important for us to understand so that we are not taken by surprise and do not blame ourselves. With this understanding, we can then stand back and think about how we'd like to work creatively with this situation so we can begin to "decontaminate" our soothing/affiliation system, to be compassionate to our fear of compassion.

In our own different contexts of meditation and psychotherapy, we commonly encounter this when people begin to engage with compassion and start to get in touch with painful emotional material—sometimes shameful or just very lonely stuff. So sometimes compassion can put people more in touch with their personal stories and suffering, and they can sometimes find themselves feeling overwhelmed or a little grief struck.

Affiliation and Emotional Fusion

A further problem arises, however, when different emotions become fused together. Consider this example: Jack's father is often aggressive to him, sometimes physically, and after being angry, sends Jack to his room. An hour later his father repents and comes to apologize to Jack and asks to be forgiven, only for the cycle to start again a week or so later. So let's consider the different types of emotions that can become fused together in this experience. First, Jack would rather be loved by his father than

163

annoy him, and so there is disappointment in what should have been a supportive and loving relationship. Second, Jack is very frightened of his father, especially if his father is physically aggressive—so his threat system becomes activated. Third, Jack is sent to his room and perhaps hides in bed or cries or tries to "switch off" so that he doesn't feel his pain. So at the very time that Jack is in a high state of threat and *needs soothing and affection*, he is actually alone, feeling cut off from comfort. Fourth, because his father was angry with him and blamed him, he might start to experience himself as being "bad," "unlovable," or a "disappoint-ment" in some way.

We now have a situation where "fear" and feelings of "loneliness" and being "unlovable" can get fused together. This could affect Jack's life in all kinds of ways, and he may struggle to deal with these fusions of different emotions. For example, if later in life, Jack is criticized, his emo-tional body memories will be activated and he might feel frightened again, as well as flooded with feelings of aloneness and being unlovable or unacceptable. This might trigger deep sadness in him and feel so over-whelming that as an adult, he doesn't want to go there ever again. He might have learned to shut this down so well as a child that now he doesn't really notice the sadness and loneliness that hides in the anxiety or the anger.

Reflecting on how unfair and aggressive his father was might acti-vate anger at the way he was treated as a child, so now Jack will have to cope with the fusion of anger, anxiety, deep sadness, and a sense of himself as being unlovable. These fusions of emotions will be very tricky to deal with. And, just to make it *even more complex*, recall how Jack's father came and apologized. The problem could now be that Jack wants to forgive his father and feel loved again and so can't deal with his anger and rage at his father for beating him. Indeed, when Jack starts to feel anger in his body, he might actually feel guilty, sad, or frightened of his anger. After all, if you want closeness and to feel lovable, the last thing you want is to have to deal with your own rage!

So this is why sometimes it's quite useful to recognize that we are multiple beings with different types of self associated with different types of feeling and body memories. None of us is a single self, and sometimes these different "selves" (angry self, anxious self, sad self, etc.) need to be listened to within us (see chapter 2). As we will see, when we work with the compassionate self and learn to make it the center of our being, it can help us engage with these tricky emotional experiences and the different types of "selves" that can flow through us in rather mixed and confusing ways. Once we recognize these fusions of emotion, it may help us become less confused by the odd assortment of emotions that can bubble up in us, and we can be more open to different textures of emotions when we engage in mindfulness and compassionate practices.

Affiliation and Anger

An often unrecognized block to compassion is rage. It can be locked in our emotional memory, and people can feel very fearful, ashamed, or guilty about it. As we said above, if you want to love and be loved, you don't really want to have to acknowledge this raging (or even sadistic) side of yourself. The problem is that we humans are evolved to form connections and linkages from the day we are born. As we keep saying, we are a highly social species and our brains are constantly being cocreated through our interactions with others. If children don't experience social connectedness and affection, it activates their threat system—and the two big emotions here are fear and anger or rage. But, of course, for a child, these emotions can become frightening and intolerable, and therefore they can get suppressed. And yet, as long as we are unable to acknowledge our rage, compassion can be blocked through the unprocessed guilt associated with the rage.[9]

Rage that begins in childhood can be especially frightening because we may have learnt to suppress these feelings so that when we start to connect with them, there can be the fear and dread of exploding into something horrible—literally being taken over by the savage parts of ourselves, as has been so well captured in books and films like *Dr. Jekyll and Mr. Hyde* and *The Hulk*. While some people find their rage a fantastic source for writing horror movies and making buckets of money, others become terrified of it because they haven't learned to see it as part of themselves and that it doesn't have to take them over; nor have they seen the deep yearning for love that sometimes lies beneath the rage.

Consider the case of Jeff, who became depressed. He described how he was feeling: "I love my wife, but there are times when I think I want to leave her, that maybe I hate her and should just go off and be on my own or find somebody else—but these are such hateful and frightening feelings. Deep inside, I think I'm actually quite an unpleasant person. So I can't see how you can talk to me about compassion when I have this rage inside of me all of the time." For Jeff, it was clear—you can only be compassionate to yourself if you have compassionate feelings for others, and a lot of the time he didn't. But for Jeff, learning to understand the source of these feelings, recognizing them as part of the threat system, and understanding that we have a tricky brain and other people have these kinds of conflicts too enabled him to hold his rage compassionately. This is not a recipe for acting out but for learning how to be reflective and assertive. This helped soften the experience for Jeff, and it allowed him to become less frightened of his anger. He began to see that beneath that anger were feelings of hurt and rejection that he had carried for a long time. Slowly he also began to pay more attention to his genuinely compassionate side rather than just letting his mind be constantly taken over by his enraged side.

Now these can be very tricky dilemmas and conflicts, and some people may require professional help; but at least if we are forewarned, it allows us to think constructively about them.

Affiliation and Slowing Down—in the Culture of Speeding Up

Compassionate values and practices flourish or wither in different cultures.[10] Political and economic systems inspire or inhibit compassion—especially as the drive for competitive edge is constantly speeding us up rather than slowing us down.[11] As we mentioned before, a good example of this is the UK's National Health Service. It is generally recognized that with reduced budgets and increased expectations, more and more is being done with less and less. Efficiency is, of course, a good thing; but, as report after report sadly testifies, these rushed and time-pressured environments actually undermine compassion and, ultimately, efficiency.[12] Clinicians end up feeling sad and stressed at the lack of time to spend with patients. Surely we can do better than this. It would be so helpful if there was an opportunity just to slow down and get ourselves into a reflective and compassionate state of mind to address these very serious issues—if we could reexamine what we mean by a caring health service that has time for people. This is one of the reasons that the Compassionate Mind Foundation is beginning to explore, with other international groups, what "compassionate leadership" might look like (see http://www.compassionatemind.co.uk). It is compassionate leadership rather than just a target-driven and output-focused leadership that can help us to develop improved services and build better working lives for all (http://www.ccare.stanford.edu/group/ccare/cgi-bin/wordpress/).

Our compassionate ability to be reflective and thoughtful, and to focus on our well-being and that of others is being increasingly eroded in schools and families too. The growth of compassion is being undermined because the values of the soothing/affiliation system are not encouraged. Simply learning how to be at peace, to be content with what we have, and to "do nothing" are rarely encouraged. Children are seldom taught to savor what comes to them through their senses. Rather we are taught to direct our thinking to "How can I do better for myself, pass more exams, get higher grades, stop falling down the ranks?" We are taught day in and day out that we must not rest on our laurels doing nothing as others will overtake us; we must always be on the move doing, innovating, and achieving. But the fact is that study after study shows that this is simply not good for our physical and emotional health. We are seriously out of balance.[13]

In traditional cultures there was often considerable value placed on simply being and connecting. Choden recalls traveling to India and being struck by a colorful family group who sat for hours on the floor of a train station—not at all worried that the train was late, simply being content where they were; chatting, connecting, and feeling safe in their little group. In contrast, the Western travelers were pacing around, constantly checking their watches, and stressing out because the train was so late. In a similar vein, while leading a retreat, Choden described the qualities of the soothing/affiliation system as being "content, safe, and connected," but one person in the group said, "What is that?" almost as if these words were part of a foreign language.

Psychology of Avoidance

As the Buddha said right at the outset, we live our lives as if we are sleepwalking, with a lack of awareness about the reality and causes of suffering within us and all around us. We distract ourselves almost all the time until something stops us in our tracks. Cancer, loss, distress, decay, and death can turn up even if we have six houses, twelve cars, three bicycles, and a pair of roller skates!

Thus far we have been exploring the fears and resistances to compassion at both an individual and cultural level. Once we understand that avoidance is part of us all to a greater or lesser extent, then we can be mindful of it and work with it in a compassionate way. Compassion allows us to begin to face up to the realities of life on this planet, and have empathy for ourselves, our emotions, and the ways our lives have been shaped in different social contexts. Compassion opens our minds to facing things as they are and taking responsibility—the very opposite of avoidance.

But suppose we are definitely not into avoidance, but quite the opposite in fact—very much motivated to be compassionate and save the world. Can that run us into trouble? Well, in fact, it can, as the story of Chenrezig will show us.

The Story of Chenrezig

We have looked at some of the blocks to compassion that can arise from Western insights, but there is considerable wisdom in Buddhism as to the ways in which compassion can become subverted. This is the opposite problem to fear and avoidance of compassionate feelings, namely being overly motivated. In the Tibetan Buddhist tradition, the archetype of compassion is the *bodhisattva* Chenrezig, who appears in a variety of forms, each carrying a particular symbolic meaning.[14] In one manifestation, he appears with a thousand arms and an eye on the palm of each hand, with which he looks out on all beings with great compassion. According to the myth surrounding his creation, Amitabha, the Buddha of limitless light, realized that he needed an expression of compassionate activity to help him free living beings who were sunk deep in confusion and suffering. So he emanated a ray of white light from his forehead from which Chenrezig miraculously appeared. Chenrezig then knelt down in front of Amitabha and made a vow to work tirelessly for the benefit of all living beings, promising he would not rest in the peace of Nirvana until all beings were free of suffering; and he also vowed that, should he break his commitment, may he shatter into a thousand pieces. Quite a commitment!

As soon as Chenrezig began his work of helping living beings, he was so struck by the deep confusion and pain in which so many were immersed that he wept profusely. Again, we see the importance of sadness as a spark that stimulates our motivation for compassion (see chapter 1). From his tears of great sadness appeared Tara, a feminine expression of compassionate activity, a fierce and quick-acting *bodhisattva* connected with overcoming fear and obstacles and instilling fearlessness in the hearts of those who invoke her. So now Chenrezig had an ally to assist him with his heroic quest. Both he and Tara worked for countless eons to free living beings from suffering and to open their eyes to the truth of their own innate wisdom and compassion that is limitless in its scope.

One day Chenrezig decided to climb to the top of the highest mountain in the universe, Mount Meru, and look down upon the different realms of existence to check on his progress. To his great dismay, despite all of his work over countless eons, the living beings sunk in misery and suffering were still innumerable. His enthusiasm and zeal suddenly evaporated, and feeling depressed and forlorn, he decided to give up his *bodhisattva* mission and rest in the peace of Nirvana. At that moment he shattered into a thousand pieces because he had broken his vow to Amitabha, and the fragments of his sublime form fell down to the foot of Mount Meru, scattering on the plain below. This stirred Amitabha from his meditative equipoise. He looked down from his heavenly abode and saw that his creation was in pieces and in great agony. And then, through the power of his enlightened mind, he re-created Chenrezig from the shattered fragments into the thousand-armed version we described above. Now Chenrezig was even more powerful than before and, once again in the presence of Amitabha, he took his vow to free living beings from suffering, not resting in the peace of Nirvana until his job was completed.

What is interesting about this myth is that it charts a process through which the heart breaks open with sadness for the immensity of suffering in life and gives birth to compassion. But what arises first can be a lofty idealism as we seek to scale the heights and achieve great things—liberate ourselves and all living beings from suffering. Then there is the disappointment as we realize that our efforts are not yielding the fruit we had hoped for. Actually it seems we can do so little against this sea of suffering—it's like using teaspoons to empty an ocean—and this realization begins the process of descent, triggered by disappointment or a sense of defeat as we tumble down from our lofty idealism and crash back down to earth. But then out of this descent and disintegration something is touched within us that initiates a process of reintegration, and out of the despair and chaos something much more powerful and authentic is born. So in the end nothing is lost, because the experience and the journey become the crucible out of which something new emerges.

At first our vision of compassion is under the influence of the drive system and is focused on outcomes—we want to see results from *our own* actions. There is nothing wrong with this approach, at least initially, as we need this system to get the process going; but at some point, a goal-oriented approach focused on outcomes will hit the wall. Just as Chenrezig fell into despair when he saw that his work over thousands of years had not achieved his goal because there was still so much suffering in the world, so too we might find something similar happening in our own lives. As therapists or spiritual teachers, we might be inspired by lofty ideals of alleviating mental suffering and "making a difference to the world"; and our initial efforts to become qualified or learn "the way" may be driven by these imperatives. But at some point, we start experiencing doubt and fatigue and cannot face hearing another tragic tale (for example, that the patient who got better this year turns up again next year with the same depressive difficulty). The hope to rescue and save the world starts to fade, and at times we may become quite cynical; we just no longer feel up to it, and our idealism is shattered. We might even contemplate doing something entirely different, such as embarking on a different career or, like Chenrezig, going on a meditation retreat in the snowy Himalayas and practice in silence, untroubled by the worries of the world!

But the meaning of this myth is to hang in there and reframe our approach; then something more authentic can start to come through. It might dawn on us that we have to look after ourselves and practice self-compassion before we can be there for others. We might begin to see that relating to suffering on a moment-by-moment basis as it arises is more realistic than having some big objective in mind. And, most importantly, we may come to see that compassion has two components (see chapter 4): first, seeing clearly the nature of suffering in the flow of life (the inner circle of attributes of the compassion circle); and, second, desiring to alleviate suffering and focusing on a kind approach that arouses warm and affectionate emotions (the outer circle of the compassionate skills). As Matthieu Ricard says in lectures and on retreats, simply staying empathic and connected with the pain can be overwhelming. It's the kindness and affectionate focus that is crucial. So the key point of the story is that compassion can become undermined if we are too goal oriented and locked into the drive system, and too absorbed in the stark reality of suffering.

Compassion as Ascent to the Angelic?

Another major misunderstanding people have with the notion of compassion is, strangely, the traits that are associated with it. As we noted in chapter 4, compassion researchers have explored the typical day-to-day use of the word "compassion" and find that it is usually linked with traits of sympathy, kindness, warmth, tenderness, and gentleness. At first glance, this would not seem to be a problem because most of us would agree that these are reasonably moral and good qualities to have—right? Unfortunately there is a "yes, but" here. If we stop for a moment and create an image of a deeply compassionate being in our minds, who comes to mind? We might generate a vision of Jesus or Mary, Florence Nightingale, Gandhi, or the Dalai Lama. Usually we see them as moving calmly, serenely, gently, with smiling faces, and rarely ruffled, anxious, or angry. They are reaching out to help the poor and sick in an angelic or godlike way. They are supposed to be tender hearted and full of loving-kindness. We can form stereotypes of people (or gods) with these traits in our minds. Now, of course, compassion does include these qualities (indeed, research shows that these are the traits most people associate with compassion); but to be honest, it's easy for us to feel a personal distance from these traits and the folks who have them, as if they are living on a different plane. We might want to be close to them but struggle to imagine ourselves becoming like them because they seem too far above us. They seem so much better than our lowly selves.

In fact, there is a difference between what we think we *should* or *ought* to aspire to and what we *think* we can aspire to (and even what we want to aspire to, if we are being truthful!). If we are not careful, compassion becomes more of an "ought" than a "can" or "want." We might even feel some shame that maybe we should be a bit more like these "higher beings"—a bit kinder, a bit more thoughtful, a bit less irritable, and a bit less self-focused. This can be inspiring, but it is important to bear in mind that since we don't like to feel shame, we can tuck these things away in our minds and try not to think about them too much—and, in any case, who wants to be goody-two-shoes all the time? In fact, research shows that if we create images or role models that are too far removed from us, rather than striving to become like them, we can avoid thinking about them at all, with the result that the whole compassionate endeavor can get somewhat buried and forgotten.

Compassion as "Cleansing and Purifying" Inner Poisons

If we think of compassion as an ascent to an angelic state where we are no longer troubled by all the messy, difficult parts of our lives, then we have probably misunderstood what compassion is all about. The key point is that compassion is not about ascent and moving above suffering; rather, it is about descent into the grittiness of suffering. We seek to cultivate compassion not to get rid of our anger, anxiety, or pleasurable desires in the first instance, but to hold them in a compassionate space and to develop the wisdom to know how to work with them. Constantly, then, we see the importance of not avoiding but engaging. Indeed, Buddhism doesn't always help much here because it sometimes refers to emotions like anger, jealousy, and lust as "mind poisons." But a poison is linked to the notion of contamination, like a toxin in the body that needs expelling. If we are sick with salmonella, for example, then of course we want to cleanse the body of the toxic substance. However, cleansing is a bad metaphor for the mind because, while you can get rid of alien toxins or bacteria, you simply can't get rid of the way the brain is built. Moreover, some of the ways in which we think about these processes as being contaminants or poisons can evoke the emotion of disgust. This can unintentionally fuel self-critical thinking and even lead to self-attacking.[15]

This "cleansing" mindset will lead us astray if we set out to try to purify our mind for the simple reason that this is impossible. In more mundane terms, the thinking goes something like this: "If you're a compassionate person, then you have to forgive people who really annoy you, or even those who have hurt you; if you're a compassionate person, you should always put other people before yourself; if you're a compassionate person, you mustn't harbor grudges or vengeful thoughts; if you're a compassionate person, then you should not drink too much and have bad hangovers. To be compassionate, you wouldn't have any of these feelings or desires, or engage in these actions."

Notice how the "shoulds," "oughts," and "have tos" creep into our thinking. In fact, as we soon see in the practice section of the book, our approach to mindfulness and compassion does not seek to get rid of anything; what it seeks to do is to understand and work with our minds *as they actually are*. If we set out to get rid of our rage, vengeance, sexual desires, anxiety, and all the other stuff that goes on in our heads, then we will be constantly monitoring if we've been successful or not, and this will undermine our mindfulness practice. Moreover, how can we understand or relate to humanity? Is it not the case that once we have struggled with these things ourselves and have come to understand our own minds, then we can understand the minds of other people better? When we feel compassion for a child who is very distressed by a broken toy at Christmas, isn't this because we remember our own sadness at such things and, through making contact with our sadness, can connect with the sadness of the young child? Is it not our ability to stay in touch with what makes us human that allows us to be compassionate?

Consider also that we use insight into our own emotions of, say, rage or jealousy to really empathize and understand the rage and jealousy of another person—if you try to get rid of these emotions, or suppress them, you will struggle to empathize with others who feel similar things. In fact, it's easy for us to forget how unpleasant and difficult certain feelings can be. Paul had this experience when waiting for an operation and reflected on the fact that he had forgotten just how intense anxiety can be in the body when one is frankly very frightened. This experience reconnected him with empathy for his patients who go through similar things.

The important thing is to find a different way of dealing with difficult feelings rather than just trying to get rid of them. The issue is not so much how our minds are the cause of our difficulties, but our reactions to what comes up in our minds. In fact, the true meaning of purification in Buddhism is not to cleanse or get rid of negative emotions themselves, but to see the inherent purity of these emotions and not get stuck in our reactions to them. This gives them the freedom to arise, display, and liberate themselves.

The Real Story of Compassion— Descent

As we have seen, when compassion is associated with a process of ascent to higher states, we can very soon come unstuck. If we are honest, we are often helpful to others because we want to be liked or feel ourselves to be likable—again perfectly understandable. But what happens if you help people and then they cheat on you or let you down in some way? What happens to your compassion then? When we realize that being compassionate is not going to serve these kinds of ego agendas, there can be a sense of disappointment and we feel let down. Just like in the story of Chenrezig, compassion is not necessarily going to give us what we want; we might not get the satisfaction of climbing to the highest peak and surveying our work with pride.

As the story of Chenrezig has shown us, what is called for is a process of "descent." This is the willingness to drop down into the unpredictable, messy humanity that we normally prefer to sanitize or avoid.

In psychotherapy this is sometimes called *entering the shadow*, or what Freud referred to as the *id*—the primitive parts of the mind we prefer to avoid. When we think about somebody being compassionate to us, we want somebody who understands exactly what it is like to be human: they understand the power of rage, what it feels like to shake with a deep fear, wanting to kill oneself because of despair and depression, the desire to assert dominance and power, the joys of love, and the passions of lust and jealousy. Genuine compassion only arises through descent into the powerhouse of the mind and knowledge of how to be in this part of our being so that these "tigers within" can guide our compassion and we can learn to be less frightened of them or not judge ourselves because of them.

So the call of compassion is *the courage to make this descent* in a compassionate way, neither rationalizing nor getting overwhelmed and turning away. We take a wise, slow step-by-step approach. This is like learning how to swim; we do not immediately jump into the deep end, but start in the shallows and gradually progress to the deeper water. In practice, this means allowing ourselves to feel what we are actually feeling—tuning in to those parts of ourselves that we tend to tune out of and opening our lens of awareness to take in more than we normally do.

There are times, however, when we are catapulted into pain. Often this process of descent can happen when an accident or tragedy slaps us in the face. It can take many forms: the death of a loved one, bankruptcy, illness, discovering your partner is having an affair, or sinking into depression. Life loses its shine, and our way of dealing with the world suddenly no longer seems to work. What is certain is that it is painful and will often be accompanied by emotions of fear, anxiety, and rage at levels of intensity that we might not be used to. We might desperately try to replay the tape in our mind and get caught up in "if only" thoughts: "If only this hadn't happened; if only I hadn't done that; if only, if only...." There might be an awareness that we cannot go back to how things were before, but the way forward is not clear either.

In the mystical Christian tradition, this is referred to as "the dark night of the soul." This process is characterized by falling down from the light of faith, belief, and hope into the dark of unknowing and doubt, where our normal life turns to ashes and everything becomes bleak. In the writings of St. John of the Cross, the dark night of the soul is one where both our mundane life and our spiritual life no longer have meaning for us—so there appears to be no refuge anywhere at all. This experience can indeed be very frightening, but spiritual thinkers of the past tend to agree that this can also be a highly creative time if we can just hold our courage. It can be a time of significant shift and reorientation at the very core of our being. It can also be a time to reach out to others.

Descent: Choden's Personal Journey

As a way of illustrating this process of descent, I (Choden) offer a personal account of how meditation practice can be linked to the drive system that aspires to enlightenment, which can then open up a whole host of complex and difficult experiences. My crisis arose some years ago when I did a traditional Tibetan Buddhist three-year, three-month retreat in Scotland. This retreat involved many hours of solitary meditation, reciting ancient texts, and doing powerful practices from the Buddhist tantric tradition. When I came later to reflect on my experiences, I wrote this:

> It felt like we were pioneers working directly at the interface of the ancient spiritual wisdom of the East as it came to the West. Every day we woke up at 4 a.m. and practiced a rigorous routine of meditation and study until 10 p.m. at night; every day was pretty much the same for the duration of the retreat. There was one period when we did not speak for six months and were not even allowed to go outside. We were doing a very powerful meditation practice that felt like immersing oneself in a crucible and undergoing a birth of fire as our inner world was being cleansed and purified. I remember thinking at one point—this is amazing, this is what I have always being looking for. And in the back of my mind I felt I was on a glorious ascent to awakening and enlightenment—this was it! And then at one point, it was as if disaster struck. It was as if the lid blew off Pandora's Box and nothing I could do could make it go back on again. I was sitting by my meditation box about to start the session, when my body flung itself involuntarily against the wall, and images of my childhood, and the pain and rage connected to it, started flooding through my mind. It was like I had suddenly dropped into another realm of my being. I had the sense that now I was in deep trouble. Images and emotions started surging through me and I found myself oscillating between great anger and sorrow. Then it was as if my whole retreat routine started to fall apart. I could not continue with the sessions. My vision of enlightenment crashed, and I was left sitting in the midst of a torrent of up-surging emotion, and all I could do was just be present and let it follow its course. It was as if my ego agendas were pushed aside and something else took over. This process carried on for about seven months. It was truly awful! However, I was very lucky to have the support of the retreat leader, who had an intuitive understanding of this process, and [the support of] my friends in retreat who were also going through their own

difficult rites of passage. Then at one point I had a dream in which I was lying down in a grave about to be buried alive and various high lamas were standing around the open grave conducting a religious ceremony and consecrating the grave. It felt like I had no option but to just lie there while this ceremony was going on and then soon I would be buried. There was a feeling of resignation—I had no option but to go through with it, but there was the sense too that this was not the end of the journey—it was more like the death of one phase in preparation for something new.

For me, coming to understand these experiences and how this can happen to other people and how we can help them has been the focus for my journey ever since. For Paul, too, in his early twenties, his own depression become a source for study and understanding the nature of the depressed mind.[16]

I am sharing this experience with you because it has significantly influenced my life and deepened my understanding of the mind and what we can go through. It was an extreme and intense experience because I had completely dedicated myself to that way of life. By no means am I suggesting that everyone needs to go through something similar to benefit from the path of mindful compassion! In fact, what I have learnt from this experience is that a more gentle and gradual path is more appropriate for most people.

Descent and the Emergence of Compassion: The Beginning of New Life

As we come to the end of part I, we would like to return to the story of Chenrezig and leave you with an important image. One of the symbols connected with Chenrezig is that of a lotus flower growing out of the mud in a beautiful lake. According to the myth, the seed of compassion lies dormant beneath the mud of the lake. It may have lain there for an entire lifetime, completely hidden and ignored. It represents our capacity to transform our own lives and the lives of many others and have a huge impact on the world. The mud represents our darker side—all those difficult, troublesome desires and emotions that afflict us on a daily basis, such as anger, desire, jealousy, and pride. It also represents our tendencies toward selfishness and neurosis that limit and preoccupy us. This is the stuff that we may want to get rid of, but this is not so easy because these emotions are part of our evolved minds. The lake symbolizes the depths of the psyche and the surface of the lake, the boundary between our unconscious experience and our conscious lives.

Now, according to the myth, what activates the seed beneath the mud and starts the process of germination is the force of compassionate motivation, namely the wish to open our hearts to the suffering of ourselves and others, and to engage with this suffering. We need to be willing to go there to enable the seed to germinate. In fact, we can think of our minds as having many potential seeds that can be germinated by different social conditions and motives. We can grow the seeds of violence and tribal hatred, if we so choose. To do the opposite is our responsibility as human beings, as we wake up to the fact that our brains are much more malleable than we may have realized and we can make choices about what we want to cultivate in ourselves. In choosing to cultivate our compassionate selves, however, we begin the process of transforming our destructive emotions and, indeed, our lives.

In the beginning, perhaps all we might know is that we are suffering and that others are suffering too. But as soon as we choose to move toward the pain, not away from it, something is touched and begins to grow within us. According to the myth, the seedling of compassion, which is the lotus flower shoot, starts to sprout; and, as we continue to practice mindfulness and compassion, it grows and finally breaks the surface of the lake. Now, although it has grown out of the mud, at the point when it blooms and breaks the surface of the lake it is completely untainted by the mud, and symbolizes the mind that opens out to the world with love and compassion.

An important part of this myth is that the lotus flower cannot exist without the mud because the mud is the manure that feeds the plant and enables it to grow. Without suffering, there is nothing to be compassionate about. This allows us to step out of shame and avoidance and to see that the difficult parts of ourselves are the very manure of transformation; so we do not need to get rid of them (and nor can we), but we can acknowledge instead that they are a source of power. In this way we can see that the awakening of compassion can sometimes depend upon the dark and difficult parts of ourselves.

Within the Tibetan Buddhist tradition, the mud is actually a source of gold. The so-called "negative" emotions of anger, anxiety, greed, and jealousy have their own innate wisdom energy. If we connect with this energy, then the emotion has the capacity to transform. For example, anger can propel us into negative images or even to lash out and hit someone who provokes our anger. But if we look at the anger directly, hold it within our awareness, and resist the pull toward action and projection, there is vitality and power within the emotion that can give us energy and clarity of mind. The wisdom aspect of anger is called *mirror-like wisdom* because it has the vividness and clarity to reflect what is arising within us, instead of being at the service of egocentric tendencies. It is like a bolt of lightning that lights up the night sky with vivid clarity. Similarly, in the case of desire, once the old-brain impulses of grasping and identification are held and understood, the energy of desire is freed up and reveals its essence to be the wisdom of discrimination, in which we are able to intelligently discriminate one thing from the next.

What is crucial here is our attitude—if we just mindlessly act out whatever anger or desirous impulses get triggered in us, they become mud; but if we look directly at these emotions and acknowledge their inner "gold," then they have the capacity to transform and become the manure for the emerging lotus flower of compassion.

Consequently, compassion is born within the depths of our being. It arises as a deep stirring beneath the mud of our everyday mind. What stirs it is the force of motivation and commitment to engage with our pain and the pain of others. But while it is important to descend and make contact with the mud, it is also important to bear in mind that the key elements of compassion are the emotions of kindness and friendliness and the genuine desire to alleviate suffering. These arise from the sense that we are all in it together—and through acknowledging the links of affiliation to everything that lives.

Compassion and the Flow of Life

There is another aspect of the story of the lotus in the mud. We (humans and, indeed, all living things) are made up of atoms and molecules that at one time might have existed at the heart of a star; we are stardust. Particular combinations of atoms and molecules give rise to DNA, which gives rise to bodies and then to brains and minds with psychologies. Consider that the psychologies that exist on this planet, the capacity for feeling, thinking, and behaving, are all part of the process of evolution and the flow of life. Five hundred million years ago, there were no living things, as far as we know, that could experience anything remotely like compassion. Rage, sexual desire, and fear maybe—but not care-focused feelings. But in the struggle for survival—*the mud of evolution*, if you like—a capacity for caring was to evolve, and this was the beginning of the seeds for compassion. It is possible to argue that from the moment the universe came into being—because of the laws of physics and chemistry and biological evolution—compassion and self-aware experience were potentials waiting to unfold. Compassion was a seed—a potential for a life at the beginning the universe itself. The self-aware, knowledge-seeking mind may be the first time that such a mind has evolved in the universe. If so, it places a huge responsibility on our shoulders to use our minds wisely and compassionately.

So, to come back to our key story about the two psychologies of compassion, compassion is not just about focusing on the mud but about nurturing the lotus flower that opens out toward the world. In other words, we attend to both of the psychologies of compassion that we mentioned in chapter 4: opening and engaging with pain (inner circle of attributes) and connecting with the positive emotional systems within us that alleviate this pain (outer circle of skills).

Key Points

- Both mindfulness and compassion are vital to the process of growth and transformation; but, while mindfulness is the servant of the awakening heart of compassion, it is the force of compassionate motivations that reorganizes the mind and sets in motion lasting change.

- Compassion is commonly misunderstood as being only about kindness, or, even worse, "niceness," and so it can wrongly be viewed as being weak or self-indulgent.

- Blocks to compassion can arise because the soothing/affiliation system closes down and people can't experience the types of affiliative emotions and insights they would need in order to develop compassion in any depth because they lack a sense of connectedness.

- Understanding the fears and resistances to compassion can arm us with ways of spotting them and not getting too caught up with them.

- Initially, compassion may be linked to the drive system and to outcomes; this is useful in the beginning to get us going, but this approach has its limitations (as Chenrezig discovered).

- Compassion is about descent into the "mud" of suffering, not ascent away from this reality.

- Once we are willing to open up to the "mud" of our experience (first psychology of compassion), we then need to attend to the growth of the lotus flower (second psychology of compassion).

Part II

THE PRACTICES

Introduction: Compassionate Motivation

In previous chapters, we saw how important motivation is for awakening compassion. This was expressed in the ancient myth of Chenrezig: being willing to descend and make contact with the "mud" of our experience and then, on the basis of this, opening up to the struggles and difficulties of others. The masters of old saw how this initiates something profound—the birth of compassion—and expressed this insight in terms of the lotus flower growing out of the mud.

In practice, this motivation is formalized in a prayer of aspiration: "May I awaken my inner potential for wisdom and compassion, and may I take active steps to bring this enlightened awareness into the world and help free beings from suffering." This is the *bodhisattva* prayer that has been the hallmark of the Mahayana Buddhist tradition for thousands of years. The form of the prayer is not what is important; what is crucial is the intention that goes behind it. And what is crucial too is the wisdom that informs this intention.

This is where modern neuroscience and psychology have much to offer the ancient wisdom traditions of the East; and in fact, if the Buddha was alive today, he might well have expressed his understanding in a different way. On the one hand, this wisdom is seeing how we are all caught in the flow of life with a complex and tricky brain we did not design and emotions that just fire through us; but then, on the other hand, it is realizing that this situation is not as solid and fixed as it might appear because we have the capacity to make choices and shape our experience from moment to moment.

From the point of view of the evolutionary model, motivation is crucial because it organizes our mind in a particular way and is one of the key attributes of the compassionate mind (see chapter 4). Motivation activates different social mentalities. If we focus on being competitive, this organizes our thinking and behavior around gain and success, whereas if we are motivated by compassion, this organizes our thinking and behavior around caring and responsiveness. For this reason it is important to formulate an authentic, heartfelt motivation, which each of us does our own way. These attributes are potentialities within us, but they require us to actively focus on them in order to awaken them. The following reflection is an aid to uncovering our motivation:

Reflection

What is my motivation?

What is my motivation or purpose for engaging with this path of training?

How do I want it to change the way that I live my life?

How do I want this to benefit the people that are close to me and in the world?

Can I express this in the form of a personal aspiration that communicates my heartfelt intention?

Outline of Practice Chapters

Having clarified our motivation, we can begin training in mindfulness and work directly with how we pay attention; this establishes a basis of stability for training in compassion (chapter 7). Through mindfulness practice, we become more familiar with how we react and learn to accept what arises in the mind from moment to moment (chapter 8). This opens up the first psychology of compassion—engaging honestly with what is present in our emotional world and that of others We then shift focus to the process of cultivating our positive emotional systems and work with the second psychology of compassion, that of alleviation and prevention. At this point we start working with the flow of compassion and compassionate imagery (chapter 9). This culminates in the awakening of the compassionate self and focusing this compassionate self on the parts of ourselves we struggle with: our angry, anxious, and self-critical parts (chapter 10). We then widen our circle of compassion to include people we might not naturally care about, like strangers and adversaries, and work directly with the self-preoccupied mind that limits the opening of the compassionate heart. Here we explore the four limitless contemplations and the "taking and sending" practice (chapter 11).

7

MINDFULNESS PRACTICE

Recognizing the Unsettled Mind

Mindfulness is the deliberate intention to observe the activity of the mind in a nonjudgmental way—to step back and notice whatever arises in the mind without reacting to it.[1] The starting point for mindfulness is simply noticing what is happening in our minds right now.

Let's begin by doing a simple exercise.

Exercise 1: Recognizing the Unsettled Mind

Sit comfortably with your back straight. For a beginner, a straight-backed chair is probably best. It's not advisable to sink into a luxurious easy chair because you might fall asleep.

Once you are sitting comfortably, simply relax, with your eyes open if possible, and experience being where you are. Feel the pressure of your body resting on the seat and ground; become aware of the space around you; notice how you naturally become aware of sights, sounds, and other sensory stimuli—perhaps the smell of cooking wafts in from next door or maybe a breeze brushes your skin.

So this practice is very simple: just allow yourself to be present, experiencing whatever happens when you sit and do nothing. Decide to sit and do nothing. Let your mind rest in the present moment, and simply be aware of where you are right now.

In a surprisingly short time you may find that you are thinking about something, even though you had decided to do nothing other than notice what occurs in your *senses* in this moment. When you realize you are "thinking," simply bring your attention back to being "here," doing nothing, just observing. Once again, before you know it, you may have drifted off into random thoughts, worries, daydreams, or ruminations. So once again, when you realize this, kindly and gently bring your attention back to being here, doing nothing.

Reflection After the Exercise

Reflect in the following way: I sat, relaxed, and became aware of what was happening in the moment. I made a decision to relax and do nothing. This "doing nothing" included not chasing after thoughts or getting lost in my imagination; but despite this decision, I almost immediately found myself thinking. Thinking began *by itself* despite my decision to do nothing, to just observe.

What does this tell me? It seems that there is a strong habit constantly active within my mind that *automatically* pulls me away from the present moment into thinking whenever my mind is not focused on a chosen topic. This habit is strong and has the power to override my conscious decision-making process. This is the unsettled mind.

Do this exercise several times until you are clear about what is meant by the unsettled mind. It is the mind that never stays still but is always on the move and has difficulty coming to rest in the present moment.

What this exercise reveals is that we can sit our body down and remain in one place, but the mind seldom follows suit even when we want it to. It immediately moves away into thinking and roves randomly from one thought to another in the grip of one emotion and then another. In many ways, this is a result of our "new brain" becoming smart. We have a brain that thinks, imagines, plans, ruminates, and regrets.

These tendencies aren't such a problem if the thoughts and emotions involved are pleasant and harmonious, but so often this is not the case. Most people seem to have a catalogue of negative and disturbing emotional themes filed in the back of their minds, such as "I am lazy," or "Something is wrong with me." When we are not involved in something that holds our attention, these files automatically drift to the front of our minds and provide themes for dwelling on negative or disturbing thoughts. Sometimes these themes are strongly activated by life events that upset us. On these occasions, extra energy is fed into them and we find ourselves dwelling on painful or disturbing issues even though we don't want to. When this happens, we discover the problem of the every-day mind: it is so accustomed to being wayward and following its own direction that even when we do not want to think about something, it does so regardless and causes us to suffer.

When we learned about the three-circle model in chapter 3, we saw that our minds are predominantly under the power of threat- and drive-focused emotions. We seek to avoid things that threaten us and to acquire things that we need to survive and be comfortable. So it is *not our fault* that our minds are always restless and on the move. We have been programmed in this way by evolution, which has designed us to be on the lookout for dangers and alert to what we need or want. We did not evolve to be like a Buddha sitting peacefully under a tree because, if this were the case, our species would have become extinct many thousands of years ago! Consequently, the purpose of our inquiry *is not* to attribute blame, or think, "I shouldn't be like this; I should control my mind better," but simply to see what is going on. This point is important because very quickly the process of inner inquiry can be undermined by the tendency to self-blame and even self-attack.

When we reflect more deeply on the unsettled mind and its implica-tions, what strikes us very quickly is that we are *not in control* of our inner world. This is something to pause and reflect on. So much of what we do externally is control oriented. We live in a culture in which much of our lives can be planned, manipulated, and changed at the push of a button on a computer screen. But we cannot control our inner world so easily. This becomes immediately obvious when we do the exercise we have just done. We observed how our mind does not obey our wishes; it drifts off and does its own thing.

We might well say: "Let the mind just do what it wants; why bother training it?" This is, in fact, the underlying message within modern consumer-oriented societies: "Let your mind go free, let it just do what it wants and have exactly what it wants, provided you stay within the con-fines of the law." But, as we have learned already, if we just let our minds "go free," they tend to follow their ingrained habits of threat and drive.

We find ourselves dwelling on painful issues again and again, criticizing and attacking ourselves, judging what we do, reliving arguments, and endlessly fantasizing about what we want, whom we desire, and what we would like to acquire. Is there any freedom in this?

Beginning to Work with Attention

By now what is becoming clear is that where our attention goes and what our mind dwells on affects our emotions and body in particular ways. It might be a wild garden with many weeds and thorny bushes or a carefully cultivated herb garden. The choice is ours. Rob Nairn refers to this process as "energy follows focus."[2] What we focus on, we give energy to, and what we give energy to, we cultivate. This principle is central to our training in mindfulness. Even though we may not be able to control what arises in our inner emotional world, what we give our attention to greatly influences what takes shape in our experience. For example, an angry thought might just arise by itself, but if we focus on it, we give it energy and it becomes a big issue in our minds; whereas if we notice it and leave it alone, it loses power over us and quickly dissipates. We can explore this principle of "energy follows focus" by doing the following exercise.

Exercise 2: Working with Attention

Sit comfortably and focus on your right foot. Explore the sensations in your toes, then your heel, and then your whole foot. Hold your attention there for about ten seconds or so. Now switch your attention to your left foot. Again, explore the sensations in your toes, then your heel, and your whole foot. Hold your attention there for ten seconds or so. Now focus on your right hand. Notice the sensations in your fingers and your thumb. Again, hold that attention for about ten seconds. Next, focus on your left hand and hold your attention there for about ten seconds. Finally, focus your attention on your lips and the sensations around your mouth.

What did you notice? Consider that when you focus on your left foot, you are not aware of your fingers or your lips, and when you refocus your attention on your fingers, the awareness of your feet disappears. What you focus your attention on in your body *expands* in your field of awareness. It is as if your attention is like a *zoom lens* or magnifying glass, a spotlight illuminating some things but leaving others in the dark. Notice too that your attention is *not fixed*; you can actually move it around *deliberately* and, when you do, different sensations flow in and out of your consciousness.

Let's look at this in terms of our emotions and feelings. As you're sitting, stop reading this book and bring to mind a time when you were laughing—maybe somebody told you a joke or you were at a party. Hold that memory in your mind and become aware of yourself laughing with your friends. Now notice what happens in your body; perhaps your face begins to smile a little. What you are bringing to mind and what your attention is drawing into the foreground are affecting you in powerful ways.

Having seen how you can bring to mind and focus on a happy thought, image, or memory, and how that made you feel a certain way, now refocus your attention and bring to mind something that you are a bit anxious about or something that has made you a little unhappy. Let your attention bring those thoughts or images into the foreground. Notice what happens to the feelings and the sensations in your body when your attention zooms in on these things and brings them into the forefront of your mind. You probably don't feel like laughing now. The point is that when you bring this memory or thought into your field of attention, the good feelings you experienced just moments before fade away. This demonstrates to us that what our attention focuses on *within our own memory systems* powerfully influences our feelings and sensations. Once you really understand the power of your attention to stimulate your body, then the value of learning to be more in control of this attention, this spotlight, or this magnifying glass becomes very clear. And sometimes it is helpful to switch attention to a more helpful focus such as compassionate images of self and others.

The purpose of this exercise is to help us recognize these things:

- Our attention is movable, not fixed, and it can be moved intentionally, as well as be taken over unintentionally by the threat and drive systems.

- Attention acts like a zoom lens, making some things bigger in our minds and blocking out other thoughts and feelings.

- Attention can have very powerful physiological effects. Bringing to mind happy memories can arouse pleasant feelings and sensations, while dwelling on unhappy things can arouse unpleasant feelings and sensations.

Once we begin to notice how easily our attention is captured by our emotions without us even realizing it, we can then learn to train our minds so that our attention brings into the foreground ideas, images, or ways of thinking that are going to be helpful to us rather than letting our attention drift around in a sea of anxiety or negative rumination. We simply need to pay attention. In fact, although it is simple, it is not so easy: our tendency to become easily distracted is powerfully ingrained, and therefore we need to engage in a sustained program of mind training.

Something important to note is that mindfulness training is not about avoiding unhappy emotions or always focusing on happy experiences. It is also about learning how to tolerate, accept, and work with difficult emotions too. These emotions are part of our experience, and often they have important messages for us if we listen and pay attention to them. However, it's also useful to recognize when we are caught up in emotions and ruminations that are not helpful so we can learn to refocus our attention on just observing them as opposed to getting caught up in the storyline that they weave.

Slowing Down and Settling

In order to be able to notice where our attention goes, and learn to redirect it, it helps to slow down. This is very important. So much of modern life takes place at high speed with conflicting priorities that require us to multitask and juggle many balls at the same time. This is often unavoidable. However, from time to time it is useful to locate gaps in our day when we can pause, slow down, and look inward, check in with how we are feeling at an emotional level, and find simple ways to calm ourselves.

An important aid for calming our mind is breathing. It is something that is happening all the time, whether we are aware of it or not, and it is something that we can turn to at any moment to reconnect us with our body and begin to slow down. Through deepening our breathing slightly and learning to regulate it, we can stimulate our parasympathetic nervous system. This helps our body to calm down and our mind to begin to settle. As we pointed out earlier, the parasympathetic nervous system triggers the soothing system, while the sympathetic nervous system is linked to the activation of the threat and/or drive systems.[3]

Some people who are very anxious or have a need to be in control can find this exercise a little anxiety provoking because they like to block out bodily feelings. So, as with all of these exercises, go at your own pace, and if you are struggling, you can move on to the next exercise. Don't force yourself to do things.

Exercise 3: Soothing Breathing Rhythm

Sit comfortably with both feet flat on the floor about a shoulder width apart and with your back straight. Your posture is comfortable but upright because the idea is to be both relaxed and alert rather than becoming sleepy, which can happen if your head drops forward. Gently, close your eyes or allow your gaze to fall unfocused on the floor. Create a gentle facial expression, an expression of friendliness, as if you are with somebody you like. Try relaxing your facial muscles by letting your jaw drop slightly, and then let your mouth turn up into a slight smile.

Now focus on your breathing, on the air coming in through your nose and down into your diaphragm, staying a short while, and then moving back out through your nose. Notice how your diaphragm moves gently as you breathe in and out. For the development of a soothing breathing rhythm, you will breathe slightly more slowly and slightly more deeply than you would normally. The in-breath is about three to five seconds, and then you pause momentarily and take three to five seconds for the out-breath. You might try to breathe a little faster and then a little slower until you find a breathing pattern that is comfortable for you and has a gentle rhythm to it, giving you the feeling of slowing down. The slow comfortable *rhythm* of the breath is key. Five to six breaths per minute is ideal but only if comfortable.

Also focus on the out-breath and the air leaving your nose with a steady rhythm. Try to ensure that the in-breath and the out-breath are even, and don't rush them. As you develop your breathing rhythm, notice the feeling of inner slowing with each out-breath. Notice how your body responds to your breathing, as if you are linking up with a rhythm within your body that is soothing and calming for you. Notice how this links to your friendly facial expression. Notice how you might feel heavier as you sit, more solid, and still in your body.

You may find that thoughts pop into your mind, which is totally okay and natural. Don't worry about it. You are not attempting to get rid of thoughts or make your mind go blank. You are, in fact, not doing anything besides focusing on the soothing breathing rhythm and not becoming involved with the thoughts that pop into your mind. You let them go free without attempting to suppress or become involved with them.

So it is perfectly okay for your mind to wander. Simply notice it happening and then gently guide your attention back to an awareness of your body and breathing, sensing the flow of air coming in and out of your nostrils—feeling your body slowing down. If you find that regulating and deepening your breathing is making you feel tense or a bit panicky, then focus instead on the grounding section of the sitting practice (exercise 6).

Now once again, check on your friendly facial expression, the gentle smile, and then continue to experience your soothing breathing rhythm. Tune in to the feeling of slowing down. Stay with this process for a few minutes, breathing slightly deeper than you would normally. When you are ready, open your eyes and if you're not going to engage with any further practices, stretch and move your body. (See http://www.coherence.com for more resources relating to breath practice.)

An important part of soothing rhythm breathing is becoming more grounded in the body. This is something we come to shortly. At this stage, however, the important point is not to see this practice as merely a form of relaxing, but rather as a way of feeling the body becoming more solid and rooted as you sit on the chair. It is a way of steadying the body and finding an inner point of stillness and calmness. In tai chi, the breath is connected with the body in such a way that we find a stable base for movement and action. Soothing breathing rhythm is similar. For example, if your feet are together with your toes and heels touching and somebody pushes you from the side, you will topple over. But if your feet are slightly apart, your weight is balanced, and you feel rooted, then a push from the side won't topple you. You have a firm base. Soothing rhythm breathing, when connected to the body, is like this—finding that position of stability, inner stillness, calmness, and preparedness. It is like the high diver preparing for a dive: first steadying him- or herself, finding a point of inner stillness and calm within, and then diving. As we saw in chapters 4 and 6, compassion is about turning toward suffering, not away from it. In this way, soothing rhythm breathing connects us to the body, and this prepares us for engaging with pain and difficulty.

An important insight from this exercise is getting used to the fact that thoughts and emotions can arise and move through our awareness without us becoming *involved* with them. For many of us, this is an unusual experience because as soon as thoughts, emotions, or mind states arise within us, we immediately identify with them as being who we are in that moment. The skill we are developing here is not so much controlling what arises in our mind—by now we realize that we cannot do this—but changing the way we *relate* to what arises. This is the heart of the mindfulness training, and it is also the foundation for training in compassion.

Generally, when people hear about meditation or mindfulness, they think that it is about emptying the mind and making it go blank, stopping thoughts, and "blissing out." All of these are misconceptions. It is a more subtle process of allowing thoughts to come and go and realizing that we do not have to engage with them. Moment by moment, we realize that we have a choice as to what to cultivate and what not to cultivate. We create a point of steadiness within. Tragically, most people do not realize that they have this choice, and they can become enslaved to habitual patterns of thinking, speaking, and acting that do not serve them, and bring them unhappiness. But even a few glimpses of this choice can initiate a fundamental reorientation in our mind as an entirely different possibility for living our life begins to open up to us.

It is as if our mind is a multistoried building with lots of figures moving around the different levels, busy with various tasks. Everything is shrouded in darkness except for a flashlight we have in our hands. So the birth of mindfulness is the realization that we are holding the flashlight in our hands and whatever we shine it on, we light up. We may not have any choice as to what house we find ourselves inhabiting and we might not be able to control the busy figures going about their work, but we can certainly control what we shine the light on.

In doing this exercise, the role of compassion is learning to be soft with ourselves, not expecting that we have to get it right, and realizing that it is understandable that our attention is going to be captured by threat and drive emotions most of the time because this is how we have been wired up. This results in a sense of patience, and even humor, realizing that this is a long process of training and that we do not need to perfect it overnight. Approaching our mindfulness training from this compassionate orientation allows our practice to ease up and be less fraught, judgmental, and goal driven.

Opening Up to Our Senses

Once we realize that we can direct where our attention goes and once we have slowed down a bit, the next step is to notice that our awareness can open up to what is all around us. When threat-based emotions like anxiety or anger seize hold of our attention, we tend to find that our field of awareness contracts and our mental world closes in around us. This often results in a feeling of inner imprisonment and tension.

When we bring awareness to this process, one of the striking things we notice is just how much we miss in our everyday lives—just how much sensory information passes us by. A bewildering contradiction of life is that we can only exist in the present moment but we are seldom in touch with it. And yet when we do allow ourselves to inhabit *this moment*, a rich experience of being alive can open up before our eyes, and we can learn to savor and appreciate so much of what previously went unnoticed. But we are so used to *not* being present, not being relaxed, and not being happy, that it might feel somewhat strange to inhabit this part of ourselves; so it takes some conscious training.

Let's begin by doing the following exercise.

Exercise 4: Mindfully Eating an Apple

Suppose you're going to eat an apple. How would you do this mindfully? First, you could look at the apple and notice its color and texture. Hold it in your hand and feel the quality of its skin. Don't rush; spend time just observing it. When your mind wanders from your focus on the apple (as it likely will), gently bring your attention back to it. In this exercise you're not judging the apple; you're simply exploring its properties. Then, take a knife and peel it or cut into it. Once again, notice the effect this has on the apple; notice the color and texture of the fruit beneath the skin. Take time to really observe it.

Next, take a bite of the apple. Now focus on your sense of taste and what the apple feels like in your mouth. Chew it slowly, feeling the texture in your mouth, noticing how the juice is stimulating your salivary glands and how the saliva feels in your mouth. Savor the taste. As you chew, notice how the apple becomes mushier. As you swallow, pay attention to the sensations of swallowing.

In this way, you have explored the apple visually, by touch and feel, by smell, by texture, and by taste. If you had dropped the apple, you would have been able to hear what it sounded like—but you don't need to do that today!

Reflection Afterward

What did it feel like to be completely immersed in the moment-by-moment activity of eating the apple? How is this different from those times when you eat an apple while thinking about something else or watching TV?

What this exercise reveals is that when we allow ourselves to be present, we reconnect with our senses—we touch, we hear, we see, and we taste. When we open to the present moment and pay attention to what's all around us, our experience of life opens up and becomes enriched. We feel the earth beneath our feet, we are aware of the changing dance of sun and clouds above our heads, we notice the smells in the rose bushes along our path, and we hear the distant call of gulls in the mountain cliffs around us. We are not tightly locked into a world of thought. We are not trapped in the loops between the old and new brain (chapter 2). Our threat and drive systems tend to trap us in thoughts and emotions that cut us off from the immediacy of present-moment experience because that is their job. However, if this happens all the time, we end up missing out on the freshness and vitality of our lives. But when we are in touch with our senses—when we allow ourselves to savor the bite of the apple—we find ourselves in living connection with our environment and those people and animals that share this moment with us. Indeed, this is why Jon Kabat-Zinn called his recent book on mindfulness *Coming to Our Senses*.[4]

What allows this process of opening up to happen is practicing the skills we have introduced so far: slowing down, noticing where our attention is, and savoring what is happening now. This gives us access to the soothing system, which is always there, like the earth beneath our feet, but which we seldom acknowledge.

Single-Focus Attention and Open-Field Awareness

When we practice mindfulness, there are always two processes happening at the same time. At one level, we are learning to be aware of what we are doing while we are doing it. This involves noticing when our attention drifts off into distraction and gently bringing it back to what we are doing. This is referred to as *single-focus attention*, and we are now acquainted with it to some extent through practicing soothing breathing rhythm. In the beginning of our mindfulness training, we direct most of our energy in this direction because our mind tends to be pulled all over the place by wild and random thoughts.

However, there is another process that runs alongside our training in noticing and redirecting our attention. This is *open-field awareness*. It refers to the process of becoming aware of the environment we are moving through and tuning in to the bigger picture even though the main focus of our attention is with what we are actually doing. We touched on this in the previous exercise of mindfully eating an apple. A good example of this is walking through a cocktail party holding a tray of glasses filled to the brim with the finest champagne. Two things are going on here: we are closely attentive to holding the tray so we don't spill the glasses of champagne all over the guests, but we are also aware of the activity in the room and all the people bustling and chatting around us so we don't bump into them. If our attention is solely focused on carrying the tray, we will very quickly bump into someone and spill the champagne; conversely if we just focus on the people around us and not the tray, the glasses might slide off. So both types of awareness are necessary—being lightly focused on what we are doing with the background awareness of what is happening all around us.

Now open-field awareness is the awareness of how we exist in relation to our environment, namely how we place ourselves in relation to the people chatting in the cocktail party, and how we respond to this environment—in this case, not bumping into them but carefully moving around them. This is where compassion arises; it emerges through the process of open-field awareness, which is the field of connection and relationship to what is happening around us. It is the awareness that we do not live in a bubble, and if we insist on doing so, we may run slap bang into somebody and spill champagne all over her beautiful dress and get fired from our jobs as cocktail waiters. So open-field awareness occurs together with single-focus attention—*both need to be present*—although, in the beginning, single-focus attention takes priority because the mind is like a puppy and needs training again and again to stay with the task at hand. However, we never lose sight of the other process, of the compassion, because it needs to be there all the time, right from the beginning.

Grounding in the Body

In order for us to stabilize the tempestuous movements of the mind, it helps to have anchors and supports that hold us in the present moment. So the next stage in our journey is learning to ground our awareness in the body. Much of the time we are so driven by the competing agendas racing through our heads that we overlook the simple fact that the mind is resident in the body and the body is always present. For this reason our body is a strong ally in mindfulness practice because it always remains present, whereas our mind can depart from the present many times in the space of a few seconds. So a big part of mindfulness practice is simply bringing our mind back to where our body is and learning to rest our attention in awareness of the body.

The process of grounding in the body is a key element of sitting practice. We look at this in more detail shortly. But right now, we explore the body scan practice because it follows on from the last exercise and establishes the foundation of body awareness and grounding for the sitting practice that follows.

Body Scan

This is a practice of progressively moving our attention through the different parts of our body, from our feet up to our head, and then back down to our feet again.[5] When we do this practice, we bring the same quality of curiosity and attention to our body as we did when we mindfully ate an apple. We gently explore the different parts of our body and become aware of the rich texture of sensations that arise and subside. In doing this practice, we build on the skills we have already developed: we slow down, notice where our attention is, bring it back to the body scan, and then move our attention through our body, opening up to and experiencing the different sensations as they arise.

We notice how the body is a complex field of energy and sensation. The practice involves precise awareness of particular body parts, the sensations on the surface of the skin, the feelings inside the body (including sensations of body organs and bones), and the movement of the breath through the body. We may notice sensations of discomfort, feelings of intensity, or sensations that are very subtle and fleeting. We may also become aware of emotional reactions, thoughts, or stories associated with different body parts. The body carries our personal histories, and our relationship to our body can be complicated.

We may start to notice more about the different ways in which we pay attention and the different qualities of awareness that are possible. We discover how our attention can be very flexible. At one moment, we are paying detailed attention to a small body part, such as our big toe. At other moments, we are holding larger areas of the body in our awareness, such as both of our legs from the ankles to the hips. We may start to notice the differences in experience if we are holding a mental image of the body in our mind's eye (what we think our left arm looks like), or if we are just experiencing the pure sensations themselves.

Through this practice, we may start to notice much about the habits of our mind. We will find ourselves often getting distracted, but when we do, we can simply acknowledge this and invite our attention back to the practice over and over again. We may notice that the mind does not really want to be present a lot of the time and we may even find that we fall asleep. Sleepiness is very common when people start with this practice. Perhaps we are just very tired, and we really notice this when we stop all of our activity for a while. It may also seem strange at first to practice wakefulness in this lying-down position.

Exercise 5: Body Scan with Compassionate Focus

Find a comfortable place to lie down, on the bed or on the floor, remembering that your intention is to foster kindness and wakefulness and not to fall asleep. If you fall asleep, then it may be that you are tired and need to rest—so pay attention to your body and what it needs. Try not to come to the practice when you are fighting off tiredness. If you like, you can do the exercise sitting upright. Ensure that you will not be disturbed while you do this practice and that you will be warm enough; cover yourself with a blanket if necessary.

Close your eyes and focus for a while on the rising and falling of the diaphragm as you breathe, and then become aware of the movement of the breath throughout the body. Feel the sense of release and letting go as each out-breath leaves the body. Then, take a few moments to become aware of your body as a whole: the outline of your skin, the weight of your body, and the sense of gravity bearing down upon it. Notice the points where your body is in contact with the surfaces it rests upon. Now place your hand on your heart as a reminder to be kind to yourself. Take three deep, relaxing breaths and then place your arms by your sides.

Imagine that your attention is infused with a warm glow of kindness and then bring your attention to the big toes of both of your feet, exploring the sensations that you find here. You are not trying to make anything happen—you are just feeling what you are feeling. Gradually broaden your awareness to include your other toes, the soles of your feet, and the other parts of your feet. Simply feel the sensations as they are and soften around them. Bring a sense of gratitude to your feet: they work so hard for us yet we pay them so little attention. Then imagine that you are breathing into both your feet on the in-breath, and breathing out from this part of the body into the space surrounding it on the out-breath.

Gradually move the warm glow of your attention up your body to your ankles, calves, knees, and thighs, simply experiencing the sensations you encounter; always being sure that your attention is tender and saturated with gratitude and respect for each part of your body. Now let the soft glow of your attention move up to your buttocks and notice if you are holding any tension in this part of the body; if so, soften around it with your awareness. Then imagine that you are breathing into this part of the body on the in-breath, and breathing out from this part of the body into the space surrounding it on the out-breath. As you breathe in, imagine that you are holding the entirety of the lower part of your body within your awareness and as you breathe out, imagine that you release this part of your body within your awareness.

When you notice that your mind has drifted off into thinking or dreaming or planning, as it will do very often, simply notice this and return to the sensations in your body—no judgment, no sense of getting it wrong, as this is just what the mind does. And then gradually move your soft attention to your abdomen, lower and upper back, shoulders, rib cage, and chest. Every now and again, pause and bring a sense of gratitude and tenderness to the part of the body you are holding in awareness, reflecting on what it does for you and how, so often, you may take it for granted.

Now bring kind awareness to your spine, gently curving through your body, and the point at which it meets the skull. Have a sense of the solid frame of your body. Then bring your awareness down your arms and into your hands, fingers, and fingertips. Notice the warmth and energy that is stored in the palms of your hands. Notice what the hands feel like at rest. And then once again imagine that you are breathing into your torso on the in-breath and breathing out from this part of the body into the space surrounding it on the out-breath.

Then gradually bring the soft glow of awareness to your head, neck, throat, and face, noting any tension held in the muscles around the forehead, around the eyes, the jaw, and the mouth. Notice how sensitive your face feels to the temperature of the air in the room. Allow your face to soften.

Now sweep your attention from your head back down to your feet again, but more quickly this time, and then bring your attention back to your breathing. Pay attention to the movement of the breath in your body as a whole—as if your whole body is breathing and is held in the warm glow of your awareness. When you are about to finish the practice, place your han on your heart again as a final gesture of kindness, and slowly start moving your body, rolling over onto one side, and then gradually getting up. This will help get the body moving again and reduce stiffness. Make sure not to jar yourself back into ordinary awareness too quickly.

Body Awareness and Compassion

This practice lays the foundation for our training in mindful compassion because we are learning to hold our experience within our awareness. At one level, the body-scan practice is concerned with progressively moving our attention through our body and noticing the sensations that arise and pass with focused attention—this is the mindfulness element. But at another level the practice is designed to help us develop our ability to stay present with difficult feelings in a warm and inclusive way, rather than moving away from what we find uncomfortable or painful—this is the compassionate element. This is important for developing our compassionate capacity, which is the ability to contain our inner emotional world as a basis for relating to it with kindness. This is in contrast to the feeling that we "cannot hold it together," in which we feel that we cannot contain the turbulent movement of our emotions and then end up dumping them on others or looking for external sources of relief like alcohol or drugs.

What helps in developing compassionate capacity is grounding our awareness in the body as an access point to the soothing/affiliation system. Threat- and drive-focused emotions tend to draw our attention into the head as the pivotal lookout point for detecting threats or seeking what we want. This can disconnect us from the body, which is often experienced as a mental image, a poor reflection of magazine icons of what looks good and attractive. And this poor self-image is often accompanied by feelings of self-loathing. However, the body scan allows us to step behind the image and experience our bodies from the inside. We learn to cultivate an awareness of the inner flow of feeling, sensation, and energy within the body.

The mindfulness element is the careful attending to the detail of our inner flow of sensation and feeling, noticing when our mind drifts away, and gently bringing it back; the compassion element is the sense of tuning in to the sensory awareness of our inner world and learning to meet the difficult edges of our inner landscape of experience with softness. With mindfulness, we move toward the flow of sensation, and with compassion, we softly engage and relax around the detail of our experience, holding it with a kindly awareness. Relating to our bodies in this way anchors us in the soothing/affiliative system because it allows for the opening up of our awareness and resting in our present-moment experience, rather than being fraught and always on the move.

Now, whenever we lose contact with this emotional system, our body gives us immediate cues—some part of our body contracts, our awareness shoots up into our head, and we start to experience the body in an objective way—somewhat at a distance as a mental image. These are signs that threat and drive emotions have seized control of our attention. In this way, the body is our friend because when we notice this, all we need to do is pause, focus on the breath, and bring our attention back to whatever feelings are occurring within our body.

For example, imagine we are shopping in a supermarket and we see somebody who offended us in some way. Immediately, we may feel a surge of anger, and a story starts to form in our mind as we remember what the person did to us. If we let ourselves just go with the story, we may find our body tensing around the shoulders, our jaw becoming tight, and may even start to feel that at any moment we may pick up a can of baked beans and throw it at the person! All the while, the story gains momentum in our head spinning round and round like a stuck record. This is one scenario. Alternatively, through learning to ground our awareness in the body, as soon as the first surge of anger arises and our memories start fueling a storyline, we can bring our attention to our body and notice where we are feeling tense and contracted, thereby tuning in to the sensations in our shoulders and jaw. We can incline our attention toward the sensations (mindfulness) and then simply feel them as they are with softness and kindness (compassion). This breaks the storyline we are caught up in and grounds our emotions in the body.

In this way we learn to rely on the body as a support and come to trust that we can contain our own emotional experience and do not need to project it outward and throw the baked beans across the aisle. This does not mean that we *suppress* the feelings of anger. Instead, we create a different relationship with them.

Sitting Practice

We are now at the point of setting up a daily sitting practice. We do sitting practice because it provides us with regular periods of training in mindfulness every day. This is not a withdrawal from life, but a way of building up the capacity from which to engage more fully with our lives. Working with the mind is not easy and changing ingrained habits takes time and consistent application. So while it is useful to incorporate mindfulness into everyday life, and indeed the reason why we do this training is to lead more mindful and compassionate lives, it is also important to devote time every day for sitting practice (even only fifteen to twenty minutes). The sitting practice is like a daily refueling point in which we recharge our batteries.

Posture

In doing sitting practice, the first thing to consider is our posture. It reflects our intention and state of mind. If we can develop a correct posture, then we will find it easier for our minds to settle. We will also feel stable and sufficiently comfortable in our bodies to maintain a meditation posture for a longer period of time. We can choose to practice sitting in a chair or on the floor. If you choose a chair, try one that is relatively upright and that allows you to place your feet flat upon the floor. Try to sit a little away from the back of the chair so your back is self-supporting. It may help to place a small cushion at the small of your back for some support.

If you choose to sit on the floor, it will help to have a meditation cushion or bench to raise your buttocks off the floor. If you use a cushion, try to sit on the front end of it. It is important that your knees are close to the ground, no higher than your buttocks, and that your thighs are sloping down toward the ground. This will support your back and maintain the hollow in the small of your back. These postures involve either crossing your legs in front of you with one heel drawn toward the body and the other leg in front of it, or kneeling using a cushion or stool with your feet behind you.

It is important to find a posture that is comfortable and that supports a wakeful and alert state of mind as you do not want to doze off. So find a posture that reflects this—upright, with your spine erect, but not rigid. Become aware of the natural curvature of your spine and the soft arch in your lower back. The head is gently poised at the top of the spine with your chin tucked in slightly. Relax your shoulders. Lower and soften the gaze of your eyes at about a 45-degree angle or gently close your eyes. The head, neck, and shoulders are vertically aligned. The chest does not sink in, but gently lifts. Imagine a golden thread pulling you up slightly from the top of your head. Rest your hands in your lap, cupped one inside the other. It can be helpful to place the tongue on the ridge behind the upper front teeth.

Key Elements of Sitting Practice

When we sit down to practice, we often find that our mind is still busily engaged with the activities of the day. So once we have settled into a comfortable posture, it can be useful to engage with the soothing breathing rhythm (exercise 3) for about five minutes to help settle the mind sufficiently to engage with mindfulness practice. This phase marks a break with the activities of the day; it clears some of the self-talk and chatter we may have carried over from our last interactions with people.

We then bring our awareness more fully into the body by doing the grounding phase. We have introduced ourselves to this stage by doing the body-scan practice above. We can very easily lose our sense of embodiment through the speedy lives we live and through the activity of the threat and drive systems that draw our attention into the head, as we explored above. Grounding our awareness in the body acknowledges the totality of who we are—we are embodied beings, not just busy heads suspended on inert bodies.

Once we have grounded our awareness in the body, we let go of any sense of needing to do anything, and just rest. It is useful at this point to give up any idea of trying to meditate, as this instills a sense of striving in the mind. A good analogy for this stage is opening our hand, which is holding a pebble, and allowing the pebble to just rest there; we neither clasp it tightly nor throw it on the ground. We just let it be there. Similarly, we allow our mental and emotional experience to be held within our body as a field of awareness—we just sit there and do nothing. Through the resting stage, we get a glimpse of the fact that the mind has a natural tendency to be at rest, like water left undisturbed, and we see how constant involvement with thinking disturbs the mind.

Resting is a way of entering the mode of *being*. Normally, much of our life is locked into the mode of *doing* and even when we stop doing things with our body, our mind never seems to stop. Through grounding and resting, we learn simply to be with whatever is present in our experience right now. It is like learning to shift down a gear. A chronic affliction of modern life is that we operate in high gear all the time and seem to have lost the ability to shift down—we have lost the ability to just *be*. Put differently, we have lost the ability to access the soothing system, and we are perpetually locked into the high-activity modes of threat and drive.

Resting is the most profound form of sitting practice, sometimes described as *choiceless awareness*. We get a glimpse of it, but due to the power of distraction, we may find that our attention is quickly carried away by thoughts. This is the point where we introduce a mindfulness support. It is a reference point for our attention to return to when we notice that we get lost in thought, and it is an anchor to hold our attention in the present moment. We normally use one of the senses as a support; in this case, we use breathing.

When we work with a mindfulness support, the important thing is to maintain the quality of resting when we focus on the support so we don't clasp tightly around the support but touch it lightly with our attention. We also remain connected with our body and the mode of being. It is not a top-down process of focusing tightly on the support and keeping thoughts away; that is a form of control that will instill tension in the mind and will suppress our emotional life. Instead it is a bottom-up process of engaging lightly with the support when we drift off, but remaining grounded in the body. So the support is always there and we know that we can return to it at any moment, but our awareness is largely grounded in the body. In this way we can see that the initial stages of slowing down, grounding, and resting are the foundations for the sitting practice, and remain in place when we work with a support.

In the beginning it can be useful to identify the stages of sitting practice in a step-by-step way, but these stages should not be seen as distinct compartments; they are a continuous flow. It is like learning to drive a car: we are taught each of the stages as if they were distinct and separate, like turning on the ignition, releasing the hand brake, putting our foot on the clutch, and moving the gears; but once we know what to do, we just get in and drive the car. Mindfulness is similar—the reason for identifying the stages is so that you become familiar with them and then find your own way of embodying the process.

Before introducing the sitting practice, there are some useful tips to bear in mind; these are relevant to all the exercises we do in this practice section of the book.

Start When Things Are Easy

If you think of anything that you would like to learn, such as swimming, playing the piano, or driving a car, it's always best to start off when things are easy. It's not a good idea to learn how to swim once you've fallen overboard in a storm, but rather to start in the shallow end of a warm swimming pool. Similarly, it is best to do these practices when you feel relatively stable and settled, and in this way you *build up capacity* to relate to the mind when things get tough.

No Time to Practice

Sometimes we find that our lives are so busy that it's difficult to put time aside to practice. This is very common. If you find that you can't set aside time for formal practice, then try to find times when you naturally have space, such as when sitting on a train or waiting for a bus. We also suggest trying to begin each day with a short practice if you can't manage any longer. Always remember that if it doesn't work out and you can't find the time to practice, this is not a reason to beat yourself up; it's just an opportunity to try again.

Practice Takes Patience

Doing practice is like training to get fit—it proceeds in a step-by-step way. If we are training to run a marathon, it's better to run a small distance the first day, a little more the next day, and so on. We don't expect ourselves to run twenty-six miles on day one! Mindfulness training is similar—it is like building up a muscle we already have that needs regular training. Sometimes people may try some of these exercises but then feel disappointed if they do not seem to work for them immediately. But life is not like this—*things take time*. So it is important to remind ourselves to be patient and work steadily on the practices. Then the benefits will gradually start to reveal themselves.

Exercise 6: Mindfulness Sitting Practice

Soothing Breathing Rhythm

Begin by settling into your posture, which is like a container for your practice. Then for a few minutes, engage with your soothing breathing rhythm, slightly deepening and slowing your breathing and allowing your awareness to flow softly with the movement of the breath, letting it soothe you and bring you more fully into the body. Then focus a little more on the out-breath and notice how when you breathe out, the body relaxes a little, and how your center of gravity begins to drop from your head into your body (see exercise 5).

Grounding

Now let your breathing fall back to its normal rhythm and bring your attention more fully into the body. Become aware of the contact and pressure where your body rests on the seat or the ground below you, and gently tune in to the sensations in the body. Do this in a relaxed and open way and allow the sensations to present themselves to you: you may be aware of the temperature of your body—warm, cold, or neutral; perhaps there is a slight pain in your right shoulder or a feeling of tension in one of your knees; or maybe there is a contraction in your stomach related to an emotion you are feeling.

Some people find that a systematic scanning of the body works best for them. If this is the case, then begin at the feet and move progressively up through the body, becoming aware of whatever sensations are present, ending up with the head, and then returning to the feet again. Others find that a random approach suits them better, in which case simply sit there and allow sensations to command your attention as they arise. Note the presence of the sensation and then relax around it until the next one appears and commands your attention. This stage does not involve analysis or investigation; you are just acknowledging the presence of sensations and relaxing around them. Notice how doing this holds your attention in the moment.

Once you have scanned your body or allowed your attention to be drawn to particular sensations, then become aware of your body as a whole, as if you are holding your whole body within your awareness. Then become aware of the space around you: notice how the body exists in space and is surrounded by it.

Resting

Now let go of any sense of trying to do anything and just be there—let go of trying to meditate. Keep your eyes open and, in a relaxed, almost casual way, allow yourself to experience whatever comes to you via your senses; but don't look at anything or listen for anything. Simply be where you are and in touch with whatever comes to you. So, for example, you may become aware of the room: objects are seen without being looked at; the same is true of sounds—you hear them because they are present but without listening in a particular way. See if you can rest in this way for a short while. When you notice that your mind drifts away and becomes involved with thoughts, which will happen very soon, then move on to the next stage, which is using breathing as a support to hold your attention in the present moment.

Breath Support

Rest your attention lightly on the natural rhythm of your breathing, and tune in to it wherever you find it most easily in your body—this could be the breath coming and going through your nostrils, your abdomen rising and falling, the sensation of the breath leaving your body, or the feeling of your whole body breathing. It does not matter where you rest your attention; what is important is to have a light touch—not shutting out thoughts and emotions, but allowing them to come and go.

So the practice is simple—breathing in, you are aware you are breathing in; breathing out, you know you are breathing out. In this way the breath is like an anchor holding your attention in the body, holding it present. When you find that your attention has drifted off into thinking, simply notice this and return your attention to the breath—no sense of succeeding or failing, just noticing and returning.

Once you come to the end of your designated practice session, spend a few moments resting without focusing on anything in particular and let go of the idea of trying to meditate. You could say to yourself: *nothing to do, nowhere to go, and nothing to achieve*. Then stretch your body and slowly get up. See if you can carry the awareness of your sitting session into the next moments of your day.

Little and Often

Although it is helpful to have a regular daily practice because this helps you become familiar with the principles of mindfulness and a wandering mind, it is also very helpful to bring mindfulness into your everyday life on a moment-by-moment basis. What is important is *to remember* to be mindful. Simply notice where your mind is at any given moment and what kinds of thoughts, emotions, and sensations you are experiencing. In fact, there is increasing evidence *that little and often* can be especially helpful. So you can practice standing at a bus stop or sitting on the train or stopping for a coffee break. To help you to do this, you could write an "M" on the back of your hand or place a small pebble in your pocket that will act as a memory cue. So practice creating as many mindful moments as you can throughout your day.

Conclusion

Sitting practice provides the foundation for the compassion practices that follow. For these practices to be effective, we need to cultivate the stability that comes from mindfulness practice. Before we can engage with difficulty, in ourselves and others, it helps to feel grounded in the present moment.

Through practicing mindfulness sitting practice, we are laying the foundations for building compassionate capacity. In particular, we are learning to access the soothing/affiliation system. We are learning to notice when our attention is captured by threat- and drive-focused emotions, and to bring it back within the domain of the soothing system. But, as we well know, this emotional system is not our default mode, so it takes practice and training to learn to step into it. This is the role of mindfulness training in this context.

Key Stages

- Clarifying our motive before we start

- Becoming aware of our unsettled mind

- Recognizing the importance of the breath

- Learning to skillfully direct our attention

- Slowing down and learning to develop a steady base in our body

- Noticing that our awareness can open up to what is all around us

- Learning to ground our awareness in the body

- Sitting meditation: Following the stages of soothing breathing, grounding, resting, and mindfulness support

8

WORKING WITH ACCEPTANCE

Habitual Reactions

When we practice mindfulness, we can often run into strong or difficult emotions. As we mentioned in chapters 5 and 6, mindfulness and compassion practice can open up space for unprocessed emotions to surface, and we may even experience things becoming more difficult when we begin to work with our minds in this way. However, this phenomenon, although very common, may be disconcerting at first. In fact, if we look at what is going on more closely, we are mostly becoming *more aware* of what has been there all along, and this increase in awareness is a sign that things are actually getting better. A useful metaphor for mindfulness practice is going into a darkened room and gradually turning up a dimmer switch so that the light reveals more and more of what is in the room. Now we see many useful and interesting things in the room, but we may also see all kinds of junk piled up in the dusty corners.

What we also begin to see is the way in which our minds follow narrow patterns of reaction and how this can ensnare and limit us. There are emotions and experiences we like, experiences we do not like, and other experiences we ignore and "tune out" of. We begin to see how we associate happiness with getting what we want and unhappiness with either not getting what we want or getting what we don't want. This was a key part of the Buddha's teaching of the Four Noble Truths that we looked at in chapter 1.

This is especially the case with our inner world. It can be a threatening place to inhabit because we are not in control of what arises and yet we often have a strong vested interest in what does arise. We can have strong preferences for how we want to feel, so when difficult emotions or mind states arise, there can be an immediate reaction and resistance. We might be sitting there meditating peacefully and thinking, "This is going to be a good day; I am in a good mood and full of energy." And then, out of the blue, an anxious mood appears and weaves a troublesome storyline that closes in on us and threatens our peace; and then we think, "Oh no, this is going to ruin my day. What can I do to preserve the feeling of peace, which I need to get through the day?"

So we can then find ourselves resisting these anxious feelings and doing whatever we can to get rid of them. In this way, our threat system is constantly on the lookout for experiences we do not want to have. But this instills a sense of conflict and stress within us, and our attempts to get rid of unwanted mind states generally backfire on us because we cannot so easily get rid of feelings and emotions.

This is because different rules apply to our inner world as compared to the outer world. If we see someone we don't like, we can find a way to avoid them, but if we feel an emotion that we do not like, it is not so easy to get away from because it is inside us and part of us. All we end up doing is either suppressing it or projecting it onto other people or situations. For example, if we feel angry or irritated, we can either find ways to push these feelings down or target people close to us as a way of offloading these feelings. But more often than not, this is like throwing gasoline on a fire; it just flares up more strongly or starts burning in a different place. And even if we do manage to get rid of what we don't want, the action of pushing it away can cause a tension in our mind and body.

Familiarization and Cultivation

In the Tibetan Buddhist tradition "meditation" has two meanings: *familiarization* and *cultivation*. First, we become familiar with what is there, and then we cultivate what is beneficial and useful. In the context of this chapter, *familiarization* means becoming aware of our ingrained tendencies to like, dislike, and tune out, and seeing how these reactions are driven by conditioned tendencies of which we are largely unaware. We then see how these habits shape how we react to our inner and outer worlds and how they can close us down. So this first stage is very important because it brings awareness to what is actually going on in our minds, and it may be startling just how unaware we may be of the powerful habits that drive us. Now, when it comes to the process of familiarization, mindfulness is the key skill we are working with because the role of mindfulness is to bring more and more awareness to these habits so we are not held in their power.

As we develop some level of stability, we are then in a position to make choices based on wise and compassionate discernment—seeing how one habit serves us and how another habit does not. This is the second meaning of "meditation" within the Tibetan Buddhist tradition. It is expressly *cultivating* wholesome habits and not feeding unwholesome ones. When the Buddha described his teaching, he summed it up in this way: not feeding what is unwholesome, cultivating what is wholesome, and taming the mind. As we become more and more familiar with what arises in the mind through mindfulness practice, we can then expressly cultivate tendencies and habits that result in the emergence of the wise and compassionate self. In this chapter, we are looking at the process of familiarization in more detail, and how to work creatively with habitual reactions that arise. On the basis of this, we move on to the stage of cultivation in the subsequent chapters, which focus more specifically on compassion practices.

To reiterate, when we practice mindfulness, we become aware of our patterns of preference and reaction. Each one of us is unique with respect to our inner environment, and each one of us has very particular patterns of preference—what we like to experience, what we do not like to experience, and what we are not interested in. When we practice mindfulness, we simply notice and bring awareness to these patterns; we do not try to stop them or block them. We become intimately aware of the mental grooves that our energies flow down, and we then learn to come to terms with our unique patterns of preference. So the process is first to see what is going on by turning up the dimmer switch and then to accept what is going on. This brings us to the main topic of this chapter.

Intention, Attention, and Acceptance

It may be useful at this point to refine our understanding of mindfulness. This will give us greater clarity as to the processes involved when we work with our minds in more focused ways. There are always three aspects to mindfulness practice: intention, attention, and acceptance. As described in the previous chapter, first, we need to form the intention to be mindful and not to get lost in thought. Then we train our attention to notice when we become distracted and to return to what we are doing in the present moment. So every time our attention drifts off, there is a period of loss of awareness and then we remember that we are trying to be mindful. Our intention wakes us up and is the agent of remembering or recollection. What then follows is a moment of noticing where our attention is, which is like waking up from a dream or from whatever mental video we are absorbed in. We then redirect our attention back to the focus of our mindfulness, perhaps washing the dishes or observing the breath.

The final element, acceptance, is very important. Every time we lose awareness and drift off, there is an acceptance of this occurrence, of distraction. If the acceptance is not there, our inner world can become harsh and judgmental, and we might find that we give ourselves a hard time in the name of mindfulness. We might even try to force ourselves to be mindful rather than creating the conditions for it. Also, if we do not accept our wayward mind that repeatedly drifts off into distraction, we can end up reacting to it instead, and this merely sets in motion another stream of distracting thoughts and loss of awareness.

Therefore each of these components needs to be in place and working together: we intend to be mindful; we lose mindfulness and get lost in thought; we notice this and accept what is happening; and then we bring our attention back to the mindfulness support. We are back with the support for a few moments, and then we get lost in thought again. Intention enables us to remember what we are trying to do; attention brings us back; and acceptance wipes the slate clean so we are not carrying any baggage of reactive thoughts into the next moment.

What is important to see here too is that acceptance is an entry point to compassion training because it is that quality of mind that acknowledges that we are not perfect and makes room for the imperfections within our experience. Without acceptance we might find that attitudes of judgment and self-criticism or dislike creep in through the back door and undermine our whole endeavor. Also, without the quality of noncondemning and being open to whatever actually happens, we might find that our practice falls prey to the threat-focused emotions of anxiety and anger: fear that we are getting it wrong, or anger that we are not doing it right. It might also fall prey to the drive-oriented emotions of getting it right and feeling we are becoming good at it. Consequently, the quality of acceptance keeps us grounded within the present moment and prevents our practice from being eroded and slipping under the power of the default modes of threat and drive. Simply being okay with whatever happens—knowing what is happening while it is happening and without judgment—cuts through all of this and keeps our efforts well rooted in the soothing system. This enables our mindfulness practice to provide a proper foundation for the compassion practices that follow.

Experiential Acceptance

We now explore the process of acceptance in more detail because it is a key part of mindfulness practice and it lays the foundation for the compassion practices that follow. Instead of reacting to the fact that our mind is perpetually distracted, we accept this fact; we give our mind permission to be the way it is, and we do not fight with this reality. We accept that our attention is not going to stay with the mindfulness support for very long and will drift off into thinking, and we accept that most of the time we are not able to be mindful because the tendency to become distracted is very strong. What this does is put us into clear alignment with what is actually going on in our inner world from moment to moment, rather than being in opposition to it.

In the academic literature on acceptance, this is described as *experiential acceptance*.[1] This means that the primary object of acceptance is our moment-by-moment experience rather than what caused the experience or the person behind it. In the example of getting angry, experiential acceptance focuses on the actual feelings of being angry rather than what triggered the anger or the predispositions of the person who became angry. This is contrasted with *experiential avoidance*, which psychologists

217

Neharika Chawla and Brian Ostafin describe as "unwillingness to remain in contact with private experiences such as painful thoughts and emotions."[2] We also suggest that this unwillingness can be outside of voluntary control, as in the case of people who are in denial or even dissociate; here it is not so much a voluntary unwillingness but rather that our minds become so disorganized and threat focused that they automatically switch off and tune out.[3] In this case, willingness is the step-by-step process of gradually recognizing and choosing to dissolve those defenses that block us from knowing. As we mentioned in chapter 5, emotional avoidance is one of the main ways in which mindfulness can be undermined, so clearly understanding experiential acceptance is very important in keeping our practice on the right track.

Before we can change something, we have to be clear about what it is that we are working with—this is the essential meaning of acceptance. If we want to scrape down and repaint a wall, we need to study closely the existing condition of the wall so we are clear where to apply our efforts and what parts we want to scrape down and clean. Similarly, if we want to work in a realistic way with our minds, we need to come to terms with what is actually going on so we can intelligently appraise what we are going to do next. If we react to our inner experiences or resist what is going on, this merely confuses the issue.

This point is important and really needs reflecting on. If we become absorbed in our reaction to a difficulty, then this is all we experience and it will then be hard to relate to the difficulty itself. The process of acceptance opens up the space around our experience so that both the difficulty and our reaction to it can be present. It is like standing in front of the wall with dark sunglasses so we cannot see any of the blemishes or cracks, when instead what we need to do is take off the sunglasses and pay close attention. This is the meaning of acceptance in the context of mindfulness practice.

Unfortunately, the English word "acceptance" has certain connotations that can cause us to misunderstand what the process is all about. As John C. Williams and Steven Lynn point out, "The etymological root of acceptance is the Latin *acceptare*, the Old French *accepter*, and finally the Middle English *accept* used by Chaucer and Wyclif in the 14th century. To accept is to receive willingly or with approval, to take toward rather than cast away...."[4] Now this is not quite what we mean by acceptance in this context. It does not mean that we condone or approve of negative states of mind; it just means that we see clearly what is going on. It also does not mean that once we accept something, we are stuck with it for good; it is not a state of resignation. Quite the contrary, it is the first step toward effective change. It also does not mean that we have to like what is going on; it just means that we do not fool ourselves about what is going on. For example, we might be experiencing bouts of low mood or even depression. Accepting this state of affairs means facing what is actually happening— not denying the depression, not condoning it, not liking it, not indulging in it, and not resigning ourselves to always being depressed. It simply means seeing clearly what is happening so we know what to do next—for example, seek help rather than shamefully hide. It is based on the understanding that reaction and resistance to what is happening merely add another level of confusion and suffering on top of whatever is already afflicting us. So reaction and resistance are like adding fuel to a fire.

We can even go so far as to say that the main issue is not so much what happens, but how we react to what happens—we might have cancer and that is very difficult, but refusing to accept it makes it much more difficult to endure or seek treatment. We may have lost our partner and that is painful, but refusing to acknowledge that this has happened, or constantly replaying the past to imagine a different outcome, turns the situation into a waking nightmare. We may be experiencing feelings of low mood and anxiety, but if we refuse to accept this because it does not stack up to how we want to see our self, it makes the situation worse. In a way, self-criticism is linked to lacking acceptance because lack of acceptance is why we are attacking ourselves. Therefore, not only is there the suffering of the problem itself, but there is also the suffering of nonacceptance of the problem, and often the latter can hurt far more.

There is a famous sutra—a teaching of the Buddha—called the sutra of the arrow.[5] According to this sutra, even the wise and the good are struck by the first arrow, which is the unavoidable pain of life, like getting sick, making mistakes, and suffering various misfortunes; but most people are struck by a second arrow that is more painful than the first arrow because it lands very close to the initial wound, and this is the arrow of nonacceptance, resistance, and struggle—not being willing to face or feel the wound of the first arrow.

In mindfulness practice, the skill of acceptance, or nonresistance, is crucial because it enables us to let ourselves off the hook and to return to the freshness of the present moment without encumbering it with layer upon layer of reactivity and struggle. So acceptance is a realistic way to approach our lives and our minds. It is a willingness *to see clearly* the facts before us, even if they are difficult to take on board. It expresses an intention of moving toward, taking in, and working with what is difficult and painful rather than moving away in denial or pushing things under the carpet. It allows us to start from where we are, not from where we might like to be, and this provides the ground from which genuine change can take place.

It is also important to remember, however, that the *alleviation* of suffering is crucial to compassion. If your hand is by the fire, then it makes sense to remove it from the source of pain. We can accept being depressed, do not need to blame ourselves for it, and fight or hate it, but that does not mean to say that we don't try to get treatment!

Two Psychologies of Compassion

In working with acceptance, we can return to the compassion circles that we described in chapter 4 as they hold the key to the process of acceptance. As discussed in this chapter, we are dealing with two distinct psychologies when it comes to compassion: on the one hand, we are called upon to open up to, engage with, and feel the pain of our experience, while, on the other hand, we need to draw on the inner resource of our positive emotional systems to hold, soften, and alleviate this pain. So the inner ring of attributes requires us to move toward the things we are anxious about or avoiding, allowing ourselves to be touched by suffering and learning to tolerate and understand it. The outer ring is concerned with skills for building our resources of inner strength and authority, connecting to our innate wisdom, and cultivating our capacity for warmth and kindness.

Mindfulness and acceptance practice play fundamental roles within each of these psychologies. In the psychology of engagement, they clearly facilitate this process so that we don't turn away and can hold what comes up. In the psychology of alleviation, mindfulness helps us to turn our attention to what is helpful and hold our focus on, say, loving-kindness.[6] Acceptance helps engagement because we don't turn away or fight our difficult experiences, but acceptance is very important with alleviation too because it helps us accept that as social beings, all of us can feel the power of compassion and kindness through connectedness. Some individuals learn to tolerate and accept *painful* things in themselves but are less comfortable with accepting their needs for *love and kindness.* They can find these feelings extremely difficult to accept within themselves because of what they can stir up, such as sadness or perhaps a realization of disconnection in the past. Even if people feel genuine compassion for others, deep in their heart they know they are blocked when it comes to accepting and experiencing compassion for themselves. So not only do we learn to accept our pain, but we also need to be open, allowing, and accepting of feelings of loving-kindness as a healing process.[7] As we noted in chapter 6, *acceptance of positive feelings* and, in particular, feelings of affiliation, can be as crucial as acceptance of negative and difficult feelings.

How Do We Practice Acceptance?

Let's now look at how to practice acceptance by working with the attributes of compassion in more detail. They are part of the compassion circle we looked at in chapter 4. As a way of illustrating the process, we will work with anxiety as an example.

Motivation

This is always the starting point. If we are not motivated to work with ourselves and try to come to terms with what we are going through, then we will struggle with the other stages. We return to this point again and again. In this context, motivation means being willing to step outside our rigid defensive ways of reacting to things and face what we are really feeling. If we are sitting meditating and feeling at peace, for example, and then there is an unwelcome knock on the door of our inner world and a feeling of anxiety threatens to intrude on our peace, motivation means being willing to turn toward what is unexpected and unwelcome. It is cultivating the willingness to face what is happening and step out of preferred avoidance. This is based on the wisdom that blocking out or denying our experience merely creates conflict in our mind and intensifies whatever we are going through.

Sensitivity

When we step out of denial, we are able to notice, pay attention to, and recognize what is actually happening in our field of experience. Returning to our example, when anxiety arises, we acknowledge it and we name it. We notice where it is in the body. In so doing, the emotion loses some of its power over us. The simple act of acknowledging takes some of the sting out of what we resist and do not like.

Sometimes we can find ourselves becoming anxious about being angry, or fearful about being fearful, and this has the effect of activating the threat system and before we know it, we are caught in a vicious circle. What we need to do is break that feedback loop and step back from it. We can do that by simply recognizing what is happening instead of automatically reacting to it.

Sympathy

As we recognize what is there, we let it touch us. We notice the thoughts and feelings "about" feeling anxious. We are not involved in a cold, detached process of observation like a scientist peering down a microscope. We allow ourselves to be moved by what we experience. In many ways this follows from the first two stages—once we are willing to face things and turn our attention toward what is happening, sympathy can naturally arise. Instead of shutting feelings of loneliness and anxiety out of our hearts by closing the door and pretending that they are not there, we open the door and let them touch us. It is like being prepared to open the door to a beggar who is looking for food and shelter and paying attention to his disheveled condition, taking his humanity and his pain on board, and not shutting off from it. In some cases, we may find that our hearts are closed to sympathy and we do not feel emotionally moved by things. In this case, we need to work more on the resources of loving-kindness and compassion, which relate to the outer circle of skills we explore in the next chapter. Also, in order to allow ourselves to be moved by something, we must learn how to tolerate it. If we cannot tolerate the sight of the beggar at the door, there is not much chance of us feeling sympathy for his condition because all we will want to do is shut the door in his face. This brings us to the next stage.

Tolerance

In practicing acceptance, a key quality is that of *allowing*. This is the meaning of tolerance in this context. Even though we may have acknowledged the presence of an emotion, we can still feel it without truly wanting to experience it. We may have opened the door to the beggar and recognized who he is, but are unwilling to let him in (in Latin, "acceptance" means "taking in"). So in this stage, we work more directly with resistance. Through resisting we are trying to stop an emotion from arising because we think we can't allow it to take hold of us or we may feel that we cannot deal with it. We might fear that if we let the beggar in, he might take over or do something. But tolerance doesn't mean that we have to jump straight into the things we are fearful of; rather, we practice a gradual process of allowing, in which we open up a little more and then a little more. But, as we have seen, trying to block our emotions adds another layer of conflict and suffering to what is already there—not only is there the feeling we are struggling with, but now also our resistance to experiencing it. This just adds fuel to the fire.

Instead, through allowing, we say to ourselves: "Okay, anxiety is present, so I will be open to it and work with it rather than trying to push it away." When we are open to things in this way, they become workable and genuine change becomes possible. However, being open to what we are experiencing does not mean jumping in the deep end or wallowing in our feelings or acting them out. It simply means giving ourselves space to feel what we are feeling by gently holding our feelings in our awareness, softening around them, and not imposing judgments on them. In so doing, we can open more fully to what we are experiencing, and this brings us more fully into the present. Instead of judging or manipulating how we feel, we can simply maintain an open presence in the face of it.

Clearly, in order to be able to tolerate and allow our experiences, we need to be able to hold them. If the feeling of anxiety is too strong, we may not be able to work with this stage because we do not have the inner resources to contain it. For this reason, the preliminary stages of mindfulness training that we covered in the previous chapter are very important for building up a sense of inner stability so that we feel able to tolerate what we are going through. In particular, if we can remember to let go of our usual preoccupations and sense how we are feeling in the body during the grounding phase, we may find it much easier to tolerate what we are going through. Furthermore, the chapters on compassion that follow build on the sense of stability that derives from mindfulness by anchoring us in the qualities of the compassionate self so that we feel confident enough to hold and engage with our difficulties.

Empathy

As we allow a difficult emotion to enter our field of awareness, the next step is to try to understand the part of ourselves that is calling for attention. In the case of anxiety, it means gently tuning in to and connecting with what it needs, what wisdom it has to offer us, and what it requires in order to be soothed. In chapter 4, we defined empathy as the ability to understand and emotionally recognize the feelings, motives, and intentions of another human being. But first we need to have empathy *for the different parts of ourselves* (see chapter 2). Now the arising of empathy depends on the previous attributes being activated—we seek to step out of denial (motivation), recognize what is present (sensitivity), let ourselves be moved by what we experience (sympathy), and allow our emotions to unfold and abide in their own way (tolerance).

An important aspect of empathy is being curious about the details of our experience so that we can learn about it and come to a wise understanding. We need to be willing to inquire into what is going on inside of us, instead of just assuming that we know what our experience is and reacting automatically. Often we think we know what we are experiencing—"I just don't like being on my own, that's all," or "This is just an old hang-up from childhood"—without understanding the complex emotional memories and bodily experiences involved (see chapters 2 and 3). If we reflect more deeply, we discover that there is more to any experience than we can know at first glance. So we need to be willing to ask ourselves "What is going on here?" and really look with an open mind, instead of thinking that we already know.

It can help if we allow ourselves to be aware of and develop empathy for the different parts of the self by inquiring into them in this way: "What is going on with my angry self?" or "What is going on with my anxious self?" The more we recognize these *multiple* aspects of ourselves, the more we can mindfully accept them as being a family of different selves. Mindful acceptance means we do not overpersonalize, overidentify with, or blame ourselves for these selves; nor do we just allow them to control the show.

In this particular context, we practice empathy by applying the four foundations of mindfulness, which derive from the teachings of the Buddha and which we touched on briefly in chapter 5. Here, we will again use anxiety as an example to illustrate the process.

- *Mindfulness of the body*: Notice where the anxiety is held within the body. There might be a contraction in the chest or tightness in the shoulders, a sickness in the stomach, shaky limbs. We then notice what kind of sensations we are experiencing in this part of the body—maybe there is tightness, tension, cold, a vibration, and so on. Notice if we are resisting these sensations. Then notice what happens if we open to them with kindness and acceptance.

- *Mindfulness of feelings*: Notice if the primary feeling is unpleasant, pleasant, or neutral. In the case of anxiety, it is likely to feel unpleasant. See if we can meet this feeling with acceptance. Then notice what layers of feeling make up the anxiety— outwardly there might be feelings of panic and restlessness, but at a deeper level, there might be feelings of vulnerability, loss, and hurt or even anger. So we notice that anxiety is not one thing, but a constellation of different feelings. We then try to meet each of these feelings with kindness and acceptance.

- *Mindfulness of thoughts*: Notice what kind of thoughts, images, stories, or beliefs are spinning around the feelings of anxiety. There could be all kinds of thoughts about the external reasons for our anxiety or judgments about feeling anxious. We could think it's bad to feel anxious or we could be locked into a mental loop of trying to think of ways to change our situation. We try to take a step back and look at these thoughts. We might ask ourselves: "Are these thoughts true or biased? Are they permanent or changing moment by moment?"

- *Mindfulness of attitude and relationship:* We notice how we are relating to our experience. Do we see the anxiety as very solid and real? Do we view it as permanent? Are we clinging to it so that it dominates how we think, feel, and behave? Are we identifying with it as who we are? This takes us to the next stage below.

Nonjudgment

Once we have inquired into the details of what we are going through, the next stage is to relate to our experience from a noncondemning standpoint. This means making space for all the different elements of our experience. In the words of Jon Kabat-Zinn,[8] it means being open to the full catastrophe of being alive, or in the words of Rob Nairn in his teaching, it means being willing to drop into our own "compassionate mess" that is both uncomfortable and yet rich in possibility. And then from the standpoint of this nonjudging attitude of mind, we inquire of every mental state or emotion that arises: "Is this really who I am, or is this just an experience that is moving through me?" In the case of anxiety, we inquire: "Has it become who I am in this moment?"

The process of identifying with something is an interesting one. If one day you suddenly get diarrhea and an attack of vomiting, you don't think you *are* the diarrhea and vomiting—you recognize that these are just temporary physiological processes going on inside you, unpleasant as they may be; and mostly you let them "run" their course (no pun intended). When it comes to disturbances of the mind, however, we have a perverse (and very unhelpful) tendency to identify with them and think that "I am an anxious or angry person," as opposed to recognizing that anger or anxiety gets triggered in us in certain circumstances and is temporary. Or we might have aggressive or sexual fantasies and then become concerned and think we shouldn't have them; so we end up fighting with them rather than seeing them as reflections of our tricky brain. Sadly, some individuals become so caught up in worrying about the contents of their mind and their fantasies that they become unwell with obsessional disorders—mild forms of which are far more common than is usually recognized, indeed so much so that the psychologist Lee Baer calls them "the imps of the mind,"[9] whereas we identify them as elements of the tricky brain.

So the point is that identifying with mind states like anxiety causes our mind to contract around them tightly so that our mental landscape becomes closed in and painful. Underlying this process is a subtle judgment and reaction to our experience—somehow feeling that it is not okay that we are going through what we are experiencing. But through making space for our experience, essentially by not judging it, our mind is able to relax its tight grip on the anxiety and a greater sense of freedom can arise. In this way, the difficult emotion is given space to unravel, work its way through us, and change.

Exercise 7: Experiential Acceptance

Step One: Turning Toward (Motive)

Follow the normal routine of soothing breathing, grounding, resting, and breath support (exercise 6).[10] If you find that a difficult thought or a certain emotion or mind state persistently arises in your mind, then actively turn toward it rather than pushing it away, treating it as something that is calling for your attention. Do this by following the steps below. As we've said before, always remember to work with emotions or mind states that are easy before you engage more difficult emotions.

Step Two: Recognizing and Labeling (Sensitivity)

Recognize what the emotion or mind state is and label it in whichever way fits best. Maybe you could label it as "loneliness," "worry," "sadness," "longing," "envy," "pride," or "lust." If there is no obvious label, then make a mental note in whatever way feels most appropriate. Mentally repeat the label two or three times in a soft, kind voice and then return to the breath as your mindfulness support. Sometimes the emotion or difficulty can exert a strong pull, in which case let your attention be drawn from your breath by the emotion, label it, and then return to your breath, going back and forth between your breath and the emotion in a relaxed, fluid way.

Step Three: Allowing (Tolerance and Sympathy)

Now actively welcome the emotion and allow it to be present. Let go of the wish for it to go away. Make space for it. Then lightly return to the breath support, but if the emotion persistently calls for your attention, then incline toward it, soften around it, and let your heart be touched by it. You can place your hand on your heart as a gesture of kindness and create a gentle friendly smile. Now switch from focusing on breathing to the emotion itself and make this the focus of your mindfulness practice. But do this in a particular way by following the next step.

Step Four: Paying Close Attention (Empathy)

First bring your attention to where the emotion or difficulty is held within your *body*. Do this by sweeping your attention from your head to your toes, and notice where the feeling expresses itself most prominently in the body. Then gently incline toward that place in your body, while continuing to breathe naturally, and just allow the sensation to be there as it is. You can place your hand over your heart again as you breathe as a reminder to be soft and kind. Allow the rhythmic motion of the breathing to soothe your body just as when you did the soothing breathing rhythm. Notice what kind of sensations you are experiencing in this part of the body—maybe there is a tightness, contraction, heat, vibration, and so on. Notice if you are resisting these sensations. Then notice what happens if you open to them with softness and acceptance.

Now bring your attention to the *emotions and feelings* connected with the experience. Notice what the primary feeling is—whether it's pleasant, unpleasant, or neutral—and then observe what layers of feeling make up the experience. You may notice that the emotion you are working with is not one emotion, but a constellation of subtle feelings. Then try to meet each of these feelings with kindness and acceptance.

Next, notice what *thoughts or beliefs* are spinning around the emotion. Take a step back and look at these thoughts: are they true or biased?

Are they permanent, or changing moment by moment?

And then notice how you are *relating* to your experience. Are you taking the emotion to be very solid and real? Are you seeing it as permanent? Are you clinging to it and focusing on it alone?

Step Five: Making Space (Nonjudgment)

Now open outward around your experience and be willing to hold whatever you are experiencing in a nonjudging awareness. In this stage, you move from paying attention to the detail of your experience to holding your experience as a whole within your awareness. Then inquire of every mental state or emotion that arises: "Is this really who I am or is this just an experience that is moving through me? Has it become who I am in this moment?"

Through practicing in this way you may come to see that the presenting emotion or difficulty is not *who you are*—it is just something moving through you. It is temporary.

When it comes to doing this acceptance practice, it is important to understand the principles and follow the stages but then to *tailor* the practice for yourself. In this way you find your own way of doing the practice that corresponds with your personality.

Cultivating the Observer

Through practicing acceptance we shift more and more into the *observing mode*. In the beginning we find that our awareness is immediately captured by thought processes. Almost as soon as thoughts and emotions arise, we find ourselves *inside them*, captive to the drama they are weaving for us. Our lives then consist of going from one thought bubble to the next. But through systematic training in mindfulness and acceptance, we can learn to distinguish between the part of us that observes and what is observed, and we learn to inhabit this observing mode more and more. We learn to step outside the thought bubble. This is a crucial shift in awareness—learning to be an objective witness of our thoughts and emotions. This does not mean that we become cold and dispassionate; it does not mean that we are no longer connected to the vitality and richness of life. In fact, we become more present and more connected to life, but we find ourselves standing in a different *relationship* to our experience. This is the key point.

In particular, through practicing the various stages of acceptance, we begin to see that what arises in our mind does not define who we are.

Increasingly, we begin to be aware of the impermanent nature of mental and emotional experience. Everything flows and changes; nothing is fixed. At some point the penny drops that we *are* witnessing this awareness. This awareness cannot be pinned down in any way; it cannot be conceptualized by the mind, and we cannot locate where it is. But every moment of the day it is there, at the very core of our being.

Learning to inhabit the observing mode is particularly important when it comes to compassion training because it enables us to step back and get some perspective on what is going on. If we are totally caught up in suffering—locked in the loop of thoughts and emotions—then there is little ground from which compassion can operate because we are totally absorbed in our suffering. So training in mindfulness and acceptance enables us step back and gain some degree of objectivity in relation to what is going on. And then, once we are in this witnessing mode, we are able to relate to what we are experiencing with kindness and compassion. This is especially important when we come to do the compassionate imagery practices, because we are learning to step into a different part of ourselves, get some perspective and distance from our ordinary self, and then learn to relate back, with compassion, to the part that might be a source of difficulty.

Key Points

- Through mindfulness and acceptance practice, we become increasingly *familiar* with the inner landscape of the mind, while through compassion practice, we learn to *cultivate* positive habits that will build harmony and well-being in our minds and relationships.

- Acceptance is a process of opening up to and not fighting our moment-by-moment experience—referred to as *experiential acceptance*.

- It is part of the first psychology of compassion: becoming increasingly sensitive and open to what we are feeling as opposed to resisting it and moving away. Bear in mind that acceptance is relevant to the outer circle of skills for alleviating suffering too. We will come to this in later chapters.

- We practice acceptance by working with the attributes of compassion (inner circle): motivation, sensitivity, sympathy, tolerance, empathy, and nonjudgment.

- Through practicing mindful acceptance, we come to inhabit the observing mode of awareness. We see that what we are experiencing changes moment by moment, and that those changes do not define who we are.

9

BUILDING
COMPASSIONATE
CAPACITY

Throughout this book, we have outlined the two distinct psychologies operating in compassion. The first psychology is concerned with the process of moving toward and opening up to suffering. This is why mindfulness is so important as a foundation for practicing compassion because it enables us to *come to land* in our own experience. The process of acceptance is important too because it enables us to disengage from the tendency to resist and struggle with what is occurring within us and to come into *clear and honest alignment* with what is actually happening. Now being willing to feel what is happening within us is no simple matter because our inner world can often be intense, complex, and fraught with conflict. Mindfulness and acceptance are important stages in this process, but they are not enough.

So we also need to develop *inner resources* that enable us to hold and contain what is happening within us so that it is not too intense or overwhelming. It is important that we do not just jump into the pain of our own experience or throw ourselves headlong at the suffering of life unprepared. We need to build up our reserves first. For example, before climbing a mountain, we need to embark on a graduated training to build up our muscles and fitness. Training in compassion is the same. This brings us to the second psychology of compassion. It is concerned with building an inner capacity from which we can effectively respond to the different parts of our inner experience, and on the basis of this, relate skillfully with the experience of others. This ability is made up of various qualities that are inherent within us but which need to be cultivated in a sustained and consistent way. In this respect, compassion involves the active stimulation of positive emotional systems and training in qualities such as kindness, strength, and courage. These in turn depend in part on stimulating our soothing/affiliation system (see "The Soothing/Affiliation System," in chapter 3) and becoming mindful, by noticing, allowing, and accepting the experiences of kindness and empathic validation that come to us from other people, as well as developing self-kindness.[1] If we are fearful of these feelings or block them, this can cause major difficulties that leave us struggling to engage with difficult experiences without the soothing/affiliation system on hand to contain them. So whereas in previous chapters we focused mostly on the first psychology of compassion, in this chapter we focus on the second psychology—building compassionate capacity. In order to build this capacity, we need to understand how compassion flows.

Compassion as Flow

Compassion can be expressed in three different ways. In the first instance, we can experience compassion being directed to us from other people, and we can become aware of the degree to which we are open to receiving other people's compassion. Quite often our minds are focused on averting threats, and we can find ourselves tuning out other people's kindness or just taking it for granted. Remember the example we gave before of going shopping one day and finding nine salespeople who are very polite and helpful but one shop assistant who's surly and rude? Which one do you talk about when you go home that night? In all likelihood you will not mention the friendly ones and will just focus on the one who was rude. In a similar way, our mind has a way of tuning out of everyday acts of kindness and friendliness. But imagine what would happen if you made a *deliberate* effort to balance your attention and bring to mind again the smiling faces and the happiness of the people who were able to help you buy a good present. Imagine what would happen in your body and your feelings if you did that regularly rather than just let your threat system run the show.

Second, compassion also flows from ourselves to others. We can feel compassion for other people when we open up to their suffering, wish them well, and *take joy* in them being happy and flourishing. These are feelings that emerge within us and are directed outward. Third, there is the compassion that we can feel for ourselves. It comes when we have a heartfelt wish for ourselves not only to deal with our tricky brains and life stories, but also to experience happiness and connectedness.

In each case the "inner circle" attributes of compassion are important. For example, when we experience compassion from other people, we sense they are motivated to help us, they are attentive to our needs, they are emotionally engaged rather than disengaged, they can cope with our distress, they can empathize with and understand what we are going through, and they are not critical and harsh. Similarly, when we feel compassion for others, we embody these same attributes in varying degrees toward others: we are motivated to help, we are attentive to their suffering, we try to relieve it if we can. The same applies when we develop compassion for ourselves. What is important is to focus on allowing the flow of feeling to go in these different directions in order to activate the positive emotional systems that feed compassion.

The flow of compassion is summarized in the following way:

- *Compassion flowing into you*: We focus our mind on opening up to the kindness of others. This is to open the mind and stimulate areas of our brain that are responsive to the kindness of others. We can experience joyful gratitude and appreciation. This is the main topic in this chapter.

- *Developing the inner compassionate self*: We focus on creating a sense of a compassionate self, just like actors do if they are trying to get into a role. This is the main topic of the next chapter.

- *Compassion flowing out from you to others*: We focus on the feelings in our body when we fill our minds with compassionate feelings for other people. This is the main topic of chapter 11.

- *Compassion for oneself*: This is linked to developing feelings, thoughts, and experiences that are focused on compassion for oneself. Life is often very difficult, and learning how to generate self-compassion can be very helpful during these times, particularly in helping us deal with our difficult emotions.

In order to get the flow of compassion going, we can start in a simple way with a series of imagery exercises that have proved very useful in working with people who experience anxiety and depression. In exercise 8, which follows shortly, we start off by imagining feeling safe and welcomed in a special place. Safeness is important because it's part of the three-circle system that we looked at in chapter 3. Learning to inhabit a place that arouses feelings of safeness is a good starting point for compassion work.

In exercise 9, we focus on receiving compassion from a color that is imbued with the qualities of the compassionate mind, whose sole intention is to heal us and soften the "inner edges" of our painful emotional patterns. For many people this is a useful first step before imagining receiving compassion from another being; they may be resistant to receiving compassion from others because they feel they don't deserve it, it alarms them, or it sets off grief and yearning processes (see chapter 6). You may prefer, however, to go straight to exercise 10, which is to imagine receiving compassion from a compassionate image that is the very embodiment of all the qualities (attributes and skills) of compassion. See which works best for you.

Working with Imagery

In chapter 8, we noted that mind training is made up of two key stages: familiarization and cultivation. Thus far we have focused on becoming familiar with our minds and establishing some degree of stability that will act as a platform for training in compassion. Now we will focus on the process of *cultivation*. A key theme of the earlier chapters of this book was that evolution has endowed us with a brain that is complex and contains many tendencies and potentialities, but we have the ability to *choose* which tendencies to cultivate given our new brain capacities for reflection and imagination. We can choose the kind of person we want to become.

A key tool in this respect is working with compassionate imagery. It is one of the skills of compassion in the compassion circle (see chapter 4). In the exercises that follow, we will direct our attention to creating particular images and sensations in the mind. These exercises are designed to help us tap into our soothing/affiliation system and cultivate our innate compassionate qualities.

Imagery is very powerful.[2] We know that *what* we imagine can have a powerful effect on our bodies and our minds. If we are hungry and see a meal, for example, this can stimulate our saliva and stomach acids. But, if we just fantasize about a meal because it's late at night and we have no money to buy one, the very act of imagining food can also stimulate our saliva and stomach acids in equal measure. Another example of how our imagination can stimulate our bodily processes is when we sexually fantasize about somebody we are physically attracted to. In this respect, our bodies respond to our imaginations in a similar way to how they would respond if the person in question was standing in front of us.

Similarly, if we are angry and we imagine arguing with somebody, this will affect our brain and bodily processes in much the same way as a real-life argument. If we put someone into a brain-scanning machine and ask them to start reliving arguments, the areas of their brain related to anger will light up. In the same way, if there are things we are anxious about or we imagine something frightening happening to us, this will stimulate our anxiety system. Conversely, if we focus on something we are looking forward to, such as imagining a sumptuous holiday in the sun, this will give us a buzz of excitement. These examples help us recognize how powerfully imagery affects our brains and bodies by stimulating particular feelings and thoughts.

It follows, therefore, that compassionate imagery can work in the same way: if we focus our minds on kindness and caring, this will affect our feelings and stimulate our bodily and mental processes in particular ways. In fact, we know from research that if we focus on feelings of caring and being cared for, this can have a range of beneficial effects on our sense of emotional well-being. Research shows that the more we focus on kindness and support for each other and ourselves, the happier and healthier we tend to be.[3]

No Clear Pictures

Some people think that they can't visualize because they are unable to create clear and lasting pictures in their minds. But this is a misunderstanding of what imagery practice is all about. Supposing we were to ask you, "What's a car?" In all likelihood, a fragmented image would pop into your mind. If we asked you, "What did you have for breakfast today?" you would have some kind of image based on memory. If we then asked you, "What kind of summer holiday do you like?" you would have a series of fleeting images based on what you like—hot or cold countries, certain activities, or just sitting by a pool. These fleeting and vague impressions are what we mean by imagery. They are very fragmented and transitory. In fact you might not have *any* clear visual image at all, just an impression; but this would be enough to give detailed information to someone inquiring about what you had for breakfast or your favorite holiday. Therefore, do not try to create vivid Polaroid pictures that are clear and sharp. If only fleeting impressions and fragments appear, these are fine. The key focus of this imagery work is on the *feelings* that we are trying to generate. Connecting to the *felt sense* is more important than having clear visual images.

Safe Place

As mentioned above, the first step is to create a sense of inner safeness and support so that the right conditions are in place to begin our training in compassion. Whenever we work on ourselves in depth, it is helpful to imagine being in an environment that feels conducive and supportive. It's the same when we settle down with a partner: we try to find a comfortable home that is warm and protective so that we have the optimal conditions to raise a family. Similarly, when we are seeking to awaken our inner compassionate self, it is useful to find the right conditions to do this.

In this exercise, we try to imagine what kind of *place* would give us feelings of safeness and calmness. This can be any place you like. It can be an actual place you visited or somewhere very familiar like a favorite room in your house or somewhere in your garden. It can also be somewhere imaginary, a place you saw in a movie or read about in a book; or it can be your own creation. It can be outside in nature or inside a safe home; it might be day or night, summer or winter—whatever conveys feelings of safeness and a sense of welcoming to you. The emotional atmosphere that we try to create is one of playfulness.

Safeness vs. Safety

It is important to make a clear distinction between safety and safeness (see "Distinguishing Safeness and Safety Seeking" in chapter 3). For example, one of Paul's clients imagined his safe place to be a bunker that was deep underground and which nobody knew about. This was in fact a place of safety that was concerned with keeping bad things out. The problem with this type of place is that while it may create a sense of relief, there may be little joy and little freedom; it's really an image that is being created by the threat system to try to keep out threats. And of course it will be like a cage or trap, because how do you get out of the bunker, how do you grow and build confidence? In some cases, however, people begin by creating a place of safety and then gradually work on becoming more open.

What we mean by *safeness* is somewhere we feel completely at ease, where we are free to explore and have a sense of expansiveness, not a place of entrapment or confinement. It is true that sometimes people like to imagine themselves under a duvet or safely snuggled up in bed, but the important thing here is that it should be a joyful place for us—and one of freedom, not one of hiding away. So the key thing with safe-place imagery is this sense of freedom rather than of keeping things out.

Intrusions

Sometimes people have a problem with "intrusions" when they do imagery work. For example, you start to create an image of a safe place and then you get an intrusion of something you really don't want—perhaps you're creating your safe place and then you get an uninvited image of a plane flying over and bombing it! Intrusions are quite common, and this is where mindfulness is helpful, because you just note the intrusion without reacting to it, and then bring your attention back to the process of visualizing your safe place. It doesn't matter how many intrusions you have; the trick is simply to notice them and return your attention to the task at hand.

Exercise 8: Creating a Safe Place

Find a place where you can sit or lie comfortably and where you will not be disturbed. Then follow the mindfulness stages of soothing breathing rhythm, grounding, resting, and breath support (exercise 6). If you do not have much time, then just engage with your soothing rhythm breathing (exercise 3) and friendly facial expression. As your mind settles, see if you can invite the image of a place in your mind that gives you the feeling of safeness and calmness. It might take a while to settle on a place, or you might hop from place to place. This is okay. Remember that you are not trying to force anything, and the very act of trying to imagine this place is helpful in itself.

As you settle on a place, then imagine looking around you—what can you see? Are there colors around you? Can you appreciate their richness? What's the quality of the light and the time of day? Now switch your attention to hearing if there are any sounds around you. Are they loud or faint? Are there any animal sounds, like bird songs for example? Now turn your attention to physical sensations and what you can feel. Notice the temperature around you and the feeling of the air on your skin. Maybe you are barefoot in your safe space; if so, notice the texture of the ground beneath your feet. Notice if you can smell anything in your safe space.

As you focus on sensory qualities, you are now going to focus on feeling qualities in relation to this place. So imagine that your safe place *welcomes you* and enjoys your being here—it is your creation, and you completely fit into this place. If there are trees nearby, they welcome you, or if you're under the duvet, it gently welcomes you too. If you are by the sea, the soft lapping waves on the sandy beach welcome you. In this way create a sense of being welcomed and wanted. While imagining this, create a soft smile of friendliness as you savor these feelings of being welcomed. Notice what happens to your feelings when you create that smile. Explore what it feels like when you imagine that this place is happy with you being there. Even if it is just a fleeting sense of where the place might be, try to create an emotional connection with it.

You can stay with this exercise for as long as you like. When you come to the end of your practice session, let the image begin to fade and then stretch and prepare yourself for carrying on with the rest of your day or moving on to the next imagery practice. Keep in mind that this safe place is your creation, and it is always available for you to return to. It is never more than a thought away. If you find yourself becoming distressed during the day, take a few deep, soothing breaths and then immerse yourself in your safe-place imagery. You can go back at any time and once again experience the sense of welcome and safeness this place offers you.

Compassionate Color

In this exercise, we go from feeling safe and welcomed to actually feeling compassion flowing into us from an external source. In this instance, the source of compassion is nonhuman, a color; but nonetheless, the color is imbued with certain qualities of mind that we will explore later—wisdom, strength, warmth, and kindness.

Exercise 9: Compassionate Color

Begin by settling into a posture that is comfortable yet alert, and then follow the mindfulness stages of soothing rhythm breathing, grounding, and resting (exercise 6). If you do not have much time, then just engage with your soothing breathing rhythm (exercise 3). As your mind settles, imagine a color or colors that you associate with compassion or that conveys a sense of warmth and kindness. This might appear as a light, fog or mist, or swirling color(s). It might only be a fleeting sense of color, but see if you can imagine this color surrounding you. Then, imagine the color entering through your heart area and slowly spreading through your body. Think of it as imbued with the qualities of wisdom, strength, warmth, and kindness. See if you can hold a soft and friendly facial expression as you do this exercise.

Now, as you imagine the color flowing through you, it is solely focused on helping you, strengthening you, and supporting you. Imagine that it flows around your body and soothes and softens any areas of difficulty, pain, or tension you might be experiencing. If blocks and barriers arise—especially those linked to feelings of not deserving this support and kindness—just recognize these as distractions and intrusions and mindfully go back to focusing on your compassionate color. Always bear in mind that we are trying to stimulate certain areas of the brain with these exercises.

Don't worry, then, if your distractions and intrusions seem overwhelming at times; just smile to yourself, go back to the soothing breathing rhythm, and try to stay with the exercise as best you can. When you come to the end of your practice session, let the image of the compassionate color fade and then stretch and try to maintain a "felt sense" of the compassionate color holding and supporting you as you go about your day.

Compassionate Image

In the next exercise we imagine compassion flowing into ourselves from a very compassionate being. This type of visualization practice is used in many spiritual and religious traditions. Over the millennia, people have used prayer as a way of contacting and opening to God (or a spiritual deity) seeking the confidence and conviction that they are fully loved and accepted by God. One of the reasons why these practices emerged and worked for people is because it is very powerful to imagine being completely loved and cared for by an idealized other.

In the Tibetan Buddhist tradition, spiritual practitioners invoke the image of Chenrezig in front of them and see this deity as the embodiment of all the wise and compassionate qualities in the universe. And then once they have created the firm conviction that Chenrezig is present and attentive to them, they make prayers to receive his grace and blessing. In reality what is happening is that they are opening up to this universal potential in *themselves*, and the process of prayer and visualization is a way of accessing these qualities. Indeed, the process of imagining an ideal compassionate other is a theme stretching back thousands of years that has deep resonance for human beings.[4]

One of the main themes of this book is that our mammalian heritage has wired our brains to respond in positive ways when we feel cared for and loved by important others. We explored this in detail in chapter 2. For some of us, however, our early caring relationships have been compromised in that we did not get the love and attention we yearned for or felt neglected in some way. So in this exercise we imagine receiving love and care from an *ideal* compassionate other. Just as when you're hungry, you imagine your favorite meal, or if you want sex, you fantasize about an ideal sexual partner, so too the very act of thinking about what you want from an ideal compassionate image begins the process of gearing your mind to what you really need. Our colleague Deborah Lee coined a term for this—"our perfect nurturer"—meaning that it's perfect for us; it gives us exactly what we need.[5]

In this section's exercise, we are working with the power of our own imaginations to create the most compassionate being we can, one beyond human frailties or limitations. Some people like to imagine a humanlike being, such as a wise person, while others prefer to imagine an animal or even something inanimate like a tree or a mountain or a mighty ocean. Others like to picture an image of light. Whatever you choose to envision is completely up to your own imagination and what feels right for you; the important thing is that your compassionate image is endowed *with a mind* that is focused on you. Drawing on the attributes of compassion, this compassionate being is completely motivated by his, her, or its compassion to help you; sensitive to your needs and emotionally in tune with your distress; able to tolerate and hold any pain and struggles you are going through; understanding and empathic; and never judgmental. It is not necessary to have a specific visual image; simply to think of such an image is enough. What is most important is the "felt sense" of the compassionate ideal other.

The key thing here is that your compassionate image is completely compassionate *to you*. In its presence, you can be yourself; there is no need to pretend to be what you are not. Your compassionate image does not judge you negatively or criticize you. It completely understands you, accepts you, and is loving toward you.

Qualities of the Compassionate Image

Wisdom

Your compassionate image is endowed with wisdom that comes from having gone through many difficulties. This wisdom is forged from this being's own life experience; it is not abstract or remote. The compassionate image understands the nature of life on Earth and how we are all caught up in the flow of life; we are caught up in something much greater than ourselves that, and we find ourselves with a brain we didn't choose that gets fired up with all kinds of emotions, fantasies, and difficulties—a brain that gets caught in loops between threat emotions like anger and anxiety. Like the Buddha, this being understands that life is full of suffering because everything is impermanent; so often we grasp at things we cannot get or try to keep hold of things we cannot keep—and this causes us suffering. It also recognizes that there are no feelings, fantasies, and motives you experience that many others before you have not experienced. We call this common humanity. We are all in the same boat; we are all created in similar ways. In essence, nothing that happens is personal. If you link this to the compassion circle, then your image has sensitivity, sympathy, and empathy that arise from deep insight into the nature of suffering.

Strength and Benevolent Authority

Your compassionate image has an inner strength and confidence that comes from its experience and understanding. It is not weak and submissive, and it is not overwhelmed by your distress. You can imagine that it truly understands you and has been through something similar, so it stands on the firm ground of experience and wisdom.

Motivation and Commitment

Your compassionate image is totally committed to your well-being, and it is not put off by your confusion or suffering. This is not a cold, detached commitment but one that is deeply textured by warmth and kindness. It is a kindness that does not in any way compromise its strength and fortitude or its ability to tolerate difficulties. If we think of the compassion circle, then it's highly motivated in a nonjudgmental way to be sensitive to your suffering the wish to alleviate this suffering.

Now, some might say that an idealized being with these qualities is not real because it is purely imaginary, so how can that be useful? But this is precisely the point: our imagination is powerful and can stimulate our emotional systems just like receiving "the real thing." Others might say that imagining an ideal compassionate figure with no human failings is unrealistic. This might be true at one level, but bear in mind that the image is *not supposed to be real*, and certainly not a substitute for real relationships. It is your creation, and you have endowed it with certain qualities. What you are doing is working with your mind in such a way that you are activating specific brain systems. It activates your own wisdom, authority, and commitment, and as your compassionate capacity grows, you will find yourself becoming more compassionate to yourself and to others. This is the meaning of the second psychology of compassion that we explore in this chapter.

Something to be aware of is that when we start working with this practice, it may stir up strong feelings inside us. It can alert us to the fact that we have felt lonely for a long time, and so we may end up feeling sad or even tearful. Bear in mind that sadness is a normal human emotion, so don't let that put you off; try as best you can to stay with your sadness and work through it. With all these practices, however, you are your own best authority, so only practice them to the extent that it feels bearable. There is no need to force things.

Exercise 10: Compassionate Image

Begin by settling into a posture that is comfortable yet alert, and then follow the mindfulness stages of soothing breathing rhythm, grounding, resting, and breath support (exercise 6). If you do not have much time then just engage with your soothing rhythm breathing (exercise 3) and friendly facial expression. As your mind settles, consider what qualities you would like your compassionate image to have: maybe complete acceptance of you no matter what; or maybe you would like your compassionate image to have a deep concern and affection for you; or a sense of kinship and belonging. For example, if you are a person who feels that you don't deserve compassion, think about what kind of image you would need in order to be helped to feel deserving of love. If you are someone who believes that you don't feel understood, then think about the kind of image you need to feel understood. You are creating a compassionate image that is ideal *for you*. Sometimes we may try to hide or suppress our feelings and fantasies, but our ideal compassionate image understands this struggle because it is so much part of being human. You can imagine your ideal compassionate image always wanting to help you become more compassionate to yourself and others, and never criticizing you.

With these thoughts in mind, let's focus on what your ideal compassionate image would look like. Would you want it to be old or young? Would it be male or female, or perhaps even nonhuman, such as an animal, the sea, or light? When you think of your ideal compassionate image, just notice what comes to mind. As you develop the practice you may find that, over time, different images come to mind. You don't have to stick to one version. Just see what happens and go with what you feel is helpful to you at any given time. What would your compassionate image sound like? If it was to communicate with you, what would its tone of voice be like? What tone of voice would you most like to hear? If your image is humanlike, what are its facial expressions? Notice how it might smile at you or show concern for you. Are there any colors that are associated with it? With these thoughts in mind, spend some time imagining your ideal compassionate image—what is perfect for you in every way; what fits your needs exactly.

Sometimes it can help if you bring to mind your safe place and imagine that you meet your compassionate image there. Imagine that it is coming toward you—it is coming to meet you, and you are going toward it. You can sense its pleasure in seeing you. Then imagine it either standing in front of you or sitting close to you. Focus on the presence of this ideal compassionate image and the sense of it being with you.

We're now going to imagine that your compassionate image has certain specific qualities. Focus first on the sense of *kindness and warmth* that you feel emanating from this image. Tune in to your own compassionate facial expression and imagine affectionate feelings while in the company of this image. Spend a few moments imagining what it would be like if you felt completely safe with this image. Remember, it doesn't matter if you do or don't feel safe—the main thing is just to imagine what it would be like if you did. Notice the feelings arising in you if you could feel safe with this compassionate image.

Now focus on its *maturity*, *authority*, and *confidence*. It is not overwhelmed by your pain or distress; and it is not put off by the strange things that go through your mind, but it may transmit the understanding that you have a very tricky brain that gives rise to these things. Spend a few moments imagining being with your ideal compassionate image, which has these qualities.

Next imagine that your compassionate image has great *wisdom* that comes through from its life path and experience. What emanates from this wisdom is a deep desire to be helpful and supportive. Imagine its wisdom enabling it to truly understand the struggles that you go through in life— your hopes and fears. It offers wisdom to you. Spend a few moments imagining being with your ideal compassionate image and feeling this great wisdom enfolding you.

Now focus on your compassionate image having a very deep *commitment* to you. Imagine that, no matter what, your compassionate image is fully committed to supporting you in becoming more compassionate to yourself, to others, and in coping with life. Imagine that its acceptance, kindness, and commitment are given freely to you; this is its sole objective, and there is nothing bad that you could do that would cause it to go away unless you really wanted it to. If you notice thoughts of not deserving, just bring your attention back to remembering that you are developing parts of your own mind and that the image you are creating is an image that is being created from your mind. Spend a few moments imagining what it feels like when you sense your compassionate image is fully committed to caring about you and helping you on your life path.

Now, while maintaining your friendly compassionate facial expression and engaging with your soothing breathing rhythm, imagine your ideal compassionate image saying the following words to you in as kind and warm a voice as you can imagine, and with a full commitment to you:

- May you be free of suffering, [say your name in your mind].

- May you be happy, [say your name in your mind].

- May you flourish, [say your name in your mind].

- May you find peace and well-being, [say your name in your mind].

Spend some time imagining that your compassionate image is looking at you with deep, heartfelt kindness and saying these things, genuinely wishing that you are free of suffering, that you become happy, that you flourish and find peace. Connect with the intention, warmth, and commitment behind the words. If you like, you can focus on just one or two of these phrases or make up similar ones that resonate with you.

Then, in your own time, let your compassionate image begin to fade. Always remember that this is your own imagination at work: you are calling on your inner capacity for compassion, and opening doors to your own compassionate abilities and feelings and the way that these can help you. These feelings are accessible to you at any time because they are part of you and they have come from you. As you learn to notice them and focus on them, they can be called upon at any time.

Try to remember to practice this each day, or as often as you can, even if it is just for a short period. Sometimes all we need to do is focus on our compassionate image and bring it to mind without necessarily going through all the stages. What is important is to connect to a *felt sense* of the image; this is often enough to give us a sense of its presence and a sense of being helped and supported.

Now some people say, "Well, suppose I encounter a murderer or psychopath, or find that I myself have a dark side—how could I experience compassion for that?" But, as we discussed in chapter 4, that is a basic misunderstanding. The first thing is that the individual you encounter didn't choose to have a brain that is capable of psychopathy or murder; nor did you choose to have a brain that succumbs to darker urges. Second, compassion doesn't mean that it's okay to be harmful to people— it definitely is not. Compassion is not saying, "Well, carry on then." Compassion is based on the understanding that people who experience these tendencies did not choose them. It is the heartfelt desire that the *source* of these destructive tendencies inside you or others ceases as you come to see your interconnectedness with all of life.

Recognizing Our Wish for Happiness

On the basis of allowing ourselves to be who we are, without pretense and shame, and slowly opening up to receiving understanding, love, and kindness from our idealized image of compassion, we can now move one step further and acknowledge our deep wish for happiness. We are generally so caught up in self-criticism and negative self-talk that we fail to acknowledge this simple truth. And yet it is something we share with every other living being. All beings yearn to be happy and to be free of suffering. In this respect we are all equal.

Exercise 11: Recognizing Our Wish to Be Happy

Begin by settling into a posture that is comfortable yet alert, and then follow the mindfulness stages of soothing rhythm breathing, grounding, resting, and breath support (exercise 6). If you do not have much time, simply engage with your soothing rhythm breathing (exercise 3) and friendly facial expression. As your mind settles, ask yourself the fo lowing questions:

- What am I looking for in my life?

- If I was lying on my deathbed and reflecting back on my life, what would I have cherished and hoped to have found?

- What would I have truly valued?

It may be useful to drop these questions into your mind without looking for a particular answer. It is like dropping a pebble into a very deep well. Just drop the question in and leave it alone. Then let your mind respond in its own language and in its own time.

If you find that the responses to these questions are superficial and relate only to sensory pleasure and the accumulation of material possessions, then drop the questions in again. See if you can uncover an inner yearning that conveys a genuine sense of well-being—something that rises up from a place deep within you, and which might express itself in a variety of different ways.

Acknowledge this aspiration for genuine happiness—for meaning, wholeness, inner peace, fulfillment—as a fundamental aspect of who you are. Recognize that this concern for your own welfare lies at the very core of your being, and simply acknowledge its presence within you.

And then, with a firm recognition of this yearning for happiness as an essential part of your being, repeat the following phrases on the out-breath:

- May I be happy....

- May I flourish in my life....

- May I find peace, well-being, and joy....

Exercises like these are used in various traditions, and a key focus is on the heartfelt wish for suffering to end and joy to arrive. The important point to realize is that none of us actually chooses to suffer, even though we often behave in ways that greatly increase our suffering. No one wakes up in the morning and thinks, "I need to suffer more today." Sometimes, of course, we believe that if we suffer, God will love us; or we put ourselves through discomfort because we know it car help us in the long run (like going to the gym). Or we may suffer because we work very hard at something that gives our lives meaning—as with people who suffer for their art or sacrifice themselves for others. But even if we suffer in these ways, the ultimate goal is always happiness and peace, and, we would say, connectedness.

If you feel you don't deserve happiness, however, look at this very carefully and ask yourself what is *behind* the fear of having happiness. Similarly, if you feel that you do not deserve to experience being loved and cared for, look at what lies behind this belief. Sometimes just by allowing ourselves to be in contact, or dialogue with, our inner compassionate image, insights can emerge into how we shut ourselves off from happiness. So often it comes down to a fear of reaching out and connecting and then being shamed, rejected, and hurt.

Key Points

- Whereas mindfulness is about becoming increasingly *familiar* with the mind and how it moves, compassion is about *cultivating* an inner capacity from which to respond to and alleviate suffering—this is the second psychology of compassion.

- Compassion is an active process that involves the flow of feeling: other to self, self to other, and self to self.

- Compassionate imagery draws on the positive emotional systems that are already within us and makes them available for engaging with difficulty and stress.

- Imagining a safe place activates the soothing system and creates the conditions for awakening our compassionate capacity.

- With the compassionate color, we imagine receiving compassion from a nonhuman source, which can be less threatening for some people in the beginning.

- The compassionate image is an idealized compassionate other that is imbued with certain qualities. We explore what it feels like to imagine receiving them.

- As we work with the compassionate image, the next step is to acknowledge our wish to be happy.

10

THE COMPASSIONATE SELF

In the previous chapter, we began to explore the second psychology of compassion, that of alleviation. We started the process of awakening the positive emotional systems that give rise to the feeling of compassion and we invited the flow of compassion into ourselves. We concluded with the simple acknowledgment that in the depths of our being we want to be happy and fulfilled in our lives; this is what we share with all other living beings. This insight helps the next step in which we imagine becoming compassionate people ourselves; it serves as the basis for the flow of compassion toward others and then to ourselves.

Cultivating Helpful Patterns

Chapters 2 and 3 explored the multiple patterns within us that can give rise to many different life possibilities, and indeed different versions of who we can be. We have hundreds, if not thousands, of potential patterns within ourselves. For the most part, the kind of person we become is arbitrary and depends on the environment we happen to be born into and the social conditions that shape us as we grow up.

As we become more mindful, however, rather than just allowing our self-identity to be shaped by random forces around us, we can begin to *choose* the kind of self we want to cultivate. This goes back to the meaning of meditation that lies at the heart of the teaching of the Buddha: to become familiar with what arises in the mind and to actively cultivate patterns that serve us in becoming happy, flourishing people. The key point is that once we become familiar with these different tendencies and potentialities that evolution and culture have given us, we are in a position to choose to cultivate the patterns that awaken the seed of compassion that lies beneath the mud in the lake (chapter 6). This is the stage we have arrived at now, namely being in a position to cultivate the compassionate self because we can appreciate that it can help us in our lives. It can have a soothing effect on our anger and anxiety, and it can also help us develop the courage to face and work with them skillfully.

In choosing to cultivate the compassionate self, we need to actively train in becoming this kind of person. For example, if you want to be a good musician, you practice playing a musical instrument; if you want to be a good driver, you practice driving. Each is a potential within us until we choose to cultivate this aspect of ourselves. The important thing is to think about what we want to become. Strangely, we seldom stop and think about this; we don't think that we can deliberately practice becoming a certain type of person, but indeed we can. We just have to decide to do so and then put in the time to practice it.

In contrast to our compassionate selves that are linked to the soothing/affiliation system, the "selves" that arise from the threat or drive systems will pop up very easily without much effort on our part. There is the angry self that thinks: *Don't mess with me!*; the ambitious self that thinks: *I want to be rich and famous*; and of course the selves from the drive system: *I must get this or that done today; so much to do.* Anger and anxiety are easy to activate, and we don't sit around thinking: *I need to practice being angry or having panic attacks!* We looked at the reasons for this in chapter 3 where we described some of our basic emotional systems. But, as we have pointed out, we do need to actively train in compassion because although the seeds exist within us, they tend to be buried in the mud of the evolved mind, covered over by all the hustle and bustle of life with all its frustrations, tragedies, and stresses.

Something important to bear in mind, however, is that becoming a compassionate person does not mean that we will escape the messiness of life. It may be tempting to think that somehow compassionate people never get angry, fearful, doubtful, confused, or even lustful—they certainly do. It is important to remember that compassion is not about getting rid of these things. Remember the distinction between compassionate ascent and compassionate descent (chapter 6).

So compassion is the ability to turn toward and engage with and work with suffering, making wise choices while accepting that sometimes our more troublesome emotions will get the better of us and take over.

Imagining Our Compassionate Self

We will work again with imagery because, as we saw in the previous chapter, visualization is a very powerful way of awakening our compassionate potential.[1] As we mentioned before, in the Tibetan Buddhist tradition the archetype of compassion is symbolized by the *yidam*, Chenrezig. *Yidam* is often translated as "deity," but this is not a useful translation because it implies that there is some external godlike figure that we address our prayers too. In fact, the literal translation of the Tibetan word *yidam* is "mind link." Through imagining Chenrezig, we are making a link to the compassionate potential *within our own mind*, which is buried beneath the mud of our conflicting emotions and confusion. We invoke this archetype by imagining it in front of us, and we make prayers and offerings to it as a way of accessing the compassionate potential *within ourselves*. There is an interesting psychology here. In the beginning we may not believe that we have "it" ourselves, and might even say to ourselves, *Oh no, I am not a compassionate person*, and prefer instead to project it onto others whom we look up to with respect: *Of course, people like the Dalai Lama are compassionate; but not me*. So, working with this psychology, the practice invites us to pray to an idealized form of compassion and then to receive the grace, protection, and love from this idealized form. This is the point we reached in the previous chapter when we imagined the compassionate image. But the next step is to imagine that the deity in front, the idealized form, dissolves into light and merges into ourselves so that now we take on its qualities. This means that we own the fact that we have these qualities within ourselves. In reality we are Chenrezig; it is our true nature. This is seen as the most important part of the process—identifying ourselves with our innate compassionate nature and developing the firm conviction that this is who we are.

Method-Acting Techniques

We can learn a lot from these forms of visualization that have existed for thousands of years. An approach that is also very useful for identifying with different versions of ourselves comes from training actors. If actors are to be convincing in their performances, they need to fully inhabit their roles, whether they're playing James Bond, a victim of crime, a drug addict, or someone else. In order to get into the role, they need to immerse themselves in the way that the character thinks, feels, and acts.[2] Instead of focusing on the technical training of an actor's voice and body, method acting requires an actor to get in touch with his or her own deepest emotions so that they can use these authentic feelings and insights to enrich the inner life of whichever character they are playing. In addition, method actors need to really understand the point of the role, the purpose and aim of the character they are trying to create.

It's this process of connecting to one's own inner resources that makes method acting useful for developing a sense of the compassionate self. You can imagine developing deep compassionate attributes and qualities and even practice expressing these qualities in your everyday life. If you were an actor learning to act a particular role, you would pay attention to key elements of your character and try to embody them yourself. This might be a character who is angry, depressed, anxious, or happy, joyful, and, of course, compassionate. You would try to *become* that character—living it from the inside—at least for a short while. You might pay attention to the way this character thinks and sees the world, his postures, his tone of voice, and the kind of things he says.

Actors will also use their memories of times when they have felt certain things and then try to recall those within themselves. All these techniques can be used when we're trying to focus on developing our compassionate self. You can focus on how much you wish to bring compassion into your life or into the world. The important point with these exercises, however, is to remember that it doesn't matter if you actually feel these qualities in you or not; instead, you simply try to *imagine what it would be like if you had these qualities*. You imagine yourself having these qualities and "feel into them." In addition, of course, you can remember times when you did feel compassion and kindness for others.

Mindfulness will help with the process of "feeling into" the qualities of the compassionate self. It allows us to pay attention to the visualization process; and, when we get distracted, mindfulness allows us to gently bring it back into focus. In addition, in sitting practice, our posture can connect us to a sense of strength and authority through becoming aware of how our body is held by the vastness of the earth beneath us, and how our mind can draw strength from this because it is held in the body just like the body is held by the earth. Whereas mindfulness connects us with these qualities in an immediate and embodied way, method-acting techniques can help to bring out these qualities as we make a connection with them.

The Qualities of Our Compassionate Self

Our focus is now on cultivating the qualities of the compassionate self. To make this personal and relevant, write down the qualities you would imagine having if you became the most compassionate "you" conceivable—you at your very best. When you look at the qualities you have written down, they might include friendliness, patience, kindness, openness, and honesty. Now all of these are tapping into your intuitive wisdom—your own deep awareness of what compassion can involve. So these will be part of your own unique personal qualities that you can imagine having when you do this exercise. However, in addition, there are some qualities that are always useful to include. We touched on these in the previous chapter when we worked with the compassionate image. It might be useful now to explore these qualities in more depth as they relate to imagining the compassionate self.

Wisdom

The first aspect of wisdom is one you now know: that we just find ourselves in the flow of life with a set of genes and a very complicated and tricky brain that evolved over many millions of years. We did not design or choose it. Furthermore, our sense of self arises from how we have experienced life and the relationships we were born into—again, we did not choose these. Working with some of what goes on in our minds—powerful emotions, mood shifts, unwanted thoughts or images, and painful memories—can be difficult. Our wisdom understands in a deep way that these things that we did not choose can be at the root of our suffering. It is the wisdom of no-blaming, just seeing clearly how things are and choosing to be kind, that becomes key.

The second aspect of wisdom arises from the Buddhist tradition. It involves seeing that things are not as solid and fixed as they appear. Our thought processes tend to solidify reality and obscure the fact that everything is fluid and changing. This is the truth of impermanence—nothing lasts, including the bad things that happen.

The third aspect of wisdom is based upon our new brain capacity to stand back, learn, and reflect on our experience. As discussed above, we can become more aware of what arises in our minds, and discern what we should focus on and what we should let go. In this context, wisdom means appreciating that we have a window of opportunity, however small, and we can choose to cultivate helpful habits and not feed unhelpful ones. Wisdom allows us to understand the unhelpfulness of self-criticism and to make choices to become more self-compassionate.

The fourth part of wisdom comes as we learn from life's journey how to do things differently or better. Wisdom is the ability to use our learning. So it is being open to our mistakes and the hurtful things we do combined with the genuine wish to improve and repair. Wisdom cannot develop without this capacity for insight into where we go wrong. This means looking at our difficulties without the avoidance that is born of shame. When we feel ashamed and critical, we can turn away from what we need to face.

Authority and Strength

We choose to see the compassionate self as the inner authority because it comes with wisdom and the ability to deal with difficult things. It is not weak but has an inner confidence and strength. The determination to face things and contain what arises in our experience is what gives us strength. To stimulate this we can breathe in a certain way or adopt a posture that helps us feel confident.

Compassionate Motive and Commitment

Of course the whole point of having this wisdom, sense of authority, and strength is because at the heart of the compassionate self is the motivation to relieve suffering. So aligning with that motive is key. This is about taking responsibility and not turning away from problems but recognizing that, although we just find ourselves in the flow of our lives and so much of what happens is not our fault, we can make a commitment to ourselves and others to work with our experience, perhaps taking small steps at a time. So commitment is not about blaming or criticizing because that is usually focused on things in the past, but it is about genuinely wanting to act in ways that are helpful. Commitment also comes from the mindfulness practice of acceptance—facing things as they are and being willing to work with our experience as we find it, rather than being sidetracked into resistance and struggle.

Warmth and Kindness

As we cultivate and make contact with our inner sense of wisdom, authority, strength, and commitment, we recognize that the emotional tone of the whole endeavor is basic kindness; that is, the heartfelt wish to relieve suffering and the sources of suffering, to create joy for oneself and others.

In the Mahayana Buddhist tradition, one of the four limitless contemplations is *maitri*, which is that sense of opening out toward our inner and outer environments with friendliness and warmth. Warmth is like an open friendliness; it is not about being "nice" but about having a genuine desire to be helpful. Again what is important is our motivation and intention to relieve suffering in a gentle but firm way even if the feelings do not immediately arise. Creating a compassionate facial expression and imagining speaking in a warm, friendly voice can help to engender this quality.

Exercise 12: Compassionate Self

Begin by settling into a posture that is comfortable yet alert, and then follow the mindfulness stages of breathing, grounding, resting, and breath support (exercise 6). If you do not have much time, then just engage with your soothing breathing rhythm (exercise 3). Bear in mind that soothing breathing rhythm is about finding a point of stillness and calm within (see exercise 3). This is particularly important with the compassionate self because it engenders that feeling of being grounded on a stable base with a sense of inner authority and security.

Notice the feeling of your body slowing down. Relax your facial muscles, starting with your forehead and then your cheeks, and let your jaw drop slightly. Allow your mouth to turn upward into a warm and friendly smile. Then just rest where you are—nothing to do. As we go through this exercise you may find your mind wandering. If so, do not worry about it; just gently bring it back to the practice you are doing.

Now, like an actor getting into a role, you are going to use your imagination to create an image of yourself at your *compassionate best*. Sometimes it can help to bring to mind a memory of when you felt very compassionate toward somebody. Recall what was going through your mind, the feelings of kindness and warmth, and your genuine wish for the person to get better or do well. It's important to focus on your compassionate feelings and not the distress that the other person might have been feeling.

Next, reflect for a few moments about the qualities you would like to have if you were to develop your compassion more fully. Remember, it doesn't matter if you don't feel as if you are a very compassionate person; the most important thing is to *imagine* the qualities of a deeply compassionate person and imagine what it might feel like if you did have them.

Now we're going to focus on the specific qualities of compassion. Start by imagining that you have *wisdom*. Bring to mind your understanding that all of us just find ourselves here in the flow of our own lives—so many complex factors have shaped who we have become, and so much of what has happened is beyond our control. See the wisdom of no blame and the value of seeing things clearly and choosing to be compassionate. Recognize that you have this wisdom right now—it is present within your life experience as a rich resource. Hold on to your friendly facial expression and consider your warm voice tone, imagining yourself expressing wisdom as you speak. For the next few moments, imagine yourself being a wise and insightful person—open, thoughtful, and reflective.

Next, imagine that from your wisdom comes a sense of *authority, strength, and confidence.* Connect to the sense of your own inner authority and dignity in your body posture. Tune in to your posture, your sense of solidness from your soothing breathing rhythm, and allow yourself to be held—body like a mountain, breath like a gentle breeze, and mind like the open sky. Draw strength from the fact that the vastness of the earth holds and supports you. Notice how you feel when you imagine yourself embodying authority and confidence. While holding your friendly facial expression and your warm voice tone, for the next few moments, think about how you would speak in a compassionate way with authority, how you would move in the world, and how you would express this confidence, maturity, and authority.

Now, on the basis of this confidence, authority, and wisdom, focus on your desire to be helpful and supportive and your wish for others to be free from suffering and the causes of suffering, to be happy, and to prosper. Hold your friendly facial expression and consider your voice tone and how you would speak in a compassionate way with *kindness.* Then become aware of any areas of tension or physical pain or emotional reaction to that tension within you and gently soften around these areas, holding them with kindness. Remember that your wisdom and strength are there as a support if things feel difficult. And so, for the next few moments, gently and playfully imagine that you have great kindness and the desire to be helpful. Notice how there is a certain calmness that comes with kindness and also a positive pleasurable feeling; it doesn't have that frenetic feeling of being agitated or frustrated. Notice how you feel when you imagine having these feelings within you.

And now, on the basis of your wisdom, strength, and kindness, imagine that you have the courage to face and work through the difficult experiences that may arise. You are willing to move toward what is difficult, without blaming or criticizing, and you are willing to take responsibility for your life. For a few moments, imagine that you are such a person, someone who is deeply *committed* and responsible for working with your own mind.

Now imagine that you are looking at yourself from the outside. See your facial expressions, the way you move in the world, and note your motivations to be thoughtful, kind, and wise. Hear yourself speaking to people and note the compassionate tone in your voice. See other people relating to you as a compassionate person and see yourself relating to other people in a compassionate way. For the next few moments, playfully watch yourself as a compassionate person in the world and others relating to you as such.

The more you practice slowing down and imagining being this kind of person in the world, the more easily you may find you can access these qualities in you, and the more easily you will find they can express themselves through you. And now, as a way of concluding this exercise, let go of trying to visualize and for a few moments, rest without focusing on anything in particular.

When you come out of this imagery practice, it can be helpful, pleasurable, and even a bit of fun to walk around as a compassionate self. In other words, notice how you walk, notice how you talk, notice how you use friendly facial expressions to greet people and how contact with you makes others feel safe. Engender a sense of authority and responsibility in creating kindness around you. You can ask yourself the following questions: How can I take more interest in people today? How can I be helpful to another human being? How can I be more mindful of other people's distress? Even if you sometimes feel that you are putting on an act, nonetheless take pleasure from the fact that you are activating a compassionate resource within you. Like learning to play the piano, it can feel a bit forced and artificial at times because it doesn't come smoothly, but with practice it can.

Remembering Our Compassionate Self

Ideally, try to practice becoming the compassionate self every day. However, many people will have the best of intentions but then forget. Days will go by, and then we suddenly remember that we would like to be practicing. So we need reminders. One effective reminder might be to hold a semiprecious stone every time you do the compassionate-self practice. Keep it in a pocket or around your neck. Each time you put your hand in your pocket, you will feel it, and that will act as a reminder for you to reconnect to your compassionate self. You can do this when you are sitting on the train or taking time out in your lunch break but also when interacting with others.

If your life is busy you can start by practicing 'compassion under the duvet." When you wake up in the morning, try to spend a few minutes practicing becoming your compassionate self. As you lie in bed, bring a compassionate expression to your face and focus on your desire to be wise and compassionate today. You have the capacity for wisdom and strength inside you, but you need to create space for it. Even two minutes a day, if practiced every day, can have an effect. However, once you get out of bed, try to maintain the compassionate feelings you were generating under the duvet. We certainly don't want you to get to the point where you say, "I'm a very compassionate person, but only under the duvet"!

You can also practice when you stand at the bus stop or when you're lying in the bath. After all, how often do we lie in the warmth of a bath and not really appreciate it because our mind is dwelling on all kinds of things—mostly worries about things we need to do? Whenever you are aware of it, even while sitting in a meeting, you can use soothing breathing and focus on becoming your compassionate self.

Doing the Work of Compassion

Now that we have begun to cultivate our compassionate potential by imagining being a compassionate self, the next step is to do the work of compassion. The Buddhist notion of *bodhicitta* requires us first to aspire to be compassionate and then to act in a way that is compassionate—mere aspiration is not enough (see chapter 4). Furthermore, as we have said repeatedly, compassion develops with training, whereas threat emotions and other motives are automatic. What is required is a step-by-step process of cultivation.

In the exercises that follow, we will work with both of the psychologies of compassion. On the one hand, we will firmly root ourselves in our compassionate qualities and activate them by imagining being a compassionate self, while, on the other hand, we will engage with difficult aspects of our experience or that of others.

Focusing Our Compassionate Self: Compassion for a Loved One

In doing the work of compassion, a first step is to identify what kindness *feels like* so we know what we are working with. This relates to the flow of compassion—getting used to compassion flowing from ourselves to others and familiarizing ourselves with this flow. In the beginning it is helpful to choose a loved one for whom we feel a relatively uncomplicated, loving connection as the object of our compassion, bearing in mind that most close relationships involve mixed feelings, which is completely normal. You could focus on your child, grandparent, partner, close friend, or even your pet. The intention here is to recognize what it feels like when positive feelings like compassion, love, and tenderness arise in us in situations where these feelings flow naturally and easily.

Also, what is important is to recognize what it feels like when we unconditionally accept another person or animal *despite his or her flaws and failings*. For example, if our child has a disability or is no good at her studies, this does not stop us loving her; in fact we might even love her more. Yet when it comes to our own flaws and failings, it is so often a completely different matter—we tend to get out the big stick and start beating ourselves.

Exercise 13: Compassion for a Loved One

Begin by settling into a posture that is comfortable yet alert, and then follow the mindfulness stages of soothing breathing rhythm, grounding, resting, and breath support (exercise 6). If you do not have much time, then just engage with your soothing rhythm breathing (exercise 3). Now imagine that you are identifying with your compassionate self. Bring to mind each of the qualities of your compassionate self and feel into them with the sense that these qualities are within you even if just a little. Remember to create a friendly facial expression and imagine you have a warm voice tone.

While connected to this compassionate mind state, bring to mind someone you care about—it could be a child, friend, partner, parent, or even an animal. Hold him in your mind's eye. Now focus your compassionate feelings on him. Name him in your mind and say the following phrases slowly on the *out-breath*:

- May you be free of suffering, [say their name].

- May you be happy, [again say their name].

- May you flourish, [and say their name].

- May you find peace, [again say their name].

Do not worry if you can't remember all of these phrases; just focus on the ones that you can relate to. The actual words or phrases are not the main issue—what is important is your heartfelt wish and the *flow of feeling*.

To enhance this practice, as you breathe out, you can imagine that you send a warm golden light from your heart that touches your loved one and eases his suffering, bringing him peace and well-being. Notice the sensations around your heart and your feelings in the body as you do this. Become aware of the feelings of *pleasure and joy* that arise in you when you imagine that he could be happy and free of suffering and find peace and happiness. So you do not focus too much on the distress he may be experiencing, but instead on your own kind and loving feelings, and the pleasure you take from his happiness.

When you have finished sending these wishes, let the image of the person you have imagined fade. Spend a few moments tuning in to the feelings that have arisen in you, noticing in particular how this feels in your body. Then for a few moments rest without focusing on anything in particular and then stretch and get up.

Focusing Our Compassionate Self: Compassion for Oneself

It is helpful to find a way to be compassionate to ourselves because if we are not able to relate to our own feelings and needs in a kind and empathic way, there may be little basis from which to relate to others with compassion, especially strangers and adversaries.

We will now introduce a series of exercises for focusing our compassionate self in different ways. First, we begin with a general exercise for relating to ourselves, and then we introduce specific exercises for working with particular aspects of ourselves. The point here is that once we learn to identify with and inhabit the compassionate self, we then *relate back* to the other parts of ourselves from this compassionate standpoint. With mindfulness practice, we learn to inhabit the observing mode, standing back and witnessing the flow of thoughts and feelings rather than being held captive in the bubble of thoughts. But with compassion we take one step further and connect with the qualities of compassion that exist within this witnessing mode. It is not just a neutral, cold observing. We tune in to the qualities of warmth and kindness. Then we relate to our angry part, anxious part, or self-critical part from this compassionate perspective.

Exercise 14: Compassion for Self

Begin by settling into a posture that is comfortable yet alert, and then follow the mindfulness stages of settling, grounding, resting, and breath support (exercise 6). If you do not have much time, then just engage with your soothing rhythm breathing (exercise 3). Now imagine that you are identifying with your compassionate self. Bring to mind each of the qualities of your compassionate self and feel into the qualities within you. Remember to create a friendly facial expression and imagine you have a warm voice tone.

Now create a picture of yourself in your mind's eye as if you're looking at yourself from the outside. You could imagine that you are watching a video of yourself going about your day. With the eyes of your compassionate self, watch your ordinary self get up in the morning and move around your room, and then get on with the day. Notice how this ordinary self is often troubled by difficult emotions or life circumstances, and how it often feels under stress and pressure, sometimes lapsing into rumination and worry, perhaps about money or nagging concerns about relationships or struggling with difficult emotions. Allow yourself to be in touch with the struggle of the person you're watching—the ordinary you—but hold to your position of inner strength and wisdom looking out through the eyes of your compassionate self with the intention of being kind and helpful.

While holding on to your compassionate self and maintaining your friendly facial expression and warm voice tone, see yourself in your mind's eye and imagine directing the following wishes to yourself:

- May you be free of suffering [and say your name—for example it might be: "May you be free of suffering, Paul," or "May you be free of suffering, Choden," really focusing on the feeling that's coming from your compassionate self to the self that you see in your mind's eye].

- May you be happy, [say your name].

- May you flourish, [say your name].

- May you find peace, [and say your name].

You can also do this exercise using the pronoun "I," thinking "May I be happy, may I be free of suffering," and so on. You may wish to try both options and see which one you prefer.

For as long as it feels comfortable, direct these feelings to yourself on the out-breath. Don't worry if you can't remember all the phrases; just focus on the ones you can remember and which you relate to. If you feel yourself getting pulled by difficult feelings when you generate compassion for yourself, then come back to resting in the awareness of your compassionate self. It is very common to experience resistance to feeling compassion for ourselves. It may be related to all manner of things like feeling we don't really deserve it, or because it brings up feelings of sadness or a yearning for closeness. Whatever resistance may arise, just notice it and mindfully return to the practice. You might even try to be compassionate to the fact that you are experiencing resistance. When you have finished sending these wishes, let the image of your ordinary self fade and spend a few moments tuning in to the feelings that have arisen in you, noticing in particular how this feels in your body. Then rest without focusing on anything in particular, stretch, and get up.

Self-Compassion Break

In his book *The Mindful Path to Self-Compassion*, Christopher Germer offers a very helpful way of contacting and bringing out your compassionate self in everyday life situations.[3] Let's suppose you have an experience of suffering, like stress, anxiety, or a low mood, or you have just had an argument. First, notice this, take a few mindful breaths to ground yourself, and slow down. Then, place your hand over your heart and say:

- This is a moment of suffering.

- Suffering is part of everyone's life.

- May I be compassionate to myself in this moment.

Repeat these phrases slowly with a compassionate voice tone and friendly facial expression. In this way, we first notice and turn toward our difficulty (rather than away from it). Next, we see that our experience of suffering is part and parcel of the human condition—we are all in the same boat. Then we focus on our compassionate intent and feeling. We can do this quick practice any time during the day when we feel anxious or stressed.

Working with the Anxious Self

In working with the compassionate self, the most important thing is to try to practice it regularly, learning to shift from being caught up in the turbulent emotions and thoughts of the everyday mind to stepping into and identifying with this compassionate part. The more we do this, the more familiar and stable it will become. Developing a sense of the compassionate self with its desire to be helpful, its sense of authority, calmness, confidence, and wisdom can be very useful when we are struggling with difficult emotions like anxiety. By doing the following exercise, we can build up capacity and skill in relating to our anxious self.

Exercise 15: Compassion for the Anxious Self

Begin by settling into a posture that is comfortable yet alert, and then follow the mindfulness stages of settling, grounding, resting, and breath support (exercise 6). If you do not have much time, then just engage with your soothing breathing rhythm (exercise 3). Now imagine that you are identifying with your compassionate self by bringing to mind each of its qualities. Remember to create a friendly facial expression and imagine you have a warm voice tone.

Now bring to mind a situation in which you felt anxious. Imagine that you are looking at the anxious part of yourself through the eyes of the compassionate self. You can let an image of your anxious self appear in front of you, or you can relate to the *feeling* of this anxious self if no image appears. Let yourself feel connected to the struggle and agitation of the anxious self while anchored in the qualities of the compassionate self: your strength is a support for the agitated, groundless part of the anxious self; your wisdom sees that this anxiety will change and how thoughts feed it and make it feel very solid and real. Then allow yourself to feel warmth for this part of you, enfolding it in loving-kindness. Then connect to your sense of commitment—really wanting to be there for yourself in a way that is constructive and does not feed rumination and self-recrimination. Imagine how you might like to help, what you might like to say to this struggling part of you to validate its feelings and to help it come through this episode.

While holding to your compassionate self and maintaining your friendly facial expression and warm voice tone, see yourself in your mind's eye and imagine directing the following wishes to your anxious self:

- May you be free of agitation and anxiety, [say your name].

- May you find stability and peace, [say your name].

The actual words and phrases are secondary; what is important is to connect to the feeling of compassion flowing from the compassionate self to your anxious self, and if the feelings do not flow easily, remain connected to your intention to be kind, committed, and so on. When you have finished sending these wishes, let the image of your anxious self fade and spend a few moments tuning in to the feelings that may have arisen in you, noticing in particular how this feels in your body. Then rest without focusing on anything in particular, stretch, and get up.

Dennis Tirch and psychologist Lynne Henderson have outlined a variety of ways you can use a compassionate focus to help you work with anxiety in different situations, such as working with anxious thinking and behavior.[4] But the important point is that while we want to soften down anxiety, we are not fighting with it or trying to get rid of it—it's about validating, accepting, and understanding it. In daily-life situations that induce anxiety, pause and engage with your soothing breathing rhythm for a few seconds, feel yourself slow down and become more grounded in your body, consciously identify with your compassionate self, and then look at the situation through the eyes of the compassionate self. You can practice this first in mildly anxiety-provoking situations, such as being in lines that are tedious and time consuming, experiencing uncomfortable feelings linked to overeating, or being in a difficult meeting. Practice in situations that are not too stressful, and in this way you will build up the ability to deal with more difficult situations.

Working with the Angry Self

For many people, anger is a difficult emotion that surges through us in response to both outer and inner triggers. There are many external situations that push our buttons and make us angry, but we can just as easily find ourselves becoming angry because of the intrusion of unexpected feelings or because we are intolerant of how we are feeling. As we saw in chapter 3, anger is a protective emotion that emanates from the threat system, closely monitoring and detecting things that threaten our inner and outer lives and stability. It is generally our first line of defense, but very often it masks deeper feelings of grief, sadness, or loneliness. It can contract the mind, shut us down, and bury these deeper feelings in the body. For this reason, it is very useful to find ways of working with our angry selves, bearing in mind that this is not easy. There are many ways that a compassion focus can help you with anger—in working with angry thoughts and behaviors, for example—which have been well outlined by the psychologist Russell Kolts.[5]

Exercise 16: Compassion for the Angry Self

Begin by settling into a posture that is comfortable yet alert, and then follow the mindfulness stages of settling, grounding, resting, and breath support (exercise 6). If you do not have much time, then just engage with your soothing breathing rhythm (exercise 3). Next, imagine that you are identifying with your compassionate self by bringing to mind each of its qualities. Remember to create a friendly facial expression and to imagine you have a warm tone of voice.

Now bring to mind a situation in which you became angry or the kind of situation in which you typically become angry. In the beginning, imagine a situation that provokes only mild anger and frustration. Using the mindfulness skill of noticing and stepping back, look at the angry part of yourself through the eyes of the compassionate self and sense how painful anger feels in your mind and body. Look at the facial expression of the angry self. What is the angry self really angry about? Are there other feelings that it's covering up, such as anxiety or sadness? If so, then maybe the compassionate self can explore those feelings as well. What would really help the angry self find peace? So you develop empathy and tolerance for your angry self without judging it. Maybe your angry self wants more recognition or to be more assertive.

Let the pain and frustration of the angry self touch you while remaining anchored in the qualities of the compassionate self: your wisdom sees how this angry outburst can be intense and all-consuming like a fire, but it is temporary and will pass; your strength allows you to remain grounded, holding the space for the angry part and letting it move through you; your warmth and kindness detect the deeper feelings that anger may be concealing like fear, sadness, or loneliness; and your commitment allows you to stand by yourself and develop the courage to go through this experience of anger and relate constructively to it.

While holding to your compassionate self and maintaining your friendly facial expression and warm tone of voice, see yourself in your mind's eye and imagine directing the following wishes to your angry self:

- May you be free of the inner turmoil stirring anger and frustration, [say your name].

- May you be in touch with the feelings that lie beneath your anger, [say your name].

- May your angry self find stability and peace, [say your name].

As with these words and phrases or similar words, let yourself feel the flow of compassion to your angry self, and if the feelings do not flow so easily, remain connected to your intention to be kind and committed. Notice what happens to the image of your angry self. When you have finished sending these wishes, let the image of your angry self fade and spend a few moments tuning in to the feelings that may have arisen in you, noticing in particular how this feels in your body. Then rest without focusing on anything in particular, stretch, and get up.

As with anxiety, keep in mind here that while we want to soften anger, we are not fighting with it or trying to get rid of it or criticizing ourselves for it. It is about validating, accepting, and understanding it, but not acting it out, because that would be unhelpful. Anger, like anxiety, can be very important for us to pay attention to because these are normal defensive emotions. With compassion we can transform anger into assertiveness and argue our case. Compassion for anger doesn't make us submissive, but wise, focused, and determined.

Also bear in mind that underneath the angry self is usually some disappointment or threat; for example, you made a mistake and that links to some memory of being criticized or rejected. The compassionate self reaches underneath the anger to ascertain the real issue, which is usually a fear of being shamed, unwanted, and rejected.

If you find yourself getting angry and frustrated in daily-life situations, pause and engage with your soothing breathing for a few seconds, feel yourself slow down and become more grounded, and then consciously shift to your compassionate self, looking at the situation through its eyes. Begin by practicing in situations that arouse mild anger, and in this way build up your capacity for dealing with more difficult situations.

Working with the Critical Self

Increasingly, research reveals that harsh self-critical thoughts and negative views of ourselves are associated with vulnerability to unhappiness, anxiety, depression, and other mental health problems.[6] A tendency toward self-criticism and self-dislike can create two major problems. First, self-criticism is usually associated with feelings of disappointment, anger, and frustration, which are threat-based emotions. So people who are routinely self-critical are constantly stimulating their threat system. Second, self-criticism blocks our ability to be self-compassionate. Indeed, even when we try to become self-compassionate, that critical voice can get in the way, passing harsh judgments by telling us that we don't deserve it or that we are not doing it properly. However, if we just fight the self-critical part of ourselves, then we can end up still being trapped in the threat system by being "critical of being critical." What is needed is to move out into the soothing/affiliation system and stimulate our feelings of compassion. If we make our compassionate self the authority within us, then this will deal with the self-critical self in a kind but firm way. Here is a way you can do this.

Exercise 17: Compassion for the Critical Self

Begin by settling into a posture that is comfortable yet alert, and then follow the mindfulness stages of soothing breathing rhythm, grounding, resting, and breath support (exercise 6). If you do not have much time, then just engage with your soothing breathing rhythm (exercise 3). Next imagine that you are identifying with your compassionate self by bringing to mind each of its qualities. Remember to create a friendly facial expression and imagine you have a warm voice tone.

Bring to mind a situation in which things were tough. Perhaps you were physically unwell or you were experiencing a bereavement or relationship conflict or you failed to achieve something that was really important to you. Tune in to the flow of self-critical thoughts and feelings.

Now imagine that you can see that part of you that does the criticizing—see it in front of you and notice what form it takes. Does it look a bit like you or something else? The self-critic can appear in all kinds of different forms. Notice the emotions it is directing at you. Be curious and note the anger or disappointment or contempt. Keep your friendly smile and try to see what's behind all the recriminating thoughts. What is your critic really frightened of? Does it remind you of anybody? Ask yourself: "Does my critic really have my best interests at heart? Does it want to see me flourish, be happy, and at peace? Does it give me a helping hand of encouragement when I struggle?" The answer is likely to be a resounding "no." The question that follows is, "Do you want to let it run the show?"

So, just as you felt compassion for your anxious and angry selves, you can do exactly the same for your critical self. Remember that looking through the eyes of your compassionate self is your sense of inner authority and the wise part of you that understands. See if you can hold the critical self with kindness, recognizing that it comes from being threatened or hurt in the past. Try to connect with the fear that lies behind it. This can be quite challenging because it can give you a sense of just how much you have been bullied by this critical self in the past and how you may have lacked an authority to restrain it. But don't go any faster or any deeper than you feel comfortable with. Now gently direct the following questions to your critical self:

- What is it that you really need?

- If you got what you needed, how would you feel?

Now imagine that you direct a flow of energy toward the critical self that takes the form of how it would feel if its needs were met. If the self-critical part needs love and attention, for example, and if it would feel at peace if it received this, then imagine that the flow of energy takes the form of *feeling at peace* in whichever way feels best to imagine. As you direct this flow of energy, you can make the following aspiration:

- May you be free of the pain that is causing you to be angry and critical of me.

Or, if you prefer:

- May I be free of the pain that is causing me to be angry and critical of myself.

As you say these words and phrases, or similar words, imagine a flow of compassion toward the self-critical part; and if the feelings do not flow so easily, then focus on the following intentions: the wisdom that sees through the self-criticism and appreciates how we are all caught up in the flow of life and undergo difficult challenges; the strength that holds and contains the anguish of the self-critical mind; the warmth that softens and connects to its underlying needs; and the courage to meet those needs rather than be drawn into a self-critical spiral.

When you have finished, let the image of your critical self fade and spend a few moments tuning in to the feelings that have arisen in you, noticing in particular how this feels in your body. Then rest without focusing on anything in particular, stretch, and get up.

This practice is derived from a Tibetan Buddhist practice that can be traced back thousands of years, with the idea that we "feed" our demons—that is, satisfy the needs they reflect—rather than fight with them.[7]

When you find yourself being sucked into a spiral of self-criticism in daily-life situations, pause and engage with your soothing breathing rhythm for a few seconds, slow yourself down, and then consciously identify with your compassionate self. Then look at your self-critical mind through the eyes of your compassionate self. Consciously connect to the needs underlying the self-critical stance and imagine meeting those needs in the way described in the exercise above. If we make efforts to work with our self-critic, this will soften it, which in turn helps us become gentler and more self-compassionate.[8]

Compassionate Behavior

Compassionate behavior includes a wide range of activities and builds up the feeling and commitment of the compassionate self. Try to do one compassionate act each day, something you normally wouldn't do. When you do this act, really focus on your intention and the feeling of compassion in doing the act. It could be a random act of kindness such as making a cup of tea for somebody, helping a work colleague, spending quality time with your children, or helping out your next-door neighbor. There is increasing evidence that developing sensitivity and compassion for others actually helps us feel better too.

Also try to carry out one compassionate act for yourself each day. Remember that compassion is not about doing things that are easy or self-indulgent like having that extra piece of chocolate cake. A compassionate act might be spending time preparing a healthy meal for yourself rather than a quick microwave one, or taking time out to do some physical exercise.

Key Points

- In this chapter we have looked at how to harness our motives, goals, and sense of self in order to create a compassionate self.

- As we saw in chapter 2, motivation and self-identity can organize our minds in different ways.

- We have considered some of the basic qualities of the compassionate self, such as wisdom, strength, warmth, and commitment.

- We have explored ways in which we can direct and focus the compassionate self using guided imagery in everyday life.

11

WIDENING OUR CIRCLE
OF COMPASSION

Now that we have connected with our innate qualities of compassion and begun to do the work of compassion for ourselves and those close to us, the next step is to widen our circle of compassion. We may find that we can easily connect with the struggles and conflicts of those we love, and extend love and compassion to them; but we may feel quite indifferent to strangers, and when it comes to people we do not like, such as competitors and adversaries, we might even feel happy that they suffer because it gives us an edge over them or justifies our desires of retribution and revenge. Indeed one of the problems with our brain is that we can actually take pleasure in inflicting suffering, especially on those we see as the "enemy." Billions of dollars are spent on creating computer games and Hollywood movies that play on exactly this theme—watching the bad guys get their comeuppance. So the next challenge on our journey is to find a way to be compassionate toward those who do not fall within our immediate circle of concern and to turn away from taking pleasure in their suffering.

Two principles lie at the heart of both the Mahayana Buddhist and evolutionary approach to cultivating compassion for others. The first is based on the simple fact that despite the many things that divide people, be it race, gender, culture, economic circumstances, or religious beliefs, we are all united when it comes to one thing—just like me, everyone wants happiness; and just like me, everyone wants to avoid suffering. Moreover, just like me, everyone wants to be loved, safe, and healthy; and just like me, no one wants to feel afraid or inadequate, or to be despised, sick, lonely, or depressed. We come to realize that whatever differences there are between people, in essence, we are all seeking the same things. Through reflecting on the fundamental equality of our self and others we are able to see beyond the differences that divide us to the common humanity that unites us. This is the basis for *identifying with others* and placing ourselves in their shoes; it is the basis for empathy, a key attribute of the compassionate mind.

The evolutionary approach informs us that all of us have been built by our genes; no one chose to be here, and no one chose to be sculpted with the values and self-identities that we have. Think for a moment about how, over the past three thousand years, tribe after tribe, group after group, nation after nation has stimulated passion and values in their people to attack, kill, maim, and torture people of other groups. The way humans constantly act out these underlying biological dramas is sheer tragedy. So no matter who our enemy is, they did not choose to be puppets in the drama of life, acting out whatever is going on inside of them. This deep wisdom allows us to stand back and begin the journey of compassion to those beyond our immediate circle of family and friends.

What is important here is to engage compassionately with the *mud of our own lives* (the complex of motives and emotions that drive us) as the basis for identifying with the struggles that others go through. Being willing to turn toward our own pain and our darker sides and consider them with compassion is the precondition for being able to relate to others in a similar way. Just as we have mud, so too do other people have mud, and through understanding and working skillfully with our own, we are in a position to offer something meaningful to others. When we begin to work compassionately with the difficult parts of ourselves—the angry or vengeful self, the anxious self, the critical self, and so on—we can appreciate how many other people are struggling in similar ways. They also struggle with feelings of anxiety and anger, and with destructive fantasies; they also experience low mood, lack of self-worth, and self-critical thoughts. By opening up to these difficult experiences in ourselves, we can sense in the depths of our being what it feels like for others. Our compassion starts to become genuine and real.

The second principle is the awareness of how interconnected life is and how interwoven our own lives are with those of others (see "Emergence and Interconnectedness" in chapter 1). We seldom pause to think about how we depend on others in so many ways. So many people from diverse cultural, economic, and religious backgrounds have been involved in producing, marketing, and distributing the simple things we take for granted in everyday life. Just think of how the food we eat arrived on our table—how many people were involved in its growth, cultivation, and distribution, and how many life-forms are consumed by us on a daily basis. Similarly, reflect on how many people and processes are involved in so many of the things we take for granted like clean water, the computer systems we use, the clothing we wear (which is often manufactured at low wages in developing countries), and the huge variety of things we consume. We are intertwined in a network of relationships that ensure our very survival and well-being.

Interconnectedness is also far more than simply recognizing our mutual dependence on the material things of life. What research has shown us is that from the day we are born, and even in the womb, the way that we interact with others affects which genes get expressed in us, the neural pathways that get laid down in our brains, and the kinds of people we become. The frontal cortex, which controls the regulation of our emotions, depends on positive social relationships to flourish. As we've noted many times throughout this book, the quality of our relationships with other people will have a major impact on the quality of our lives, values, and sense of self. These reflections are the basis for cultivating *gratitude and appreciation of others*.

Four Limitless Contemplations

- Loving-kindness (*maitri*)—wish for all beings to have happiness and the causes of happiness

- Compassion (*karuna*)—wish for all beings to be free of suffering and the causes of suffering

- Sympathetic joy (*mudita*)—rejoicing in the well-being and happiness of others and appreciating the positive things in life

- Equanimity (*upeksa*)—abiding in an impartial state of mind in which we do not grasp after what we like, reject what we do not like, and become indifferent to what does not interest us

Within the Buddhist tradition, the process of widening one's circle of compassion to include others is practiced by way of these four limitless contemplations. Each of these qualities complements the others and is part of a balanced system. Loving-kindness refers to feelings of warmth and friendliness toward our inner and outer worlds. Where it meets pain, it becomes compassion, and this draws on the particular qualities that we have explored in chapter 10 when we worked with the compassionate self. But remember, if we focus too much on pain and difficulty, there is a danger we will feel overwhelmed. This is where joy is important, and it starts with learning to appreciate and savor the simple things in our lives. This joy informs our compassion practice too—compassion is not just about becoming aware of suffering and trying to relieve it in others; it is also about rejoicing in the possibility of others being happy and free of suffering.

But equanimity is crucial. It is the axis around which the other qualities turn. Equanimity is an impartial state of mind. This does not imply that we are indifferent to what happens and that we are not moved by anything. It means we seek to care equally for all beings. In practice, it involves working with our tendencies to favor those we love, reject those we do not like, and ignore those who fall between these two extremes. So we work on opening up to those we dislike and paying attention to those we might normally ignore. It is based on the first principle we mentioned above, namely, the fundamental equality between all beings when it comes to avoiding suffering and seeking happiness. Without it, our love and compassion is limited—we tend to think just about ourselves and those close to us, and not about strangers or adversaries. Now this is perfectly normal; and, from the point of view of evolution, we are actually conditioned to protect those close to us. It is not an evolutionary prerogative to be concerned about all sentient beings, as our inbuilt drives are toward the survival and procreation of those who are part of our clan and genetically linked with us. But, as we have mentioned throughout this book, we have a "new brain" that can imagine and cultivate a different possibility. This is something that the Buddha realized thousands of years ago, but it is something that we today need to work on, and this is the focus of this chapter.

Practicing Compassion for Others

We will start by practicing equanimity because it exposes our likes and dislikes. This opens up the ground for the other qualities to take root; otherwise they remain partial and limited. We will do a practice that involves three processes: aspiring, dissolving, and equalizing. It is adapted from a practice devised by the psychologist and Buddhist author Aura Glaser.[1] In doing this practice, we will work with various categories of people: people we feel closely connected to, people we feel neutral toward, people we have difficulty with such as adversaries or competitors, and then all people everywhere. But, in order for these practices to work, it is important to bring to mind actual people and think about how they go about their lives; otherwise the practices remain conceptual and abstract and may not become real and meaningful.

Aspiring

In accordance with the four limitless contemplations, we can start by making aspirations for these people to be happy (loving-kindness), free from suffering (compassion), and to find joy in their lives (sympathetic joy). Aspiration is important because it connects us with compassionate motive, which is one of the key attributes of compassion that organizes our mind (attention, feeling, thinking, and behaving) in a particular way (chapter 4). So this is where we begin.

Now it is easy to meditate on the thought, "May my friends, family, colleagues, and everyone who I love and care about have happiness." When you imagine them being happy and smiling, this may give you a warm feeling. The feeling of compassion might flow naturally and easily for these people because they fall within our circle of love and concern. It might be more tricky to think, "May the person who offended me, may the colleague who hurt my feelings, may the family member who is avoiding me—may all of these people have happiness and be free from suffering." This is because evolution has designed our brains to want to fight or avoid those who threaten or hurt us. We might find that we run into all kinds of resistances; in fact, we might not want to be compassionate to these people at all. As Aura Glaser points out

> [I]t can feel like what we are really saying is, "May all beings have happiness, and may they all be free from suffering—but really only those I like and not those I dislike." We might sincerely love "all beings" in a general way when we're sitting on our meditation cushions, but actual, or even imagined, encounters with real people show us with unfailing honesty where we get stuck.[2]

Being open and honest about this is all part of the process. What is important here is to become aware of our anger, or that gut-level resistance, revulsion, or prejudice, without running away from it and without condemning ourselves or justifying it. This is where mindfulness is important. We can tune in to how these reactions feel in our body so we become thoroughly acquainted with these habits of resistance and holding. We do not have to *pretend* to be compassionate or go on some witch-hunt to force ourselves with a "must, should, or ought" because that will achieve little. Instead, we can learn to hold our resistances kindly and remain connected to our intention: "At this moment, I cannot open my heart to this person who hurt me, but I form the aspiration that one day I will be able to open my heart more fully than today." And remember, the first step to compassion is simply to understand that even our worst enemy does not want to suffer; they did not choose to be here with the brain and set of values that they have.

It is important to be clear at this point what we mean by wishing our enemies well. Matthieu Ricard has pointed out that if we are confronted by a tyrant or torturer, or somebody who is doing harm, then this is not about wishing them to be happy by continuing with their bad behavior.[3] Instead, compassion is wishing that the *root cause* of what is driving them to behave in destructive and harmful ways would cease. It is also based on the wisdom that cultivating anger and hatred toward an enemy *hurts us* and does not address the root cause of the situation.

Dissolving

A key observation of the Buddha's was that the more we live our lives simply following our tendencies to go for what we want, avoid what we do not want or like, and tune out of what does not interest us, the more our inner world starts to contract around a tight, embattled "me," and the more we suffer. We all know that sensation of going about our daily lives feeling stressed and preoccupied, with a tight knot of contraction in our bodies as things start to close in. But, as we have seen in previous chapters, there is no blame in this; we are evolved to be like this sometimes, so it is not our fault. But of course, it is our responsibility to do something about this condition because we are a species with a new brain that gives us a capacity for awareness and insight that no other animal has, and it's from this that we develop the wisdom not to be a slave to our evolved, socially constructed minds.

So bringing to mind the various categories of people we mentioned above, we work with each in a vivid and real way. We bring a friend to mind and notice our patterns of attachment and approval, thinking about what we like about them and becoming aware of our opinions, feelings, and bodily sensations as we do this; then we think about an adversary, bringing to mind an individual who pushes our buttons and noticing the things that irritate us, and what we do not like about them. We then do the same for a neutral person, thinking perhaps of a bus driver or the person who serves us cappuccinos every day at the café.

Now we consciously *shift our perspective* and think about how other people see and feel about these very same people. To someone at her work, the person who is your friend might be seen as hostile and aggressive, and she might well be the object of hatred. Likewise, you may see your adversary in the eyes of their family, to whom she or he might be adorable. Then we see the neutral person from the point of view of someone who loves them. What this immediately reveals is that the way we perceive people may have more to do with how they *behave* toward us, rather than an *intrinsic* quality within them. It is more to do with us and our perceptions than it is to do with them. Again, we are not trying to force anything here or wring out some feeling of compassion. All we are doing is acknowledging that how we feel is related to how we see things—*it is to do with us*. Now this is empowering.

Equalizing

Through reflecting in this way, we create some space in our mind to accommodate people's behavior and notice how it triggers positive and negative reactions in us, all of which are perfectly understandable. We see how this does not detract from their basic humanity or ours. In this way the simple truth of equality reveals itself: beneath the surface, we all want the same thing, however unskillfully we may behave at times. When we work with people with mental health problems who may engage in aggressive behavior or self-harming, it's important to recognize that deep inside, they too want happiness and to love and be loved; it's just that their threat system is so overly active that they don't know how to do it. When we choose to see through the surface layer of reactivity, instead of feeling separate from others, we see how similar to them we really are. We do this by acknowledging the fundamental truth we outlined above—just like me, everyone wants to be happy, and just like me, everyone wants to avoid suffering. This does not mean that we need to condone people's negative behavior—we might well need to take action against someone if their behavior infringes our rights—but we can still respect the humanity of that person. Furthermore, we do not need to suppress our negative reactions and gloss over them with some false sense of compassion—they can remain there in full view. But what we can do is allow ourselves to make contact with the poignant vulnerability that lies at the heart of the human experience. This is the birth of the compassionate heart—this is what causes the seed to germinate beneath the mud and the seedling of compassion to grow.

Aura Glaser aptly sums it up:

> Aspiration allows us to continually extend the reach of our heart. Dissolving softens the fixations and defenses that keep us habitually caught in accepting some of life and rejecting the rest. And equalizing brings us back again and again to the naked truth of our shared humanity and shared heart. Together, these practices of equanimity move us closer to ourselves, closer to life, and closer to the heart of compassion.[4]

Let's now do an exercise to practice the stages of aspiring, dissolving, and equalizing.

Exercise 18: Widening Our Circle of Compassion

Begin by settling into a posture that is comfortable yet alert, and then follow the mindfulness stages of soothing breathing rhythm, grounding, resting, and breath support (exercise 6). If you do not have much time, then just engage with your soothing breathing rhythm (exercise 3). Now imagine that you are identifying with your compassionate self. Bring to mind each of the qualities of your compassionate self—wisdom, strength, warmth, and commitment—and imagine that these qualities are present within you. Remember to create a friendly facial expression and imagine you have a warm voice tone.

Someone Who Is Close

Now bring to mind someone you hold dear and imagine that she is sitting in front of you or going about her daily business. This can be a visual image or a felt sense of her being present. This might be a parent, child, partner, or even an animal for whom you feel a natural flow of love and care. Now think of a time when this person (or animal) was going through a difficult phase. Notice how you feel a sense of concern based on your feelings of tenderness and care, and how there is a natural movement of compassion, wanting to reach out and help alleviate her suffering.

While holding to your compassionate self and maintaining your friendly facial expression and warm voice tone, imagine directing the following heartfelt wishes to this person:

- May you be happy and well, [say their name].

- May you be free of suffering and pain, [say their name].

- May you experience joy and well-being, [say their name].

Connect to the flow of compassion toward your loved one and pay attention to the feelings that arise in you when you focus on your heartfelt wish for her to be happy and free from suffering. If the feelings do not flow easily, then remain connected to your intention to be kind, supportive, and committed.

Now shift perspective and reflect for a moment on how it may be very natural for you to feel love and care for this person, but to someone at work, for example, your loved one might be seen as hostile and aggressive and may even be the object of loathing. And then reflect on how, for the vast majority of people, your loved one is merely part of a faceless crowd. So you see how your feelings arise out of your particular relationship; they are not qualities intrinsic to that person.

And now reflect that just like you and your loved one, the people who do not like her and the people who are indifferent to her all want to be happy and free from suffering. In this respect they are all equal. Then let the image of the loved one fade, and spend a few moments tuning in to the feelings that may have arisen in you, noticing in particular how this feels in your body.

Someone Who Is Neutral

Now think of someone who you neither like nor dislike, but have some form of contact with on a daily basis. It might be a bus driver, the person who serves you coffee as you walk to work, a classmate, or someone you see on the train every morning. Bring to mind an actual person. Think that, just like you, this person has dreams, hopes, and fears. Just like you, this person finds herself in the flow of life and struggles with her emotions, life circumstances, and setbacks. Just like you, this person struggles with feelings of anxiety and anger and self-critical thoughts; she is hurt by rejection and boosted by love.

Now imagine this person facing suffering in some way: perhaps dealing with conflict at work, struggling with addiction or depression, or feeling lonely and unloved. Then allow your heart to feel tenderness and concern for this person and make the following heartfelt aspirations:

- May you be happy and well, [say their name].

- May you be free of suffering and pain, [say their name].

- May you experience joy and well-being, [say their name].

Notice how you feel when you express these wishes. Perhaps there is a natural flow of care and concern, or perhaps you feel indifferent or even irritated by the exercise. If you notice yourself feeling shut down, irritated, or resistant, simply be curious about this and notice where you feel this in your body. Is there tightness in your face, jaw, or shoulders, or tension and contraction in some other part of your body? Try to be gentle and honest, not suppressing the emotions you are feeling. Try looking "from the balcony," so to speak, as an observer of how your threat and compassion systems are clashing in some way. Then affirm your intention that although you cannot open up to this person right now, you make the wish that one day you may open your heart more fully.

Now shift perspective and think about how this person to whom you feel indifferent loves and cares for some people; there are people who look forward to seeing her when she comes home from work; there are things in her life that she cherishes. In this way, reflect that your indifference or neutrality is *about you* and the way you see things; it is not intrinsic to her.

And now reflect that just like you, this person wants to be happy; and just like you, this person wants to be free of suffering and pain. Just like you, she wants to be loved, safe, and healthy; and just like you, she does not want to be despised, lonely, or depressed. Let the poignancy of this person touch you. Then let the image of this person fade and spend a few moments tuning in to the feelings that may have arisen in you, noticing in particular how this feels in your body.

Someone Who Is Difficult

Now think of someone you dislike, and who may have done you some harm, someone who is an adversary or competitor, or someone you know but have little time or regard for. Bring a particular person to mind and imagine that he is present in front of you, focusing on the felt sense of his presence. Despite what this person has done, just like you, he has hopes and aspirations for his life. Just like you, he finds himself in the flow of life with a complex brain and a difficult array of emotions that pull him this way and that. Just like you, this person struggles with feelings of anxiety and anger and self-critical thoughts.

Now imagine this person facing suffering in some way, perhaps dealing with conflict at home or at work, struggling with addiction or depression, or feeling lonely and unloved. Maybe you can even see that one of the reasons he is difficult is because inside he is suffering; he may be insecure and angry at the way his life is. Then allow your heart to feel tenderness and concern for this person and make the following heartfelt wishes:

- May you be happy and well, [say their name].

- May you be free of suffering and pain, [say their name].

- May you experience joy and well-being, [say their name].

Notice how you feel when you make these wishes. Is there a natural flow of tenderness and care toward this person, or does your heart feel contracted and resentful, not really wanting this person to be happy and free of suffering? Simply notice how you are feeling—there is no right or wrong way to feel. Be curious and tune in to how you are feeling in your body—is there tightness in your face, jaw, or shoulders, or tension and contraction in some other part of your body? Maybe you feel the very opposite of compassion, and that is completely okay. Just affirm your intention that one day you may open your heart more fully than today.

Now shift your perspective and reflect that other people might see your adversary in a very different light. He might be adored by some even though you cannot stand the sight of him. He might be a loving parent at home and very tender with animals. In this way, reflect that your feelings and reactions may have a lot more to do with you than they have to do with him. This does not mean to say that you have to condone his negative actions. If you find this step too difficult, then return to the aspiration stage and aspire to one day see past your initial reactions and wish him well.

And now, once again, reflect that just like you, this person wants to be happy; and just like you, this person wants to be free of suffering and pain. Just like you, this person wants to be loved, safe, and healthy; and just like you, he does not want to be despised, lonely, or depressed. Let the humanity of this person touch you. In essence, he is just like you. Then let the image of this person fade and spend a few moments tuning in to the feelings that may have arisen in you, noticing in particular how this feels in your body.

Opening Out to All Others

Now bring to mind the three types of people you have been working with—someone close, someone you feel indifferent toward, and someone who is difficult. Recall that they all share the same basic yearning to be happy and free from suffering; they are all actors in the flow of life. In this respect, they are exactly the same. Now contemplate people you know, going through them person by person. Begin with friends and then move on to people you have less connection with such as those who serve you coffee or sell you the morning newspaper as you walk to work. Then gradually open this up to include adversaries and those you find difficult. Imagine that, just like you, these people want happiness and don't want suffering; just like you, these people do not want stress; just like you, these people want safety and ease; just like you, they want to be loved. The more personal you make it, the more powerfully it will move you. Now gradually expand your awareness to take in other people who live or work near you, those in your neighborhood and your town, those who live in the same country and continent, and finally all living beings everywhere. And now, imagining all beings everywhere, you can conclude with the aspiration of the four limitless contemplations:

- May all living beings be happy and create the causes of happiness.

- May they all be free from suffering and the causes of suffering.

- May they all experience great joy and well-being untainted by suffering.

- May they come to rest in an impartial state of mind.

Focus mainly on your heartfelt wishes flowing out in all directions and becoming more and more expansive. And then foster a sense of appreciation for all these countless living beings upon whom our lives depend in so many ways, in this way seeing life as an interconnected web. Then let the visualization fade and spend a few moments tuning in to the feelings that may have arisen in you, noticing in particular how this feels in your body. Then rest, without focusing on anything in particular; stretch, and get up.

Dissolving and Equalizing "On the Spot"

Walking down the street or sitting in a café can be a good time to observe how easily we close down or open up. We see how quickly we become judgmental of others and how all kinds of emotions follow on from this. Before we know it, we're taking sides. It doesn't take much to trigger our reactions. There's attraction to the person we find beautiful, irritation at children in the street making a lot of noise, or contempt for a dirty vendor on the side of the street. Try to notice when you feel attraction or irritation and catch it before it solidifies into a fixed mindset. It is important to do this with honesty and kindness, not suppressing the emotions you are feeling, simply noticing them but then not feeding them.

Instead of going through our day caught up in our own world, we can take a few minutes to focus on the practice of equalizing. It is so simple and direct, and yet it can really open our eyes and touch our hearts to consider others in this way. When you meet another person, think: "Just like me, he wants to be happy and he doesn't want to suffer; just like me, these people walking past me in the street are caught up in the drama of the flow of life."

Self-Preoccupation

Opening our heart in this way is not easy. It challenges our deeply ingrained instinct to place "me" at the center of our world and only to be concerned with ourselves and those who are close to us. We might have run into this tendency when we experienced resistance to widening our circle of compassion in the last two exercises. For this reason, we need additional skills to address this tendency. A classic Mahayana Buddhist text called *The Seven Points of Mind Training* says that all compassion training comes down to one thing—overcoming self-centeredness and focusing instead on the welfare of others. It is referred to as the *sacred mystery that leads to true happiness.*

It is important, however, to clarify exactly what is meant by self-centeredness. It does not mean that we should not have an ego. In fact, a strong and healthy ego is necessary to live effectively in the world and to undertake the path of compassionate mind training. It also does not mean that we should not be concerned with our own happiness. As we have seen, self-compassion is necessary both for our own well-being and as the basis of compassion for others.

What we are talking about here is the process of self-preoccupation— being sucked into habitual tendencies to grasp at things we like, push away things we do not like, and ignore what does not interest us. But, as we have seen in earlier chapters, we are set up by evolution to grasp at things we need and avoid things that are threatening. It is not our fault that our minds work in this way. The issue here is not so much that it is wrong or bad to have a sense of self or to experience emotions like anger, anxiety, desire, and craving. The issue is more about how much we choose to feed these tendencies once we become aware of them. We experience many different kinds of impulses and emotional tendencies moving through our minds, none of which are our design or fault; but given our new-brain propensities, we have the capacity to choose what to focus our energy on. This is a central theme of this book. The key point is that if these tendencies are left unchecked, the mind can solidify around its defenses so that our energies become inwardly focused and everything is about "me" and what "I" want or do not want.

This is especially the case with emotional wounds and early life pain. Our minds can contract around painful feelings and experiences as a defensive strategy, and we can end up shutting feelings out that threaten our sense of stability and control. In this way, we can become deeply defensive and isolated people—defended against our emotions and armored against people and situations that threaten to trigger these emotions. We can find ourselves inhabiting an increasingly contracted world with very clear likes and dislikes that relate to how we like to feel, what we like to do, and who we like to spend time with. This is the deeper meaning of *dukkha* as taught by the Buddha.

Tonglen: Taking and Sending

A practice that goes to the root of self-preoccupation is called *tonglen*. This is a Tibetan word that means "taking and sending." "*Tong*" means "sending out" or "letting go," and "*len*" means "receiving" or "accepting." The practice originated in India and was brought to Tibet in the eleventh century by the Indian master Atisha. It forms part of *The Seven Points of Mind Training* and is a core meditation practice within each of the main Tibetan Buddhist lineages.[5] It has become popular in the West in large part due to the writings and teachings of Pema Chödrön, a Tibetan Buddhist nun who lives in the United States.[6]

The idea is that we take in the suffering and pain of others and then we send them all our joy, well-being, and peace. Whenever we see or feel suffering, we breathe it in with the notion of completely feeling it, accepting it, and transforming it. Then we breathe out loving-kindness, release, and openness. Many people recoil at this idea because this is the last thing they want to do. They might think that things are bad enough as it is without taking on the suffering of others. Our normal tendency is to hold onto the good and keep away from the bad, whereas *tonglen* reverses this tendency—we give away the good and welcome the bad. In this respect, *tonglen* is counterintuitive and goes against the grain.

Our immediate instinct might be that *tonglen* is harmful—we will take on the negativity and pain of others, and it will be toxic. In fact, what is happening is that when we take on the suffering of others, especially those we do not like, we are not really taking on their suffering in a literal sense; rather, we are taking back our own resistances and aversions. We are acknowledging the huge amount of energy that is associated with resistance and aversion and we are gradually reclaiming this lost energy. In so doing we are breaking down the walls between ourselves and life around us. We are allowing our hearts to open and be more responsive to the suffering of others. This is the real meaning of this practice.

In this way, *tonglen* works directly with the process of self-preoccupation. The underlying principle of *tonglen* is that what really causes us problems is not so much difficult emotions or troublesome people and life situations, but how we react to these things—how we shut them out of our minds and hearts. We have worked with this already when we looked at the practice of acceptance in chapter 8. But *tonglen* goes further and works in an active way with these reactions. *Tonglen* helps us become more deeply aware of how our mind closes down and contracts when we push things away—either people or emotions—and we notice how this makes us suffer. Just recall the last time you saw someone you did not like and how you may have instinctively closed down and even felt a tension in your body. With *tonglen*, we actively open up to discomfort and resistance and draw it toward us by breathing it in rather than following the normal pattern of closing down and pushing it away; and we then open outward with kindness and spaciousness as we breathe out. In this way, we are working directly with the tendency of the mind to contract inwardly, shut down, and disconnect from the flow of life.

This practice brings together the two psychologies of compassion. In earlier chapters, we used the example of a doctor who needs to be in tune with the suffering of her patient to wisely understand the problem and make the correct diagnosis, but then needs to shift her attention to prescribing medicine or carrying out surgery to relieve the suffering. First, there is an opening up to suffering that requires us to be able to hold it and feel it (first psychology) and then a shift of focus to the alleviation of suffering through the positive emotions of loving-kindness and care (second psychology).

This distinction is captured superbly in the practice of *tonglen*. On the in-breath, we are drawing pain toward us, being sensitive to it, and letting it touch our hearts; and then on the out-breath, we are conveying our intention to relieve suffering by giving out loving-kindness, joy, and spaciousness. In this way, the practice of *tonglen* actively moves between these two psychologies, using the breathing as the medium of awareness.

Practicing Tonglen

We have laid the foundations for doing this practice in the preceding practice chapters. The soothing breathing rhythm helps us to slow down and bring the mind back to the body, in this way grounding us in the moment. Breathing is important because it is the basis for visualizing suffering coming in through the in-breath and relief from suffering going out with the out-breath. Furthermore, we do the practice from the perspective of our compassionate self. This is very important. If we do it from the point of view of our everyday, fallible, and limited selves, we could feel that it is all too much. So we identify with the compassionate self and bring to mind its qualities of wisdom, strength, warmth, and commitment.

We begin the practice of *tonglen* by engaging with the pain and difficulty in our own experience. Throughout this practice section, we need to start with *self*-compassion for the practice of compassion to be authentic. Just as we did in the previous chapter, we work with ourselves in a general sense, and then we work with particular aspects of ourselves that cause us difficulties, such as the anxious self, the angry self, and the critical self. Afterward, we move on to doing *tonglen* for others; we start again with those who are close to us, relating to a mild difficulty at first, and then we move on to working with strangers and adversaries, and finally opening the practice out to all beings everywhere.

Exercise 19: *Tonglen* for Your Self

Begin by settling into a posture that is comfortable yet alert, and then follow the mindfulness stages of soothing breathing rhythm, grounding, resting, and breath support (exercise 6). If you do not have much time, then just engage with your soothing breathing rhythm (exercise 3).

Now imagine that you are stepping into and identifying with your compassionate self. Bring to mind each of the qualities of your compassionate self—wisdom, strength, warmth, and commitment—and imagine that these qualities are fully present within you. Remember to create a friendly facial expression and imagine you have a warm voice tone.

Imagine that directly in front of you is the ordinary part of you that is struggling, perhaps feeling lonely, fearful, misunderstood, angry, or troubled by physical illness or grief. As you look toward your ordinary self and become aware of the suffering you've been carrying, pay attention to the detail of your experience, almost as if you are watching a film of yourself going about your day. Let the pain and conflict of your ordinary self touch you and hold it with a warm and compassionate concern. Be curious and interested in what you are going through without judging or condemning it. If you notice any resistance to opening up to yourself in this way, just become aware of this resistance and hold it gently in your awareness.

Now consider that the suffering of the "ordinary you" takes the form of a dark cloud and with each in-breath, imagine that you breathe it in. As the cloud of suffering enters your being, imagine that it loosens the tight knot of self-contraction around your heart, revealing the wisdom and compassion at the center of your being. As you exhale, imagine that you freely give out understanding, joy, and kindness, in the form of light, to the suffering part of you. Continue this giving and receiving with each breath for as long as you like. If you find yourself going numb, blanking out, or not being able to connect, then make this the focus of your practice, breathing *this* in on the in-breath and breathing your release from this on the out-breath. However, always go gently and do not force yourself if it causes upset.

If you find it difficult to imagine a dark cloud, or if this feels too heavy or literal, then practice in a more feeling-oriented way. While rooted in your compassionate self, imagine being in contact with the pain of your ordinary self, and then, on the in-breath, focus on opening up to this pain and letting it touch your heart, drawing it toward you rather than pushing it away. Then imagine that as this pain touches your heart, it transforms—a bit like hot air being transformed into cool air by an air conditioner. So you are opening up on the in-breath, opening up on the out-breath, with no sense of anything getting stuck. There is no need to visualize too ardently—just set up the process and trust that the breathing does the work. What is important is the intention of drawing suffering toward you and breathing out release from suffering on the out-breath, and then trusting that this process runs by itself.

As you continue the practice, imagine that the ordinary part of you is gradually relieved of suffering and filled with well-being and joy. Each time you conclude, consider that the "ordinary you" is freed of some of the burden of its pain and distress and is more able to tolerate and work through what remains. Any pain you take in never stays there because it is always transformed into light or joy. Now let go of visualizing and just rest without any focus. If you notice any feelings of well-being or spaciousness, tune in to where you feel them in the body and allow yourself to appreciate and rest in these feelings. Then rest without any focusing on anything in particular, stretch, and get up.

You can work with *tonglen* for yourself in this general way and then you can focus on specific aspects of yourself that you may be struggling with, such as your anxious self, your angry self, and your critical self. Consequently, this practice follows on directly from the practices of the compassionate self we introduced in the previous chapter.

Exercise 20: *Tonglen* for Others

Begin by settling into a posture that is comfortable yet alert, and then follow the mindfulness stages of soothing breathing rhythm, grounding, resting, and breath support (exercise 6). If you do not have much time, then just engage with your soothing rhythm breathing (exercise 3).

Now imagine that you are identifying with your compassionate self. Bring to mind each of the qualities of your compassionate self—wisdom, strength, warmth, and commitment—and imagine that these qualities are fully present within you. Remember to create a friendly facial expression and imagine you have a warm voice tone.

Imagine that sitting in front of you is someone in your life you know to be suffering. Bring to mind the details of his appearance and what he is going through, opening yourself to this person's pain and letting it touch you. Be curious and interested in what he is going through without judging or condemning it. Then form a strong intention to release the person from his suffering and its causes.

Now imagine breathing in the other person's suffering in the form of a dark cloud and visualize it being drawn into your heart region, where it dissolves the tight knot of contraction in your heart and reveals the fullness of your compassionate potential. Remember that all the suffering gets transformed in your heart region; none of it gets stuck in there. As you breathe out, imagine that you are sending the other person all your healing love, warmth, energy, confidence, and joy in the form of brilliant light. Again, if you find the image of a dark cloud too strong, then focus on the flow of feeling—being aware of the person's pain, opening up to it on the in-breath, letting it touch you, and opening out on the out-breath, giving out feelings of spaciousness, loving-kindness, and care.

Continue this practice of "giving and receiving" with each breath for as long as you wish. If you find yourself feeling blocked or going numb, then shift your focus to these feelings in yourself and make them the focus of the practice, breathing in for yourself and all other people in a similar situation. If this still feels difficult then go back to focusing on soothing breathing rhythm and resting in your compassionate self, bringing to mind the qualities of the compassionate self.

At the end of the practice, consider that your compassion has dissolved all of the person's suffering and its causes, filling him with peace and happiness. If you notice any feelings of well-being or spaciousness in yourself, tune in to where you feel them in your body and allow yourself to appreciate these feelings. Then rest without focusing on anything in particular, stretch, and get up.

* * *

As your *tonglen* practice becomes stronger and more stable, you can gradually imagine others who are suffering—colleagues, patients, relatives, or even strangers—and practice taking in and transforming their suffering and giving them your happiness, clarity, understanding, forgiveness, and love. The *tonglen* practice can follow on from the practice of widening our circle of compassion (exercise 18, above). It is particularly useful when we run into resistance to opening up to strangers and adversaries because it provides a way to directly work with this resistance.

An important aspect of *tonglen* is to imagine that when we breathe in the suffering of someone, we imagine that we also breathe in the suffering of all other people who suffer in a similar way. For example, if a loved one is suffering from grief and loss, we then imagine that we take in the grief and loss of both our loved one and all others who suffer in this way. This has the effect of expanding our field of awareness to include other people in similar situations. But it is always important to start with a specific person or situation and then expand outward to others; otherwise the practice can become too abstract.

Tonglen on the Spot

You can also practice *tonglen* in everyday-life situations. This is often when it is most effective. For example, if you're walking down the street and you notice someone in pain or distress, on-the-spot *tonglen* means that you do not just close down and rush away. Clearly, if there is something you can do in a concrete way, like offering money or help, do what is appropriate; but if this is not the case, you can approach the situation using *tonglen*: let the humanity of this person touch you, breathe in their distress with the wish that they be free from suffering, and then send them warm wishes and feelings of happiness on the out-breath. If you find that the other person's pain brings up fear or resistance in you, then do *tonglen* for these feelings and reactions in yourself. The idea behind this practice is to work through your own blocks and resistances so that you can relate to changing life situations in a fresh and open way.

Here is another example. If you have missed a train and feel irritated and upset, imagine on the in-breath drawing into your own irritation all the frustration of others who are angry and irritated about late transport. Imagine it is transformed in your heart and then breathe out relief for the frustration of others on the out-breath. This has the effect of expanding outward and counteracting the tendency to contract inward around our own irritation and distress.

Also, when you experience moments of joy and happiness, there is an opportunity to practice *tonglen*. In these moments, practice breathing out your joy and happiness and share them with all beings everywhere, cultivating the wish that they too may feel joy and happiness in this moment, just like you do.

Through practicing *tonglen* in everyday-life situations, we bring together all the practices we have been learning. When encountering difficult people and adverse situations, there is an instinctive tendency to want to ward these things off and shut down and just focus on maintaining our own head-space and well-being in that moment. But, as we have seen, this has the opposite effect—it closes us down and sows the seeds of self-preoccupation and rumination; we are feeding our threat system. The approach we have been learning is to open up to life: to pay attention, let the world in, and cultivate a warm holding space that can accommodate more and more. This is the first psychology of compassion. And then, through slowing down and connecting with our breathing— even a few mindful breaths—we step into our compassionate self and give out loving-kindness, generosity, and warmth. This is the second psychology of compassion. In this way, everyday-life situations present an opportunity to bring together all the elements of our mindfulness and compassion practices and begin the process of gradually widening our circle of compassion.

Conclusion

Tonglen is about reconnecting to life. We are part of life and yet we easily cut ourselves off from it. There are many reasons why we do this, but disconnecting in this way hurts because we are going against the truth of being connected; and yet opening up to life and relating holds the potential for being hurt too. So *tonglen* invites us to take a risk. It invites us to open up to feeling the pain—and the joy—of being alive. It also invites us to let the natural energy of loving-kindness and care flow in response to the pain we experience. This is the true meaning of the two psychologies of compassion. So what it brings us back to is the fact that opening up to pain and responding with love and care are natural processes of being alive; we are not introducing anything new. We are simply acknowledging the reality of being part of an interconnected process called life. The breathing is a symbol of this process: life flows in and life flows out and we have the choice whether to be in accord with it or to resist, but if we resist, it comes with a price—we suffer.

Key Points

- The two key principles for widening our circle of compassion are identification and appreciation.

- The four limitless contemplations provide a balanced framework for widening our circle of compassion.

- Training in impartiality and equanimity is crucial for ensuring our compassion is not limited and biased. There are three key elements to it: aspiring, dissolving, and equalizing.

- We practice this in relation to loved ones, people we feel neutral toward, people who are difficult, and then all beings.

- *Tonglen* works with our tendency toward self-preoccupation in an active way and it employs the two psychologies of compassion.

CONCLUSION: THE COMPASSIONATE JOURNEY

So we have come to the end of our journey together. Ours—and we hope yours—continues with some of the practices in this book. We started our travels way back in time, millions upon million of years ago, in fact, and explored the way our brain has come to be the way it is. We saw how its textures and shapes, which give rise to our values and sense of self, are influenced by the genes we get from our parents and the social world in which we grow up. In one type of social environment, we could become violent or develop a sense of entitlement because of inherited wealth, but growing up in a different environment might instill a desire for justice, peacefulness, and unlocking the secrets of well-being. This is the challenge of our humanity: to understand our minds better and to cultivate the conditions that support our ability to nurture ourselves, others, and the planet we live on. Indeed, around the world there is increasing recognition of the importance and power of compassion-based psychologies in supporting mental health, harmonious social relationships, and endeavors toward justice and fairness. The compassionate mind takes an interest in others and the consequences of its behavior on others. The compassionate mind offers a way of working with the complex emotions and motivations that we inherit from our human and prehuman ancestors.

We are enthusiastic about the way in which psychological science is interacting with ancient spiritual insights to deepen and broaden our understanding and application of compassion. But the task ahead is not easy. We have seen that the human brain is wonderful but also potentially very dangerous. It gave rise to culture, art, and medicine; it has landed people on the moon and given us mobile phones and computers. However, without care, it can also build factories that churn out weapons to maim and kill people in the millions; it can build torture chambers; it is consumed by tribal prejudices; it can be aggressive and violent even to an individual's own partners and children; it can ruminate on frightening things; and it can drive us insane and lead us to commit suicide. As we begin to understand more about our brains, we come to realize just what a responsibility we have to become familiar with, understand, and then train our minds and not let them run riot in the way that they so easily do. Without training, the powerful drives of the pleasure-seeking, resource-demanding drive system and the anxious and aggressive threat system can run the show.

Thankfully these are not particularly new insights. Although evolution has given us new angles of understanding, we can turn to age-old traditions to learn how to train our minds, particularly with practices such as mindfulness and compassion, which have the capacity to transform our destructive emotions. We can find and nurture the lotus in the mud. We begin by becoming attentive to the self-monitoring and self-critical parts of ourselves. We adopt a friendly attitude to them, becoming mindful of when and how they arise, where they came from, and what their function is. We then work on softening the blaming and shaming that locks us into the threat system. As we have mentioned many times in this book, we become accustomed to accessing the soothing/affiliation system as this opens up feelings of loving-kindness and a genuine wish to be supportive, helpful, and in harmony within ourselves and with others. We pay attention to our bodies, facial expressions, the rhythms of our breaths, and our tones of voice, and we acknowledge our wisdom. All along, we are guided by the understanding that we are all on a journey that none of us chose, but we just find ourselves here doing the best we can.

The practice section started with the ancient Buddhist premise that the compassionate mind is the mind that transforms. We noted too that mindfulness is crucial to this process because it enables us to see just how chaotic our minds are and how much our attention is pulled here and there by thoughts and feelings that arise involuntarily. When we sit and try to just be fully present, we realize how difficult it is because our thinking brain is always planning, anticipating, imagining, remembering, and so on. Moreover, recognizing that what we focus on significantly affects how we are and what we feel impresses upon us the need to train the flashlight of our attention. In this way, mindfulness is the ground upon which we can build compassionate attributes and skills within ourselves. In learning how to choose what to cultivate, we can focus on our innate caregiving motives so they flourish and become a guiding force for the kind of mind we wish to have and the self we want to become. Angry self, anxious self, and wanting self will turn up relatively automatically, whereas compassionate self requires our attention, training, and cultivation. But, as we have said, we can *train to become the self we want to be.*

In one way or another, many spiritual philosophies of old (e.g., Stoicism) have understood this and have offered different solutions. Contrary to many misconceptions, cultivating a compassionate mind does not weaken us or undermine our drives; rather it directs our lives and drives in a particular way. Indeed, it can invigorate and energize us. The compassionate mind makes it possible to have a relationship with ourselves that is genuinely friendly, supportive, and encouraging on this difficult journey called life.

So practice what you can when and where you can. Practice in the bath, while waiting for a bus, or when spending a few minutes under the duvet before you get up—as often as you can—remembering to bring to mind the self you want to become. If you can put time aside to train in mindful compassion, it can reap huge dividends in your life.

But go gently with an attitude of openness, curiosity, and patience. Always keep in mind that we have all found ourselves here with this tricky brain and social conditioning. So we can start each day, seeing it as a great opportunity to be kind and helpful to ourselves and others and to make this journey in life a little easier.

FIND OUT MORE

Books

Mindfulness

Williams, M. and D. Penman. (2011) *Mindfulness: A Practical Guide to Finding Peace in a Frantic World*. London: Piatkus.

There are many books on mindfulness. Three classics are

Hanh, Thich Nhat. (1991) *The Miracle of Mindfulness*. London: Rider.

Kabat-Zinn, J. (2005) *Coming to Our Senses: Healing Ourselves and the World Through Mindfulness*. London: Piatkus.

Nairn, R. (1999) *Diamond Mind: A Psychology of Meditation*. London: Shambhala.

The Dalai Lama

The Dalai Lama is the spiritual head of Buddhism, which can be seen as both a spiritual approach and a basic psychology. Buddhism is particularly useful for its psychology and insights built up over thousands of years of meditation and introspective observation.

The Dalai Lama. (1995) *The Power of Compassion*. London: Thorsons.

The Dalai Lama. (2001) *An Open Heart: Practising Compassion in Everyday Life*, ed. N. Vreeland. London: Hodder & Stoughton.

Other Books

Bikshu Sangharakshita (2008) *Living with Kindness: The Buddha's Teaching on Metta*. London: Windhorse Publications.

Gilbert, P. (2010) *The Compassionate Mind*. London: Constable & Robinson; Oakland, CA: New Harbinger.

Henderson, L. (2011) *Improving Social Confidence and Reducing Shyness Using Compassion Focused Therapy*. London: Constable & Robinson; Oakland, CA: New Harbinger.

Lee, D. (2012) *The Compassionate Mind Approach to Recovering From Trauma*. London: Constable & Robinson; Oakland, CA: New Harbinger.

Kolts, R. (2012) *The Compassionate Mind Approach to Managing Your Anger*. London: Constable & Robinson; Oakland, CA: New Harbinger.

Tirch, D. (2012) *The Compassionate Mind Approach to Overcoming Anxiety*. London: Constable & Robinson; Oakland, CA: New Harbinger.

CDs

Some useful CDs that will guide you are

Chödrön, P. (2007) *How to Meditate: A Practical Guide to Making Friends with Your Mind*. Boulder, CO: Sounds True. Chodron offers a very comprehensive program based on mindfulness.

Kabat-Zinn, J. (2005) *Guided Mindfulness Meditation*. Boulder, CO: Sounds True. You can find more of Kabat-Zinn's work by typing his name into a search engine.

Websites

Compassion: Bridging Practice and Science

http://www.compassion-training.org

From 2011 to 2013, a group of international researchers and practitioners came together under the leadership of the Max Planck Institute's Professor Tania Singer to develop an internationally available resource on compassion. The result was a very large e-book that is free to download at the website provided above.

Compassionate Mind Foundation (UK)

http://www.compassionatemind.co.uk

In 2007, Paul Gilbert and a number of colleagues set up a charity called the Compassionate Mind Foundation. On this website, you'll find various essays and details of other sites that look at different aspects of compassion. You'll also find a lot of material that you can use for meditation on compassion. Foundations using the basic model outlined here are now being developed around the world.

Compassionate Wellbeing

http://www.compassionatewellbeing.com

This is run by Hannah Gilbert for the dissemination and teaching of compassion in different contexts.

Compassionate Mind Foundation (USA)

http://www.mindfulcompassion.com

This is run by Dr. Dennis Tirch. You will find various downloads that can be used for guided practice and meditation.

Center for Compassion and Altruism Research and Education

http://www.stanford.edu/group/ccare/cgi-bin/wordpress/

This center provides extensive information with lecture and videos on all facets of compassion—a truly excellent resource.

Mindfulness Association

http://www.mindfulnessassociation.net

Choden is one the founders of the Mindfulness Association, a nonprofit organization that has been set up to provide secular mindfulness, compassion, and insight training. Its compassion training draws on the evolutionary matter of Paul Gilbert, and it offers teacher training in mindfulness. It works in association with the University of Aberdeen, offering a Master's program in Mindfulness Studies (MSc).

Mind & Life Institute
http://www.mindandlife.org
The Dalai Lama has formed relationships with Western scientists to develop a more compassionate way of living. More information on this can be found on this website.

Mindful Self-Compassion
http://www.mindfulselfcompassion.org
This is run by Christopher Germer. You will find various downloads that can be used for meditation.

Samye Ling
http://www.samyeling.org
Samye Ling is a traditional Buddhist monastery in the Scottish Borders. It runs various retreats (including three-year ones) and provides for those who are interested in a Buddhist way of life and study. Choden studied here for many years. This is also where the MSc in Mindfulness and Compassion is run in liaison with the University of Aberdeen.

Self-Compassion
http://www.self-compassion.org
This is run by Dr. Kristin Neff, one of the leading researchers into self-compassion. You will find various downloads that can be used for meditation.

Breathing

For more information about breathing and how breathing affects our bodies, visit:
http://www.coherence.com

Building Compassionate Societies

Community Development Framework No Community Left Behind:
http://www.nocommunityleftbehind.ca

Community Foundation
http://en.wikipedia.org/wiki/Community_foundations

Community Foundation Network
http://www.communityfoundations.org.uk

Compassion in World Farming
http://www.ciwf.org.uk

Compassion in Elementary Schools: Ideas for a school-wide theme and lesson plans
http://www.vsb.bc.ca

Principles for Responsible Investment
http://www.unpri.org/principles

Restorative Justice Council
http://www.restorativejustice.org.uk

Restorative Justice 4 Schools
http://restorativejustice4schools.co.uk

SureStart
http://www.education.gov.uk/childrenandyoungpeople/earlylearning
andchildcare/delivery/surestart/a0076712/sure-start-children's-centres

NOTES

Introduction

1 Phillips, A. and Taylor, B. (2009) *On Kindness*. London: Hamish Hamilton.

2 The Dalai Lama (1995) *The Power of Compassion*. London: Thorsons; and The Dalai Lama (2001) *An Open Heart: Practising Compassion in Everyday Life* (ed. N. Vreeland). London: Hodder & Stoughton. See also Geshe Tashi Tsering (2008) *The Awakening Mind: The Foundation of Buddhist Thought: Volume 4*. London: Wisdom Press.

3 Ibid.

4 There are some very useful and easily accessible books available now for thinking about mindfulness. Probably the best known is Kabat-Zinn, J. (2005) *Coming to Our Senses: Healing Ourselves and the World Through Mindfulness*. New York: Piatkus. Another popular one with many useful exercises is Siegel, R.D. (2010) *The Mindfulness Solution: Everyday Practices for Everyday Problems*. New York: Guilford. Some books also link mindfulness and compassion in very interesting and important ways, e.g., Germer, C. (2009) *The Mindful Path to Self Compassion: Freeing Yourself from Destructive Thoughts and Emotions*. New York: Guilford. Another book that does this is Siegel, D. (2010) *Mindsight: Transform Your Brain with the New Science of Kindness*. New York: Oneworld.

5 You can see Matthieu Ricard talking about this research at http://www .huffingtonpost.com/matthieu-ricard/could-compassion-meditati_b _751566.html.

6 Jeffrey Sachs (2011), in his important book *The Price of Civilization: Economics and Ethics after the Fall*. London: Bodley Head, articulates how self-focused behaviors, especially those that focus on competitive edge in

getting ahead of others regardless, are seriously distorting economic and world resource distribution systems. It's a world where the strong get stronger and the weak weaker. Increasingly now economists are recognizing that trickle-down economics of unbridled self-focused competition is seriously damaging not only for our economies but also for our minds (see Twenge, J.M., Gentile, B., DeWall, C.N., Ma, D., Lacefield, K. and Schurtz D.R. [2010] Birth cohort increases in psychopathology among young Americans, 1938–2007: A cross-temporal meta-analysis of the MMPI. *Clinical Psychology Review*, 30, 145–154).

7 Self-compassion has become an important focus in Western approaches to well-being. The reason the West has become so interested in self-compassion is because we are very individualistic and competitive, and therefore self-critical and shame prone. Although there are different approaches to self-compassion based on different models, key figures in this area are Neff, K. (2011) *Self Compassion: Stop Beating Yourself Up and Leave Insecurity Behind*. London: Morrow; and Germer, C. (2009) *The Mindful Path to Self Compassion: Freeing Yourself from Destructive Thoughts and Emotions*. New York: Guilford. My (2009) book *The Compassionate Mind* (London: Constable & Robinson), is also focused on self-compassion in some sections.

8 Phillips, A. and Taylor, B. *On Kindness*.

9 My research unit has become very interested in the concept of the fear of compassion—Gilbert, P., McEwan, K., Matos, M. and Rivis, A. (2011) Fears of compassion: Development of three self-report measures, *Psychology and Psychotherapy*, 84, 239–255. doi: 10.1348/147608310X526511; and Gilbert, P., McEwan, K., Gibbons, L., Chotai, S., Duarte, J. and Matos, M. (2011) Fears of compassion and happiness in relation to alexithymia, mindfulness and self-criticism, *Psychology and Psychotherapy*, 84, 239–255. doi: 10.1348/147608310X526511.

10 Geshe Tashi Tsering (2008) *The Awakening Mind: The Foundation of Buddhist Thought*, Volume 1. Boston: Wisdom Press.

11 Ardelt, M. (2003) Empirical assessment of a three-dimensional wisdom scale, *Research on Aging*, 25, 275–324, suggests that wisdom has many facets—there is an ability to thoughtfully reflect on the way things are (e.g., the human condition), an ability to feel a certain way and of course a *motivation* to understand, "to know and learn" with an openness to the new. Wisdom also enables us to actively reason and think about things when we integrate our knowledge and experience. There are also studies looking at the way wisdom operates in our brain: Meeks, T.W. and Jeste, D.V. (2009) The neurobiology of wisdom, *Archives of General Psychiatry*, 66, 355–365. At the time of going to press Christopher Germer and Ronald

Siegel, two leading writers on mindfulness and compassion, have just published their landmark edited book (2012) *Wisdom and Compassion in Psychotherapy: Deepening Mindfulness in Clinical Practice*. New York: Guilford.

1 Waking Up

1   Geshe Tashi Tsering (2005) *The Four Noble Truths: The Foundation of Buddhist Thought*, Volume 1. Boston: Wisdom Publications.

2   Ibid.

3   Bodian, S. and Landaw, J. (2003) *Buddhism for Dummies*. Chichester: Wiley & Sons Ltd. Don't be put off by the title because actually this is a really accessible and knowledgeable book.

4   Whitfield, H.J. (2006) Towards case-specific applications of mindfulness-based cognitive-behavioural therapies: A mindfulness-based rational emotive behaviour therapy. *Counselling Psychology Quarterly*, 19, 205–217.

5   Ibid.

6   Geshe Tashi Tsering, *The Four Noble Truths*.

7   Once again Bodian and Landaw's *Buddhism for Dummies* offers an excellent and short review of this approach. For more detailed explorations see Geshe Tashi Tsering (2008) *The Awakening Mind: The Foundation of Buddhist Thought*, Volume 4. Boston: Wisdom Publications.

8   For a fascinating read on emergence see Johnson, S. (2002) *Emergence: The Connected Lives of Ants, Brains, Cities and Software*. London: Penguin.

9   Christakis, N. and Fowler, J. (2009) *Connected: The Amazing Power of Social Networks and How They Shape Our Lives*. London: HarperCollins.

10 Belsky, J. and Pluess, M. (2009) Beyond diathesis stress: Differential susceptibility to environmental influences. *Psychological Bulletin*, 135, 885–908. doi: 10.1037/a0017376.

11 A very accessible and fascinating book if you're new to the area would be Gerhardt, S. (2007) *Why Love Matters*. London: Routledge. For more comprehensive coverage of the power of relationships to affect us in our bodies and brains Paul's favourites are Cozolino, L. (2007) *The Neuroscience of Human Relationships: Attachment and the Developing Social Brain*. New York: Norton; and Cozolino, L. (2008) *The Healthy Aging Brain: Sustaining Attachment, Attaining Wisdom*. New York: Norton.

12   Cacioppo, J.T. and Patrick, W. (2008) *Loneliness: Human Nature and the Need for Social Connection.* New York: Norton

13   Zimbardo, P. (2008) *The Lucifer Effect: How Good People Turn Evil.* London: Rider.

14   Johnson, *Emergence.*

15   Christakis and Fowler, *Connected.*

16   Pinker, S. (2011) *The Better Angels of Our Nature: The Decline of Violence in History and Its Causes.* New York: Allen Lane.

17   Gerhardt, S. (2010) *The Selfish Society: How We All Forgot to Love One Another and Made Money Instead.* London: Simon & Schuster. See also Twenge, J. (2010) *The Narcissism Epidemic: Living in the Age of Entitlement.* London: Free Press.

18   Twenge, J.M., Gentile, B., DeWall, C.N., Ma, D., Lacefield, K. and Schurtz, D.R. (2010) Birth cohort increases in psychopathology among young Americans, 1938–2007: A cross-temporal meta-analysis of the MMPI. *Clinical Psychology Review,* 30, 145–154. Part of this may be because we are becoming more self-centered and less community oriented.

19   Ballatt, J. and Campling, P. (2011) *Intelligent Kindness: Reforming the Culture of Healthcare.* London: Royal College of Psychiatry Publications. An excellent argument for a compassionately organized and delivered NHS.

2 Evolved Mind and Motivations

1   Bolhuis, J.J., Brown, G.R., Richardson, R.C. and Laland, K.N. (2011) Darwin in mind: New opportunities for evolutionary psychology. *PLOS: Biology,* 9, 7, e1001109. doi: 10.1371/journal.pbio.1001109. This gives a good review of some of the most recent adaptations and evolutionary changes that have taken place in the past hundred thousand years or so. We humans are still changing and evolving.

2   Schimpf, M. and Tulikangas, P. (2005) Evolution of the female pelvis and relationships to pelvic organ prolapse. *International Urogynecology Journal,* 16, 4, 315–320. doi: 10.1007/s00192-004-1258-1. This is a good example of how an advantage in certain areas—being able to stand up and also have bigger brains—can actually cause serious problems for us!

3   Nesse, R.M. and Williams, G.C. (1995) *Evolution & Healing.* London: Weidenfeld & Nicolson. This is an excellent book to introduce you to the basic concepts of how evolution can cause us all kinds of problems rather

than perfecting wellness. Professor Nesse has been at the forefront of this work, and you can find out much more if you visit his website: http://www.personal.umich.edu/~nesse/.

4 Sapolsky, R. M. (2004) *Why Zebras Don't Get Ulcers*. St. Martin's Press.

5 A therapy developed by Stephen Hayes and his colleagues called Acceptance and Commitment Therapy has focused on how people's emotional difficulties are linked to their efforts to avoid emotions, hence the importance of "acceptance." Hayes, S.C., Follette, V.M. and Linehan, M.N. (2004) *Mindfulness and Acceptance: Expanding the Cognitive Behavioral Tradition*. New York: Guilford. Also, if you search for Acceptance and Commitment Therapy on the internet you will find many discussions about these issues. The problems of dealing with emotions have also been well explored by emotion therapists such as Leslie Greenberg (see Pascual-Leone, A. and Greenberg, L.S [2007] Emotional processing in experiential therapy: Why "the only way out is through." *Consulting and Clinical Psychology*, 75, 875–887. doi: 10.1037/0022-006X.75.6.875); and a very useful and helpful exploration of how mindfulness and compassion and help emotion regulation can be found in Leahy, R.L., Tirch, D. and Napolitano, L.A. (2011) *Emotion Regulation in Psychotherapy: A Practitioner's Guide*. New York: Guilford.

6 If you are interested in looking more deeply into the various different interacting parts of the brain, then look up Nunn, K., Hanstock, T. and Lask, B. (2008) *Who's Who of the Brain: A Guide to Its Inhabitants, Where They Live and What They Do*. London: Jessica Kingsley. And if you're thinking about how researchers are looking at brain processes in terms of some of the Buddhist concepts, then you may well enjoy Hanson, R. and Mendius, R. (2009) *Buddha's Brain: The Practical Neuroscience of Happiness, Love, and Wisdom*. Oakland, CA: New Harbinger. If you want to find out more about how the evolved brain gives rise to and influences our emotions, then a good read is LeDoux, J. (1998) *The Emotional Brain*. London: Weidenfeld & Nicolson.

7 Gilbert, P. (1989) *Human Nature and Suffering*. Hove: Psychology Press. Gilbert, P. (2000) Social mentalities: Internal "social" conflicts and the role of inner warmth and compassion in cognitive therapy. In Gilbert, P. and Bailey, K.G. (eds) *Genes on the Couch: Explorations in Evolutionary Psychotherapy* (pp. 118–150). Hove: Brenner–Routledge. Gilbert, P. (2005) Social mentalities: A biopsychosocial and evolutionary reflection on social relationships. In M.W. Baldwin (ed.) *Interpersonal Cognition* (pp. 299–335). New York: Guilford.

8 Simon-Thomas, E.R., Godzik, J., Castle, E., Antonenko, O., Ponz, A., Kogan, A. and Keltner, D.J. (2011) An fMRI study of caring vs. self-focus

during induced compassion and pride. *Social Cognitive and Affective Neuroscience*, Advance Access, 6 September, p. 1. doi: 10.1093/scan/nsr045. There is now also some excellent research work showing that the kind of self-identities we pursue can have quite a major impact on our well-being and quality of relationships. Crocker, J. and Canevello, A. (2008) Creating and undermining social support in communal relationships: The role of compassionate and self-image goals. *Journal of Personality and Social Psychology*, 95, 555–575.

9 Ornstein, R. (1986) *Multimind: A New Way of Looking at Human Behavior*. London: Macmillan, p. 9.

10 Coon, D. (1992) *Introduction to Psychology: Exploration and Application*, sixth edition. New York: West Publishing Company, p. 1.

11 Gilbert, *Human Nature and Suffering*; Social mentalities: Internal "social" conflicts and the role of inner warmth and compassion in cognitive therapy; Social mentalities: A biopsychosocial and evolutionary reflection on social relationships.

12 Carter, R. (2008) *Multiplicity: The New Science of Personality*. London: Little Brown.

13 James, W. (1890) *Principles of Psychology*, Volume 1. New York: Henry Holt and Company, pp. 309–310. Retrieved from http://jbarresi.psychology.dal .ca/Papers/Dialogical_Self.htm.

14 Taylor, C. (1989) *Sources of the Self: The Making of the Modern Identity*. Cambridge: Cambridge University Press.

15 McGregor, I. and Marigold, D.C. (2003) Defensive zeal and the uncertain self: What makes you so sure? *Journal of Personality and Social Psychology*, 85, 838–852.

16 Leary, M. (2003) *The Curse of the Self: Self-Awareness, Egotism, and the Quality of Human Life*. New York: Oxford University Press. See also Leary, M.R. and Tangney, J.P. (eds) (2002) *Handbook of Self and Identity*. New York: Guilford.

17 Shame is one of the most problematic personal experiences because we can be very aggressive to avoid shame, but also shame can make us very submissive, appeasing, depressed, and anxious. The reason is because shame threatens rejection and even persecution by others, and these, from an evolutionary point of view, are serious. Indeed shame can throw our brains into an intense sense of threat. You can read more about shame in Tracy, J.L., Robins, R.W. and Tangney, J.P. (eds) (2007) *The Self-Conscious Emotions: Theory and Research*. New York: Guilford. And see Gilbert, P. (2007) The evolution of shame as a marker for relationship security. In

Tracy, J.L., Robins, R.W. and J.P. Tangney (eds) *The Self-Conscious Emotions: Theory and Research* (pp. 283–309). New York: Guilford.

18   McGregor, I. and Marigold, D.C., Defensive zeal and the uncertain self (see note 14).

19   Leary, M. *The Curse of the Self*; see also Leary and Tangney, *Handbook of Self and Identity*.

20   Hanson, R. and Mendius, R. (2009) *Buddha's Brain: The Practical Neuroscience of Happiness, Love, and Wisdom.* Oakland, CA: New Harbinger.

21   Simon-Thomas et al. An fMRI study of caring vs. self-focus during induced compassion and pride.

22   Robin Dunbar has been at the forefront of helping us understand the evolutionary pressures that led to the development of this fantastic new brain which can think, reason, anticipate, ruminate, etc. It turns out that the pressure was actually social and that much of it was to do with developing affiliative and cooperative relationships. A good introduction to some of this can be found in Dunbar, R.I.M. (2010) The social role of touch in humans and primates: Behavioral function and neurobiological mechanisms. *Neuroscience and Biobehavioral Reviews*, 34 260–268. doi: 10.1016/j. neubiorev.2008.07.001.

23   Simon-Thomas et al. An fMRI study of caring vs. self-focus during induced compassion and pride.

24   Cacioppo, J.T. and Patrick, W. (2008) *Loneliness: Human Nature and the Need for Social Connection*. New York: Norton.

3 Emotional Systems

1   Haidt, J. (2001) The emotional dog and its rational tail: A social intuitionist approach to moral judgment. *Psychological Review*, 108, 814–834. This is a very helpful review of the complexity of our emotions.

2   Leahy, R.L., Tirch, D. and Napolitano, L.A. (2011) *Emotion Regulation in Psychotherapy: A Practitioner's Guide*. New York: Guilford offers a very good overview of how some psychotherapists think about emotions and ways in which people can learn how to develop their understanding and abilities to cope with their emotions. For more technical interest, see Kring, A.M. and Sloan, D.M. (2010) *Emotion Regulation and Psychopathology: A Transdiagnostic Approach to Aetiology and Treatment*. New York: Guilford.

3 Two books that explain why our emotions are tricky for us and how mindfulness can be helpful are Siegel, R.D. (2010) *The Mindfulness Solution: Everyday Practices for Everyday Problems*. New York: Guilford; and Siegel, D. (2010) *Mindsight: Transform Your Brain with the New Science of Kindness*. New York: Oneworld.

4 A very important paper underpinning some of these ideas to follow is Depue, R.A. and Morrone-Strupinsky, J.V. (2005) A neurobehavioral model of affiliative bonding. *Behavioral and Brain Sciences*, 28, 313–395. Another key researcher in the field is Panksepp, J. (1998) *Affective Neuroscience*. New York: Oxford University Press. If you want to follow his work and find out how he sees emotional systems in slightly different ways, you can download one of his papers: Panksepp, J. (2010) Affective Neuroscience of the Emotional BrainMind: Evolutionary perspectives and implications for understanding depression. *Dialogues in Clinical Neuroscience*, 12, 383–399 (http://www.dialogues-cns.org).

5 Ibid.

6 LeDoux, J. (1998) *The Emotional Brain*. London: Weidenfeld & Nicolson offers a very readable account of how the brain processes information, especially threatening information.

7 For more on the compassionate mind approach to anxiety with many exercises see Tirch, D. (2012) *The Compassionate Mind Approach to Overcoming Anxiety: Using Compassion-Focused Therapy*. London: Constable & Robinson. Also see Lynne Henderson (2011) *Improving Social Confidence and Reducing Shyness Using Compassion-Focussed Therapy*. London: Constable & Robinson.

8 For more on the compassionate mind approach to anger with many exercises see Kolts, R. (2012) *The Compassionate Mind Approach to Managing Your Anger: Using Compassion Focused Therapy*. London: Constable & Robinson.

9 Haidt, The emotional dog and its rational tail.

10 Gilbert, P., Clarke, M., Kempel, S., Miles, J.N.V. and Irons, C. (2004) Criticizing and reassuring oneself: An exploration of forms, style and reasons in female students. *British Journal of Clinical Psychology*, 43, 31–50. Disgust and psychopathology was also the subject of a special edition of the (2010) *International Journal of Cognitive Therapy*, 3.

11 Gilbert, P. (2009) *The Compassionate Mind*. London: Constable & Robinson.

12 LeDoux, *The Emotional Brain* (see note 6).

13 Tobena, A., Marks, I. and Dar, R. (1999) Advantages of bias and prejudice: An exploration of their neurocognitive templates. *Neuroscience and Behavioral Reviews*, 23, 1047–1058. Gilbert, P. (1998) The evolved basis and adaptive functions of cognitive distortions. *British Journal of Medical Psychology*, 71, 447–64.

14 See note 4.

15 Pani, L. (2000) Is there an evolutionary mismatch between the normal physiology of the human dopaminergic system and current environmental conditions in industrialized countries? *Molecular Psychiatry*, 5, 467–475.

16 Twenge, J.M., Gentile, B., DeWall, C.N., Ma, D., Lacefield, K., Schurtz, D.R. (2010) Birth cohort increases in psychopathology among young Americans, 1938–2007: A cross-temporal meta-analysis of the MMPI. *Clinical Psychology Review*, 30, 145–154. Part of this may be because we are becoming more self-centered and less community oriented.

17 Gilbert, P., Broomhead, C., Irons, C., McEwan, K., Bellew, R., Mills, A. and Gale, C. (2007) Striving to avoid inferiority: Scale development and its relationship to depression, anxiety and stress. *British Journal of Social Psychology*, 46, 633–648; Gilbert, P., McEwan, K., Irons, C., Broomhead, C., Bellew, R., Mills, A. and Gale, C. (2009) The dark side of competition: How competitive behaviour and striving to avoid inferiority are linked to depression, anxiety, stress and self-harm. *Psychology and Psychotherapy*, 82, 123–136.

18 Leahy et al. *Emotion Regulation in Psychotherapy*; Gilbert et al. (2007); Gilbert et al. (2009).

19 Gilbert et al. Striving to avoid inferiority; The dark side of competition (see note 17).

20 Depue, R.A. and Morrone-Strupinsky, J.V. (2005) A neurobehavioral model of affiliative bonding. *Behavioral and Brain Sciences*, 28, 313–395. This paper articulates and reviews important concepts of contentment and the ability to be "at peace."

21 Ibid.

22 Gilbert et al., Striving to avoid inferiority; The dark side of competition (see note 17).

23 Pani, Is there an evolutionary mismatch? (see note 15).

24 The evolution of caring behavior and the way in which parents came to look after and care for their children is now well-established psychology: see Geary, D.C. (2000) Evolution and proximate expression of human parental investment. *Psychological Bulletin*, 126, 55–77. We also know

something about the evolution of specific physiological systems and the brain for caring: see Bell, D.C. (2001) Evolution of care-giving behavior. *Personality and Social Psychology Review*, 5, 216–229; Depue and Morrone-Strupinsky, A neurobehavioral model of affiliative bonding. We also know that there have been some very fundamental adaptations in the autonomic nervous system which allow animals to get close together for affiliative purposes without overactivating their fight flight system: see Porges, S. (2003) The Polyvagal theory: phylogenetic contributions to social behaviour. *Physiology & Behavior*, 79, 503–513; Porges, S.W. (2007) The polyvagal perspective. *Biological Psychology*, 74, 116–143.

25 Ibid.

26 John Bowlby's three classic books on attachment sparked a revolution in child development research and are still a good read today: (1969) *Attachment: Attachment and Loss*, Volume 1. London: Hogarth Press; (1973) *Separation, Anxiety and Anger: Attachment and Loss*, Volume 2. London: Hogarth Press; (1980) *Loss: Sadness and Depression: Attachment and Loss*, Volume 3. London: Hogarth Press. Today, research on attachment relationships has advanced enormously, and you can get a good overview of the research and developing field from Mikulincer, M. and Shaver, P.R. (2007) *Attachment in Adulthood: Structure, Dynamics, and Change.* New York: Guilford.

27 Cozolino, L. (2007) *The Neuroscience of Human Relationships: Attachment and the Developing Social Brain*. New York: Norton.

28 Ibid.

29 Depue and Morrone-Strupinsky, A neurobehavioral model of affiliative bonding (see note 20).

30 Porges, The Polyvagal theory (see note 24).

31 Rockliff, H., Gilbert, P., McEwan, K., Lightman, S. and Glover, D. (2008) A pilot exploration of heart rate variability and salivary cortisol responses to compassion-focused imagery. *Journal of Clinical Neuropsychiatry*, 5, 132–139.

32 Dunbar, R.I.M. (2010) The social role of touch in humans and primates: Behavioral function and neurobiological mechanisms. *Neuroscience and Biobehavioral Reviews*, 34, 260–268. doi: 10.1016/j.neubiorev.2008.07.001.

33 MacDonald, K. and MacDonald, T.M. (2010) The Peptide that binds: A systematic review of Oxytocin and its prosocial effects in humans. *Harvard Review of Psychiatry*, 18, 1–21. A rather older outline that's still very readable is Carter, C.S. (1998) Neuroendocrine perspectives on social attachment and love. *Psychoneuroendocrinology*, 23, 779–818.

34 Rockliff, H., Karl, A., McEwan, K., Gilbert, J., Matos, M. and Gilbert, P. (2011) Effects of intranasal oxytocin on compassion-focused imagery. *Emotion*, 1, 1388–1399. doi: 10.1037/a0023861.

35 Belsky, J. and Pluess, M. (2009) Beyond diathesis stress: Differential susceptibility to environmental influences. *Psychological Bulletin*, 135, 885–908. doi: 10.1037/a0017376.

36 Cozolino, The Neuroscience of Human Relationships (see note 27).

37 Panksepp, J. (1998) *Affective Neuroscience* (Oxford: Oxford University Press) sees the play systems as a separate and important mammalian system in the brain. We believe that play is indeed extremely important for the process of affiliation with low threat and open attention. Whether or not we should focus on it as a special system or a particular combination of drive and soothing systems, however, is open to research and debate. There seem to be key brain areas for play, playfulness, and pretend.

38 Dunbar, The social role of touch in humans and primates (see note 32).

39 Ibid.

40 Pani, Is there an evolutionary mismatch?; Twenge et al., Birth cohort increases (see notes 15 and 16).

41 Cozolino, L. (2008) *The Healthy Aging Brain Sustaining Attachment, Attaining Wisdom*. New York: Norton. This is also brilliantly articulated by one of the pioneers and leaders in social neuroscience in Cacioppo, J.T. and Patrick, W. (2008) *Loneliness: Human Nature and the Need for Social Connection*. New York: Norton. So there is indeed now considerable evidence that social relationships and a sense of community are key to many health indices; see, for example, Holt-Lunstad, J., Smith, T.B. and Layton, J.B. (2010) Social relationships and mortality risk: A meta-analytic review. *Public Library of Science Medicine*, July, 7, 7, e1000316.

4 Emergence of Compassion

1 Two excellent books by the Dalai Lama are his (1995) *The Power of Compassion*. London: Thorsons; and (2001) *An Open Heart: Practising Compassion in Everyday Life* (ed. N. Vreeland). London: Hodder & Stoughton. Research around the world is now showing that when we train ourselves in compassion we actually change not only our thoughts and feelings but also physiological processes including processes in our brains. For a fascinating study and review of the literature see Klimecki, O.M., Leiberg, S., Lamm, C. and Singer, T. (2012) Functional neural plasticity and

associated changes in positive affect after compassion training. *Cerebral Cortex*, advance publication (1 June). doi: 10.1093/cercor/bhs142.

2 There are many good Buddhist texts on the nature of *Bodhicitta*, e.g., Geshe Tashi Tsering (2008) *The Awakening Mind: The Foundation of Buddhist Thought*, Volume 4. London: Wisdom Publications. However, a scholarly and fascinating book that explores the relationship of the concepts of *bodhicitta* and Western concepts of archetypes and a "modern psychology of motives" is Leighton, T.D (2003) *Faces of Compassion: Classic Bodhisattva Archetypes and Their Modern Expression*. Somerville, MA: Wisdom Publications. This was a great find for Paul. See also Vessantara (1993) *Meeting the Buddhas: A Guide to Buddhas, Bodhisattvas and Tantric Deities*. New York: Windhorse Publications.

3 Geshe Tashi Tsering, *The Awakening Mind*, p. 1 (see notes 1 and 6; chapter 1).

4 Spikins, P.A., Rutherford, H.E. and Needham, A.P. (2010) From homininity to humanity: Compassion from the earliest archaics to moderns humans. *Journal of Archaeology, Consciousness and Culture*, 3, 303–326.

5 Goetz, J.L., Keltner, D. and Simon-Thomas, E. (2010) Compassion: An evolutionary analysis and empirical review. *Psychological Bulletin*, 136, 351–374. doi: 10.1037/a0018807.

6 Feldman, C. and Kuyken, W. (2011) Compassion in the landscape of suffering. *Contemporary Buddhism*, 12, 143–155. doi: 10.1080/14639947.2011 .564831.

7 Neff, K. (2011) *Self-Compassion*. New York: Morrow.

8 The Dalai Lama, *The Power of Compassion, An Open Heart*; Geshe Tashi Tsering, *The Awakening Mind*.

9 Feldman and Kuyken, Compassion in the landscape of suffering, p. 143, italics added (see note 6).

10 Ibid., p. 145.

11 Matthieu Ricard gives a lovely explanation of this and the concept of "altruistic love": http://cultureofempathy.com/References/Experts/Matthieu -Ricard.htm. If you follow the links on the internet you will also find many other excellent talks by Matthieu Ricard. See too Ricard (2007) *Happiness: A Guide to Developing Life's Most Important Skill*. London: Atlantic Books.

12 Geshe Tashi Tsering, *The Awakening Mind* (see note 3).

13 Phillips, A. and Taylor, B. (2009) *On Kindness*. London: Hamish Hamilton, p. 4.

14   Ibid., p. 5.

15   Ibid.; Ballatt, J. and Campling, P. (2011) *Intelligent Kindness: Reforming the Culture of Healthcare*. London: Royal College of Psychiatry Publications.

16   Phillips, A. and Taylor, B., *On Kindness*, p. 27 (see note 12).

17   Ibid.

18   Ballatt and Campling, *Intelligent Kindness* (see note 14).

19   Neff, K. (2011) *Self-Compassion: Stop Beating Yourself Up and Leave Insecurity Behind*. New York: Morrow. Kristin has been at the forefront of developing the concept of self-compassion and you can find references to all her work—along with some questionnaires you can fill in to look at your own levels of self-compassion—on her Self-Compassion website: http://www.self-compassion.org. Other important books that combine mindfulness and self-compassion are Germer, C. (2009) *The Mindful Path to Self-Compassion: Freeing Yourself from Destructive Thoughts and Emotions*. New York: Guilford; and Siegel, D. (2010) *Mindsight: Transform Your Brain with the New Science of Kindness*. New York: Oneworld.

20   Gilbert, P. (1989) *Human Nature and Suffering*. Hove: Psychology Press; Gilbert, P. (2005) Compassion and cruelty: A biopsychosocial approach. In P. Gilbert (ed.) *Compassion: Conceptualisations, Research and Use in Psychotherapy* (pp. 3–74). London: Routledge. Gilbert, P. (2009) *The Compassionate Mind*. London: Constable & Robinson.

21   Fogel, A., Melson, G.F. and Mistry, J. (1986) Conceptualising the determinants of nurturance: A reassessment of sex differences. In A. Fogel and G.F. Melson (eds), *Origins of Nurturance: Developmental, Biological and Cultural Perspectives on Caregiving*. Hillsdale, NJ: Lawrence Erlbaum Associates Inc.; Ehlers, A., Hackmann, A. and Michael, T. (2004) Intrusive re-experiencing in post-traumatic stress disorder. Phenomenology, theory and therapy. *Memory*, 12, 403–415.

22   Gilbert, *Human Nature and Suffering*; Compassion and cruelty; *The Compassionate Mind* (see note 19).

23   Gilbert, P., McEwan, K., Matos, M. and Rivis, A. (2011) Fears of compassion: Development of three self-report measures. *Psychology and Psychotherapy*, 84, 239–255.

24   Gilbert, *Human Nature and Suffering*; Compassion and cruelty; *The Compassionate Mind* (see note 19).

25   See note 10.

26 Gilbert, *Human Nature and Suffering*; Compassion and cruelty; *The Compassionate Mind*.

27 See note 2.

28 Phillips, A. and Taylor, B., *On Kindness*, p. 29.

29 Although this was published in 1989 in *Human Nature and Suffering* it was derived from ongoing research at the time. Particularly impressive was a paper by Wispe, L. (1986) The distinction between sympathy and empathy. *Journal of Personality and Social Psychology*, 50, 314–321. There is also the important Decety, J. and Ickes, W. (2011) *The Social Neuroscience of Empathy*. Cambridge, MA: MIT Press. The first chapter by Bateson is especially useful because he points out the complexity and multiple meanings given to empathy. Another key researcher in this area is Eisenberg, N. (2002) Empathy-related emotional responses, altruism, and their socialization. In R. Davidson and A. Harrington (eds), *Visions of Compassion: Western Scientists and Tibetan Buddhists Examine Human Nature* (pp. 131–164). New York: Oxford University Press.

30 Karp, D. (2001) *The Burden of Sympathy: How Families Cope with Mental Illness*. Oxford: Oxford University Press. This is a very moving book based on 60 interviews with families coping with relatives with a mental illness and reveals how complex sympathy is in everyday lived experience. Caregiving that is felt to be obligatory in some way or the need of the other exceeding the resources one wants to put into caring can, however, be stressful and detrimental to health; see Vitaliano, P.P., Zhang, J. and Scanlan, J.M. (2003) Is caregiving hazardous to one's health? A meta-analysis. *Psychological Bulletin*, 129, 946–972.

31 Ballatt and Campling *Intelligent Kindness* (see note 14).

32 Researchers such as Nancy Eisenberg draw distinctions in our reactions to pain and suffering, such as empathy, sympathy, and personal distress. To be compassionate means we can not just turn away when distressed by confronting suffering. Eisenberg, N. (1986) *Altruistic Emotion, Cognition and Behaviour: A New View*. Hillsdale: NJ: Lawrence Erlbaum. Eisenberg, N. (2002) Empathy-related emotional responses, altruism, and their socialization. In R. Davidson and A. Harrington (eds), *Visions of Compassion: Western Scientists and Tibetan Buddhists Examine Human Nature* (pp. 131–164). New York: Oxford University Press.

33 Ballatt and Campling *Intelligent Kindness* (see note 14).

34 Willingness and motivation are very important in many therapies such as existential psychotherapy; see Yalom, I.D. (1980) *Existential Psychotherapy*. New York: Basic Books, which has a fascinating chapter on willingness. Also some of the newer therapies focus on willingness: Hayes, S.C.,

Strosahl, K.D. and Wilson, K.G. (2004) *Acceptance and Commitment Therapy: An Experiential Approach to Behavior Change*. New York: Guilford. Christopher Germer and Ronald Siegel also address this in (2012) *Wisdom and Compassion in Psychotherapy: Deepening Mindfulness in Clinical Practice*. New York: Guilford.

35 Rifkin, J. (2009) *The Empathic Civilization: The Race to Global Consciousness in a World in Crisis*. Cambridge: Polity Press. You can see a short but brilliant Royal Society of Arts YouTube sketch of these key ideas at: http://www.youtube.com/watch?v=l7AWnfFRc7g. To explore research on different types and degrees of empathy see Baron-Cohen's (2011) *Zero Degrees of Empathy*. London: Allen Cane.

36 Ibid.

37 Rogers, C. (1957) The necessary and sufficient conditions of therapeutic personality change. *Journal of Consulting Psychology*, 21, 95–103.

38 See note 28.

39 Margulies, A. (1984) Toward empathy: The uses of wonder. *American Journal of Psychiatry*, 141, 1025–1033. This is a paper that had a major impact on Paul many years ago.

40 Elliott, R., Bohart, A.C., Watson, J.C. and Greenberg, L.S. (2011) Empathy. *Psychotherapy*, 30, 43–46. doi: 10.1037/a0022187. And for fascinating research see Neumann, M., Bensing, J., Mercer, S., Ernstmann, N., Ommen, O. and Pfaff, H. (2009) Analyzing the "'nature'" and "'specific effectiveness" of clinical empathy: A theoretical overview and contribution towards a theory-based research agenda. *Patient Education and Counseling*, 74, 339–346.

41 Nickerson, R.S. (1999) How we know—and sometimes misjudge—what others know: Imputing one's own knowledge to others. *Psychological Bulletin*, 125, 737–759.

42 Bering, J.M. (2002) The existential theory of mind. *Review of General Psychology*, 6, 3–24.

43 Western, D. (2007) *The Political Brain*. New York: Public Affairs.

44 Stopa, L. (ed.) (2009) *Imagery and the Threatened Self: Perspectives on Mental Imagery and the Self in Cognitive Therapy*. London: Routledge.

45 Ringu Tulku Rinpoche and Mullen, K. (2005) The Buddhist use of compassionate imagery in Buddhist meditation. In P Gilbert (ed.) *Compassion: Conceptualisations, Research and Use in Psychotherapy* (pp. 218–238). London: Brunner–Routledge. Vessantara (1993) *Meeting the Buddhas: A*

Guide to Buddhas, Bodhisattvas and Tantric Deities. New York: Windhorse Publications.

46   Phillips and Taylor, *On Kindness*; Ballatt and Campling *Intelligent Kindness* (see note 14).

47   See notes 1 and 2.

48   See note 10.

49   Gilbert *The Compassionate Mind* (see note 19).

50   Ibid.

51   Ibid.

52   Phillips and Taylor *On Kindness* (see note 12).

53   Ibid.; Ballatt and Campling *Intelligent Kindness* (see note 14).

54   Oliner, S.P. and Oliner, P.M. (1988) *The Altruistic Personality: Rescuers of Jews in Nazi Europe.* New York: Free Press.

5 The Challenge of Mindfulness Practice

1   Gethin, R. (2011) On some definitions of mindfulness. *Contemporary Buddhism*, 12, 263–279. doi: 10.1080/14639947.2011.564843. In 2010 the journal *Emotion* (vol. 10, part 1) published a special edition on mindfulness with many excellent papers discussing the problems of defining mindfulness, the methods of measuring mindfulness, and differences in training. This is an excellent resource for those who want to go into this area more deeply.

2   Kabat-Zinn, J. (2005) *Coming to Our Senses: Healing Ourselves and the World Through Mindfulness.* New York: Piatkus, p. 108.

3   Siegel, R.D. (2010) *The Mindfulness Solution: Everyday Practices for Everyday Problems.* New York: Guilford, p. 27.

4   Nairn, R. (1998) *Diamond Mind.* London: Kairon Press, p. 30.

5   Kabat-Zinn *Coming to Our Senses* (see note 2).

6   Brewer, J.A., Worhunsky, P.D., Gray, J.R., Tang, Y., Weber, J. and Kober, H. (2011) Meditation experience is associated with differences in default mode network activity and connectivity, *Proceedings of the National Academy of Sciences*, 108(50), 20254–20259. http://www.pnas.org/cgi/doi/10.1073/pnas.1112029108.

7 Siegel, D. (2010) *Mindsight: Transform Your Brain with the New Science of Kindness*. London: Oneworld. See also Germer, C.K. and Siegel, R.D. (2012) *Wisdom and Compassion in Psychotherapy: Deepening Mindfulness in Clinical Practice*. New York: Guilford.

8 Four foundations of mindfulness (see http://www.dhagpo-kagyu.org/anglais/science-esprit/chemin/medit/etat_esprit/mindfullness2.htm for a fuller description).

9 Holmes, K. (2010) An introduction to Buddhist mindfulness. Unpublished paper, Samye Ling Tibetan Centre, Scotland.

10 Maex, E. (2011) The Buddhist roots of mindfulness training: A practitioner's view. *Contemporary Buddhism*, 12, 165–175. doi: 10.1080/14639947.2011.564835. There are many excellent papers in this issue. Also Feldman, C. and Kuyken, W. (2011) Compassion in the landscape of suffering. *Contemporary Buddhism*, 12, 143–155. doi: 10.1080/14639947.2011.564831 makes similar points in relation to mindfulness and compassion.

11 Hofmann, S.G., Sawyer, A.T., Witt, A.A. and Oh, D. (2010) The effect of mindfulness-based therapy on anxiety and depression: A meta-analytic review. *Clinical Psychological Review*, 78, 169–183. doi: 10.1037/a0018555. See also Davis, D.M. and Hayes, A.A. (2011) What are the benefits of mindfulness? A practice review of psychotherapy-related research. *Psychotherapy*, 48, 198–208. doi: 10.1037/a0022062—this is an excellent summary of key issues and findings. Grossman, P. (2010) Mindfulness for psychologists: Paying kind attention to the perceptible. *Mindfulness* (published online Spring; Springer). doi: 10.1007/s12671-010-0012-7.

12 Lutz, A., Brefczynski-Lewis, J., Johnstone, T. and Davidson, R.J. (2008) Regulation of the neural circuitry of emotion by compassion meditation: Effects of meditative expertise. *Public Library of Science*, 3, 1–5.

13 Williams, M., Teasdale, J., Segal, Z. and Kabat-Zinn, J. (2007) *The Mindful Way Through Depression: Freeing Yourself from Chronic Unhappiness*. New York: Guilford. These authors have done considerable research on mindfulness and depression, but this self-help book is the most accessible. For those interested in the research on processes in mindfulness and change see Kuyken, W., Watkins, E., Holden, E., White, K., Taylor, R.S., Byford, S., Evans, A., Radford, S., Teasdale, J.D. and Dalgleish, T. (2010) How does mindfulness-based cognitive therapy work? *Behaviour Research and Therapy*, 48, 1105–1112.

14 Gethin, On some definitions of mindfulness (see note 1).

15 Holmes, An introduction to Buddhist mindfulness (see note 9).

16 Brewer et al., Meditation experience is associated with differences in default mode network activity and connectivity (see note 6).

17 Neff, K. (2011) *Self-Compassion: Stop Beating Yourself Up and Leave Insecurity Behind.* New York: William Morrow. Germer, C. (2009) *The Mindful Path to Self Compassion: Freeing Yourself from Destructive Thoughts and Emotions.* New York: Guilford.

18 Recent research on mindfulness for depression suggests that one of the mediators of the benefits might be via the development of self-compassion; see Kuyken et al., 2011. Professor Kuyken, one of the leading authorities on research into mindfulness and depression, believes that keeping to the straightforward mindfulness focus without specific compassion training is important to this work, but we think that specific compassion focusing is necessary, especially when helping people with fears of compassion. However, we could be wrong and so these are fascinating debates which require much more research.

19 Maex, The Buddhist roots of mindfulness training, p. 171. (see note 10).

20 Watson, G., Batchelor, S. and Claxton, G. (1999) *The Psychology of Awakening: Buddhism, Science and Our Day-to-Day Lives.* London: Routledge.

21 Many psychotherapists recognize that some people are very frightened of feelings of warmth, closeness, and affiliation; they block out feelings of kindness for all kinds of reasons. We have just started doing research on this and have found that fear of compassion is linked with problems with mindfulness: see Gilbert, P., McEwan, K., Gibbons, L., Chotai, S., Duarte, J. and Matos, M. (in press) Fears of compassion and happiness in relation to alexithymia, mindfulness and self-criticism. *Psychology and Psychotherapy*; Gilbert, P., McEwan, K., Matos, M. and Rivis, A. (2011) Fears of compassion: Development of three self-report measures. *Psychology and Psychotherapy*, 84, 239–255. doi: 10.1348/147608310X526511.

22 The concept of acceptance is tricky and has a long history. You can find an excellent review of the issues in Williams, J.C. and Lynn, S.J. (2010) Acceptance: An historical and conceptual review, *Imagination, Cognition and Personality*, 30, 5–56. doi: 10.2190/IC.30.1.c.

23 The point here is that at a moment-by-moment level, awareness is free of the constructs that move through it which are built by genes and social conditioning. A good analogy is the sky and clouds. The sky is like awareness that is inherently free and open, and the clouds are like our social conditioning and genetic make-up. The true meaning of acceptance is to make space for the clouds and not fight them as this places us in alignment with the sky, which is the deeper truth.

24 Cacioppo, J.T. and Patrick, W. (2008) Loneliness: Human Nature and the Need for Social Connection. New York: Norton.

25 Kabat-Zinn, *Coming to Our Senses* (see note 2).

26 Hayes, S.C., Strosahl, K.D. and Wilson, K.G. (2004) *Acceptance and Commitment Therapy: An Experiential Approach to Behavior Change*. New York: Guilford. See also Germer and Siegel *Wisdom and Compassion in Psychotherapy*.

27 Nairn, *Diamond Mind* (see note 4).

28 Watson et al., *The Psychology of Awakening* (see note 20).

29 Neff, *Self-Compassion* (see note 17).

6 The Lotus in the Mud

1 Hofmann, S.G., Sawyer, A.T., Witt, A.A. and Oh, D. (2010) The effect of mindfulness-based therapy on anxiety and depression: A meta-analytic review. *Clinical Psychological Review*, 78, 169–183. doi: 10.1037/a0018555. See also Davis, D.M. and Hayes, A.A. (2011) What are the benefits of mindfulness? A practice review of psychotherapy-related research. *Psychotherapy*, 48, 198–208. doi: 10.1037/a0022062—this is an excellent summary of key issues and findings. Grossman, P. (2011) Mindfulness for psychologists: Paying kind attention to the perceptible. *Mindfulness* (published online Spring; Springer). doi: 10.1007/s12671-010-0012-7. See also Hofmann, S.F., Grossman, P. and Hinton, D.E. (2011) Loving-kindness and compassion meditation: Potential for psychological interventions. *Clinical Psychology Review*, 31, 1126–1132. doi: 10.1016/j.cpr.2011.07.003. This is a very helpful paper that looks at the links between mindfulness, compassion, and loving-kindness.

2 For a fascinating discussion of the links between mindfulness and compassion training in relationship to Western psychology, see the Dalai Lama and Paul Ekman's (2008) *A Conversation with the Dalai Lama and Paul Ekman*. New York: New York Times Books.

3 The Dalai Lama (2001) *An Open Heart: Practising Compassion in Everyday Life*. London: Hodder & Stoughton, p. 85.

4 Cacioppo, J.T. and Patrick, W. (2008) *Loneliness: Human Nature and the Need for Social Connection*. New York: Norton.

5   Pauley, G. and McPherson, S. (2010) The experience and meaning of compassion and self-compassion for individuals with depression or anxiety. *Psychology and Psychotherapy*, 83, 129–143. See page 140.

6   Gilbert, P., McEwan, K., Matos, M. and Rivis, A. (2011) Fears of compassion: Development of three self-report measures. *Psychology and Psychotherapy*, 84, 239–255. We have pursued this research and looked at compassion in relationship to mindfulness and alexithymia as well. Gilbert, P., McEwan, K., Gibbons, L., Chotai, S., Duarte, J. and Matos, M. (in press) Fears of compassion and happiness in relation to alexithymia, mindfulness and self-criticism. *Psychology and Psychotherapy*. Some people respond to compassion as if it is a threat. See: Rockliff, H., Karl, A., McEwan, K., Gilbert, J., Matos, M. and Gilbert, P. (2011) Effects of intranasal oxytocin on compassion-focused imagery. *Emotion*, 11, 1388–1396. doi: 10.1037/a0023861.

7   Gilbert, P. and Irons, C. (2005) Focused therapies and compassionate mind training for shame and self-attacking. In Gilbert, P. (ed.) *Compassion: Conceptualisations, Research and Use in Psychotherapy* (pp. 263–325). London: Routledge. See also Gilbert, P. (2010) *Compassion-Focused Therapy*, CBT Distinctive Features Series. London: Routledge.

8   Affectionate relationships are crucial to so many aspects of our minds, and the data is very clear on this. There are two excellent books: Cozolino, L. (2007) *The Neuroscience of Human Relationships: Attachment and the Developing Social Brain*. New York: Norton; and Cozolino, L. (2008) *The Healthy Aging Brain: Sustaining Attachment, Attaining Wisdom*. New York: Norton. If you want more information about how important affiliative behaviour is and how it has driven human evolution, look at Dunbar, R.I.M. (2010) The social role of touch in humans and primates: Behavioral function and neurobiological mechanisms. *Neuroscience and Biobehavioral Reviews*, 34, 260–268. doi: 10.1016/j.neubiorev.2008.07.001.

9   One of the best-known books on body memory and its link to mental-health problems is Rothschild, B. (2000) *The Body Remembers: The Psychophysiology of Trauma and Trauma Treatment*. New York: Norton. However, many people who work with trauma now recognise the importance of how our automatic bodily reactions can arise; see Van der Hart, O., Steele, K. and Nijenhuis, E. (2006) *The Haunted Self: Structural Dissociation and Treatment of Chronic Traumatization*. New York: W.W. Norton.

10 Gilmore, D.D. (1990) *Manhood in the Making: Cultural Concepts of Masculinity*. New Haven, CT: Yale University Press—This is a wonderful book for capturing how identities get shaped by their social environments.

Pinker, S. (2011) *The Better Angels of Our Nature: Why Violence Has Declined*. New York: Allen Lane.

11 Sachs, J (2011) *The Price of Civilization: Economics and Ethics After the Fall*. London: Bodley.

12 Ballatt, J. and Campling, P. (2011) *Intelligent Kindness: Reforming the Culture of Healthcare*. London: Royal College of Psychiatry Publications. An excellent argument for kindness and proper NHS organisation.

13 Gerhardt, S. (2010) *The Selfish Society: How We All Forgot to Love One Another and Made Money Instead*. London: Simon & Schuster. See also Twenge, J. (2010) *The Narcissism Epidemic: Living in the Age of Entitlement*. London: Free Press.

14 Vessantara (1993) *Meeting the Buddhas: A Guide to Buddhas, Bodhisattvas and Tantric Deities*. New York: Windhorse Publications.

15 In fact the emotion of disgust and its link to "getting rid of and purification" is now understood to be linked to some of our psychology of moral feelings in very complex and important ways. This is too big a topic to take up here, but interested readers can explore this for themselves—seeing once again how our evolved minds can shape us in ways that are sometimes surprising—and it directs us to great caution in how we feel and think about moral issues. Oaten, M., Stevenson, R.J. and Case, T.I. (2009) Disgust as a disease-avoidance mechanism. *Psychological Bulletin*, 135, 303–321. doi: 10.1037/a0014823. Russell, P.S. and Giner-Sorolla, R. (2011) Social justifications for moral emotions: When reasons for disgust are less elaborated than for anger. *Emotion*, 11, 637–646. doi: 10.1037/a0022600. A very fascinating book, exploring the whole nature of morality and suffering, is Shweder, R.A., Much, N.C., Mahapatra, M. and Park, L. (1997) The "big three" of morality (autonomy, community and divinity) and the "big three" explanations of suffering. In A.M. Brandt and P. Rozin (eds), *Morality and Health* (pp. 119–169). New York: Routledge.

16 Gilbert, P. (2009) *Overcoming Depression: A Self-Guide Using Cognitive Behavioral Techniques*, third edition. New York: Basic Books. Paul is also working on a specific compassionate mind approach to depression which is due for publication in 2014.

7 Mindfulness Practice

1 See chapter 5, note 1 (page 327).

2 Nairn, R. (1998) *Diamond Mind*. Cape Town: Kairon Press. Rob was one of Choden's teachers and therefore some of what is presented here, including

the exercise "Recognizing the Unsettled Mind," which opens the chapter, is derived from his teachings and work. See also Mindfulness Based Living Course (2011) by Mindfulness Association Ltd. (http://www.mindfulness association.net).

3   Farhi, D. (1996) *The Breathing Book: Good Health and Vitality Through Essential Breath Work.* New York: Holt. A new, excellent book with a guided-practice CD for training in breathing is Richard Brown and Patricia Gerburg (2012). *The Healing Power of the Breath.* Boston: Shambhala.

4   Kabat-Zinn, J. (2005) *Coming to Our Senses: Healing Ourselves and the World Through Mindfulness.* New York: Piatkus.

5   There are now many CDs to purchase and also YouTube demonstrations of body-scan mindfulness. Examples by Jon Kabat-Zinn, Ron Siegel, and Mark Williams can be recommended.

8 Working with Acceptance

1   Hayes, S.C., Strosahl, K.D. and Wilson, K.G. (2004) *Acceptance and Commitment Therapy: An Experiential Approach to Behavior Change.* New York: Guilford. Williams, J. C. and Lynn, S.J. (2010) Acceptance: An historical and conceptual review. *Imagination, Cognition and Personality,* 30, 5056. doi: 10.2190/IC.30.1.c. This is a full and excellent summary of the concept of acceptance in Buddhism and other schools of thought.

2   Chawla, N. and Ostafin, B. (2007) Experiential avoidance as a functional dimensional approach to psychopathology: An empirical review. *Journal of Clinical Psychology,* 63, 9, 871–890 (p. 871).

3   It is important that we don't see "willingness" as simply a choice because sometimes we really have such a struggle with our tricky brains, and things that are causing this trouble are outside awareness—so we can't be willing or unwilling because we are not aware of the problem. In fact we now know quite a lot about these processes, which are sometimes called "dissociative" (see Dell, P.F. and O'Neil, J.A. [2010] *Dissociation and the Dissociative Disorders: DSM-V and Beyond.* London: Routledge). Often we are not quite sure why we feel what we feel and being dissociated from the causes of our suffering is more common than has been recognised in the past (see Carter, R. [2008] *Multiplicity: the New Science of Personality, Identity and the Self.* London: Little Brown).

4   Williams and Lynn, *Acceptance,* p. 3 (see note 1).

5   Sallatha Sutta, The Arrow; translated from the Pali by Thanissaro Bhikkhu: http://buddhasutra.com/files/sallatha_sutta.htm.

6 Hofmann, S.F., Grossman, P. and Hinton, D.E. (2011) Loving-kindness and compassion meditation: Potential for psychological interventions. *Clinical Psychology Review*, 31, 1126–1132. doi: 10.1016/j.cpr.2011.07.003. This is a very helpful paper that looks at the links between mindfulness, compassion, and loving-kindness.

7 Ibid.

8 Kabat-Zinn, J. (2005) *Coming to Our Senses: Healing Ourselves and the World Through Mindfulness*. New York: Piatkus.

9 Baer, L. (2001) *The Imp of the Mind: Exploring the Silent Epidemic of Obsessional Bad Thoughts*. New York: Plume Press. This is an excellent book for people who are troubled by the kinds of thoughts and feelings that are coming into their minds.

10 Kabat-Zinn, *Coming to Our Senses* (see note 8).

9 Building Compassionate Capacity

1 Neff, K. (2011), *Self-Compassion: Stop Beating Yourself Up and Leave Insecurity Behind*. New York: Morrow. Kristin Neff has been at the forefront of developing the concept of self-compassion, and you can find references to all her work—along with some questionnaires you can fill in to look at your own levels of self-compassion—on her Self-Compassion website: http://www.self-compassion.org. Other important books that combine mindfulness and self-compassion are Germer, C. (2009) *The Mindful Path to Self-Compassion: Freeing Yourself from Destructive Thoughts and Emotions* (New York: Guilford); and Siegel, D. (2010) *Mindsight: Transform Your Brain with the New Science of Kindness* (New York: Oneworld). In our approach it is important to learn to recognize and accept the affiliative feeling of kindness—to be aware when someone is kind and let it in—and then to work with the blocks to kindness, which are often linked to past emotional memories that are difficult.

2 In Buddhist tantric practice, imagery is very important because it enables practitioners to connect to their inner capacity for wisdom and compassion that is obscured by their habit patterns shaped by conditioning. Leighton, T.D. (2003) *Faces of Compassion: Classic Bodhisattva Archetypes and Their Modern Expression*. Somerville, MA: Wisdom. This was a great find for Paul. See also Vessantara (1993) *Meeting the Buddhas: A Guide to Buddhas, Bodhisattvas and Tantric Deities*. New York: Windhorse Publications. He goes into much detail about how you would build up visualisations and how powerful this is for the practitioner in awakening the inner capacity for wisdom and compassion.

Imagery is now used a lot in psychological therapy. An interesting book is Stopa, L. (ed.) (2009) *Imagery and the Threatened Self: Perspectives on Mental Imagery and the Self in Cognitive Therapy.* London: Routledge. A fascinating book that uses imagery for exploring and developing hypnotic techniques is Frederick, C. and McNeal, S. (1999) *Inner Strengths: Contemporary Psychotherapy and Hypnosis for Ego Strengthening.* Mahwah, NJ: Lawrence Erlbaum Associates.

3   Gilbert, P. (2010) *Compassion-Focused Therapy*, CBT Distinctive Features Series. London: Routledge. See pages 9–12 for a short review.

4   See note 2.

5   Lee, D.A. (2005) The perfect nurturer: A model to develop a compassionate mind within the context of cognitive therapy. In P. Gilbert (ed.) *Compassion: Conceptualisations, Research and Use in Psychotherapy* (pp. 326–351). London: Brunner–Routledge. A new book on the compassionate mind approach to trauma is Lee, D. and James, S. (2012) *The Compassionate Mind Approach to Recovering from Trauma.* London: Constable & Robinson.

10 The Compassionate Self

1   See chapter 9, notes 1 and 2.

2   Chubbuck, I. (2004) *The Power of the Actor: The Chubbuck Technique.* New York: Gotham Books. There are many books on method acting and some very good YouTube demonstrations that can give you some basic insights. Recent research has also shown that we can practice imagining a certain type of self and this can have a huge impact on our confidence and emotions. See, for example, Meevissen, Y.M.C., Peters, M.L. and Alberts, H.J.E.M. (2011) Become more optimistic by imagining a best possible self: Effects of a two week intervention. *Journal of Behavior Therapy and Experimental Psychiatry*, 42, 371–378; and also Peters, M.L., Flink, I.K., Boersma, K. and Linton, S.J. (2010) Manipulating optimism: Can imagining a best possible self be used to increase positive future expectancies? *Journal of Positive Psychology*, 5, 204–211.

3   Germer, C. (2009) *The Mindful Path to Self-Compassion: Freeing Yourself from Destructive Thoughts and Emotions.* New York: Guilford.

4   Tirch, D. (2012) *The Compassionate Mind Approach to Overcoming Anxiety: Using Compassion Focused Therapy.* London: Constable & Robinson. See

also Lynne Henderson (2011) *Improving Social Confidence and Reducing Shyness Using Compassion-Focused Therapy*. London: Constable & Robinson.

5 Kolts, R. (2012) *The Compassionate Mind Approach to Managing Your Anger: Using Compassion-Focused Therapy*. London: Constable & Robinson.

6 Zuroff, D.C., Santor, D. and Mongrain, M. (2005) Dependency, self-criticism, and maladjustment. In J.S. Auerbach, K.N. Levy and C.E. Schaffer (eds) *Relatedness, Self-Definition and Mental Representation: Essays in Honour of Sidney J. Blatt* (pp. 75–90). London: Routledge; Gilbert, P., Clarke, M., Kempel, S., Miles, J.N.V. and Irons, C. (2004) Criticizing and reassuring oneself: An exploration of forms, style and reasons in female students. *British Journal of Clinical Psychology*, 43, 31–50.

7 Allione, T. (2008) *Feeding Your Demons*. New York: Little, Brown. This is a fascinating book drawing on an ancient Buddhist approach to identifying inner "demons" such as the self-critical mind, and then learning to identify what they need and heal them as opposed to just rooting them out.

8 See chapter 10 of Gilbert, P. (2009) *The Compassionate Mind*. London: Constable & Robinson. Gilbert, P. and Irons, C. (2005) Focused therapies and compassionate mind training for shame and self-attacking. In P. Gilbert (ed.) *Compassion: Conceptualisations, Research and Use in Psychotherapy* (pp. 263–325). London: Routledge.

11 Widening Our Circle of Compassion

1 Glaser, A. (2007) The hidden treasure of the heart, *Shambhala Sun*, July: http://www.shambhalasun.com/index.php?option=com_content&task=view&id=3106&Itemid=24.

2 Ibid.

3 Matthieu Ricard: http://cultureofempathy.com/References/Experts Matthieu-Ricard.htm.

4 Glaser, A., The hidden treasure of the heart.

5 Dilgo Khyentse Rinpoche (2006) *Enlightened Courage: An Explanation of the Seven-Point Mind Training*. Snow Lion Publications.

6 Chodron, P. (2005) *When Things Fall Apart: Heart Advice for Difficult Times*. New York: Element Books.

Paul Gilbert, PhD, is world-renowned for his work on depression, shame, and self-criticism. He is head of the mental health research unit at the University of Derby and author of *The Compassionate Mind* and *Overcoming Depression*.

Choden was a monk for seven years within the Tibetan Buddhist tradition, Choden (aka Sean McGovern) completed a three-year, three-month retreat in 1997 and has been a practicing Buddhist since 1985. He is originally from South Africa, where he trained as a lawyer and where he learned meditation under the guidance of Rob Nairn, an internationally renowned Buddhist teacher. He is now involved in developing secular mindfulness and compassion programs drawing upon the wisdom and methods of the Buddhist tradition, as well as contemporary insights from psychology and neuroscience. He is an honorary fellow of the University of Aberdeen and teaches on their postgraduate study program in mindfulness (MSc) that is the first of its kind to include compassion in its curriculum.

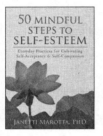
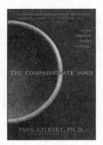
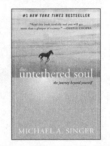
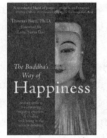
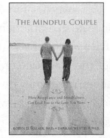
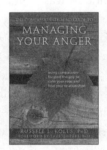